CONFESSIONS

OF A

PARAMEDIC

A True Story By

Sharon M. Holbert, AZ CEP, NREMT-P, Ret.

Published by Sand Dancer Publishing, Arizona - 2011

Copyright © 2011 by Sharon M. Holbert

Published by Sand Dancer Publishing
P.O. Box 4630, Page, Arizona 86040-4630
www.sand-dancer.com

ISBN – 13:978-1466442474
ISBN - 10:1466442476

DEDICATION

This book is dedicated to the memory of my father, G. Cleo Mercer for his contribution to who I am and what I have achieved in my life. He always told me "You can do it Sis!"

I also what to acknowledge my husband Maurice and sons David and Stephen, who supported me in my career as an EMT-Paramedic. Without their cooperation and encouragement I could never have followed this career path and this book could not have been written. I want to give special thanks to Stephen who edited my book and assisted me in getting this book published.

Table of Contents

PREFACE

I lived two lives at once. I would be serving dinner to my husband and two sons or sitting in a parent teacher conference and ten minutes later I was at the scene of a horrible car accident, a shooting or in command of a house fire. I had to switch on and off my two separate personalities. One life as a wife and mother and the other life of a rural Emergency Medical Technician (EMT), Assistant Chief of the Page Arizona Fire Department and Rescue Chief in charge of thirty-two EMTs. I was cross trained as a Firefighter/Engineer and The PFD had a response area of two thousand, five hundred square miles. The first half of my career was with the fire department. The second half of my career was as a Paramedic, Arizona and New Mexico certified, as well as National Registry. I worked on the remote Navajo Reservation, the size of the State of West Virginia.

It was a juggling act of unbelievable proportions. It was a struggle, like trying to swim against the current of a rapid flowing river. So, why did I do it? I admit it. I was a trauma junkie. I craved the sound of my pager going off, I lived to ride through the streets with lights and sirens blaring. I loved the personal challenge when faced with the difficult decisions required of Emergency Medical Service (EMS) personnel. I liked helping people. I also liked being in the middle of whatever was going on. I found the danger and the excitement stimulating.

Emergency Medical Services (EMS) is a demanding occupation. It is exciting, intense and rewarding, but it can be stressful. My husband would never ask, "What did you do today?" He was afraid I would tell him, ". . . well, there was this severed arm . . . ." He worked long hours and had a lot of responsibility in his job. When he came home he just wanted to relax, not listen to the details of my day. I found myself needing a confidant. I needed an outlet, a way to vent, critique, and contemplate what I had just experienced, the good and the bad. I decided to start writing about the "calls" (aka "runs") as a form of therapy. To write experiences down on paper, to be completely honest, helped relieve stress. It is similar to the person lying on a couch and telling a psychiatrist or therapist their deepest thoughts. I had no intentions of ever publishing my therapeutic journal.

When I decided to write a book I was surprised to find I had enough stories to fill four or more books. Well, after all, it was a thirty-two year career. I found it hard to pick and choose which stories to include in this book. I started with the beginning of my career and then added interesting stories that spanned the years. This is a little bit of beginning, middle, and end of career stories. I tried to make it a collection of different

7

types of runs (or calls). Some reflect the life of a volunteer, firefighting, an Assistant Chief of a Fire Department, and a Professional Paramedic.

I don't go into many details of patient care, as this isn't a "how-to" book. This book is more about sharing with you, the medical and non-medical reader my career as a Basic-EMT and later as a Paramedic. It shows what it is really like in the back of an ambulance with another person's life in your hands. It shows the challenge serving in the remote four corners region presents to the EMS responders. Their families, friends, volunteers, and professionals will find this book informative and entertaining. It's my personal experiences involving my co-workers, interesting patients, strange, dangerous and humorous situations. It tells the true story of the impact this career has on my personal and professional life and the life of the medic's with which I have worked.

EMS is a man's world where eighty-two percent of all EMS personnel are male. At the time I entered the profession the numbers were even higher. Equality on the home front had not been achieved by most couples. Even when both people worked there was usually a form of traditional roles played by the couple. It presented a greater challenge for a wife and mother who had to juggle the traditional female role's responsibilities, particularly during my *volunteer* years. If a male EMT-Paramedic was late coming home his children were still tucked in bed and his dinner was in the oven. When I was late, there was a revolt at home. I juggled family and work demands and I sometimes dropped the ball and other times performed with distinction. Even after the children grew up and my husband's work demands allowed him to mellow a bit, it still wasn't easy.

EMS work is exciting and challenging but can take a physical and emotionally personal toll on the rescuer. EMS personnel work in all types of weather, kneeling, bending, heavy lifting, risk of noise induced hearing loss from sirens and back injuries from lifting patients. They are exposed to diseases such as Hepatitis and AIDS, as well as violence from drug addicted patients or the mentally unstable. No one can hold a dead baby in their arms and not be affected. I am different because of what I have seen and done over the years. Is that good or bad? I don't know. But I am different now.

I started out as a EMT-Basic and some of the stories will reflect that level of training. Later I went back to school to become a Paramedic (EMT-P or aka CEP). There is a difference in skill level between and EMT and Paramedic. An EMT-B is a skilled professional, trained to identify, treat medical emergencies, package and transport the ill or injured. An EMT-B spends one semester, about one-hundred and thirty-five actual hours of classroom training and ten hours observation time in the emergency room of a hospital. A Paramedic is an EMT-B with at least two years of experience that has completed roughly two-thousand hours of additional Advanced Life Support training. An EMT provides a good basic level of care and that is sufficient in about ninety-five percent of the emergency calls. It's the five percent of patients that face airway issues, cardiac difficulties, or other immediate life threatening problems that require administration of drugs Advanced Life Support procedures, that make a paramedic essential in EMS.

Early in my career, I was honored to serve with the best group of volunteers in Arizona, the Page Ambulance Group of Emergency Services (PAGES). Later, I worked professionally as a full time Paramedic in a number of locations and settings alongside dedicated people giving everything they had to help the ill and injured. Some people I have worked with are exceptional examples of the best people in EMS. They exhibited bravery by "walking where angels fear to tread" to help a complete stranger. They watched my back, helped me become what I am and taught me many life lessons. Over the years lasting friendships were formed. I want to publicly acknowledge them. They are Dave Auge, Mona LeGate, Cindy Maynard, George Gasaway, Janet Marley, Sylvia Hall, Linda Jensen, Charlene Gustaveson, Glenn Thompson, Jim Hall, Terry Carnell, Noah Brock, Tim "Tato" Tahanni, Marsha Bratcher and Robert Schwartz.

Unfortunately some EMS workers, just like the general public, are flawed. I have been partnered with a Neo-Nazi who worshiped Hitler. Some were addicts of alcohol or prescription drugs while others were poorly skilled, lazy or just hateful and/or sexists. Some were racists and for the record not all racists are white. Some supervisors and most Fire Chiefs left a lot to be desired. I'm not picking on fire chiefs, it's just that in my experience this was the perfect example of the Peter Principle: *"workers are promoted to their highest level of incompetence."* In this book I don't name everyone, sometimes due to poor memory or inadequate documentation. Other times I know my co-workers would feel awkward about the praise or at times angry at the criticism. To keep this book true to the facts, good or bad, as best preserved in my memory, I have decided to simply change the names of everyone. This will protect the innocent and not so innocent.

I have edited the stories to protect patient confidentiality and to comply with the Federal HIPA law. Sometimes I changed the sex, age, time of day, location or minor details when it wasn't an important element to the story to further protect the patient's identity. In two stories I have combined two EMS providers into one to help facilitate the telling of the story, but the details are unaltered. I used very little literary license, usually it wasn't necessary. In a small town and with long transport times, there is opportunity to get the *rest of the story*. The stories were interesting and didn't need embellishment. I am certain others may remember an incident in this book from their own personal perspective and their recollections may differ from mine. Perhaps in the future they will write their own memoirs and I can enjoy a different prospective on a familiar story.

To the best of my ability, the stories told here remain truthful and are told from my personal memories, notes, official documentation and the therapeutic journal I wrote to unwind after calls. The thoughts and feelings are mine and mine alone. I do not pretend to represent other EMS workers. The following stories are not presented in any particular order, but reflect my skill level and work environment at the time of the incident and cover a long and rewarding career.

INTRODUCTION

There are 1.1 million EMT's and Paramedics in the United States. About 280,000 men and women serve in the urban environment, representing only 18% of all EMT's and Paramedics. Out of the 280,000 urban medics only around 15,600 (about 6%) are women. Television programs, Hollywood and many books show Emergency Medical Service (EMS) personnel serving in the large metropolitan areas. Their stories are exciting and very interesting, but there is another kind of EMS 911 responders serving the rural communities make up about 82% of all EMT's and around 75% of all Firefighters. Their story has remained untold, until now. Some providers are volunteers while others are full time professionals. The emergency is the same, whether it's the broken leg or car accident, whether it happens in the middle of a huge city or a deserted section of highway in the middle of nowhere. Medical treatment is the same, but everything else is different.

In New York City the response time from phone call to arrival of the ambulance for 90% of the "911' calls is within ten minutes. If they need police backup, another ambulance, helicopter, bomb squad, swat team, or a fire truck, they just call and within minute's backup arrive. It's an entirely different story in the rural southwestern United States. Some 911 providers have three to ten-thousand square miles or more to cover, timely backup is often an hour or more away or completely non-existent. Often rural ambulance crews in northern Arizona will find themselves in a situation where there are multiple patients, no radio or cell phone reception, dirt roads and savage weather. They have to handle the situation with the limited resources available often with a two person

10

crew. The Golden Hour (optimal time for the best patient outcome) is only wishful thinking.

Many of the ambulance calls in this book involve the City of Page, Arizona and the Navajo Reservation. I was Rescue Chief for nine years, supervising the ambulance responses and cross trained in Incident Command, including Fire Response, Hazardous Materials, Rope Rescue, Vehicle Extrication, Arson Investigation, Disaster Response and Radiological Emergencies. PFD served around fifty miles in any direction and over two hundred miles of narrow, two lane highways, 89, 89-A, and 98. Page is a city of around ten thousand people. It's an isolated community just eight miles south of the Utah border. The closest larger cities are Flagstaff, Arizona about one hundred and forty miles to the south and St. George, Utah about the same distance to the west. Flagstaff and St. George have a population of about fifty-thousand. To reach a larger city a person from Page would have to drive almost three-hundred miles south to reach Phoenix Arizona or around the same distance west to Las Vegas Nevada.

It may sound as if there wouldn't be enough 911 calls to fill a book but that could not be further from the truth. Because of its location, Page is a tourist community. It sits in the middle of the "Grand Circle". The circle contains ten US National Parks, three Navajo Nation Tribal Parks, and a number of recreation and wilderness areas, various historical sites, many ancient ruins and a lake with two-thousand miles of shoreline (more than the entire west coast). This accounts for the four million tourists from all over the world that visit the area every year. In addition to Page's ten-thousand citizens, over 25,000 Native Americans on the reservation and a number of small communities in southern Utah see Page as their commercial center. Many work here. Some drive a two-hundred mile round trip to shop in Page's Wal-Mart Super Center.

I also worked in the Page Hospital ER, a local doctor's clinic, two industrial clinics and taught the EMT class for two local community colleges. For years I worked as a paramedic on the Navajo Reservation or "Rez" as it is known locally. It is roughly 27,000 square miles, the size of West Virginia. I worked as one of the 7.5% Anglos in Tuba City and Kayenta. Most of the roads are dirt. The narrow two lane highways are often open range and livestock roam freely. I once responded to a reported *man not breathing* and it was a seventy-five mile one way trip with half the journey on a narrow winding highway and the second half on a washboard dirt road. As you can see, the term "rural" takes on a different meaning in relationship to many other parts of the country. Now for the first time the true story of Rural EMS in the American Southwest is told.

WHAT AM I DOING HERE? (How It All Began)

The sun shined brightly in the clear blue sky of northern Arizona. Park Service had requested Page Fire assist with a two car head-on inside the Lake Powell Recreation area. The accident was on a very narrow paved road that curved around the base of a hill. The employee trailer park sat on top of the hill overlooking Lake Powell. The location is about ten miles from Page. We arrived at the scene and found a mess. I could see a car and a small pickup had hit head on. The truck was slightly damaged, but the car had rolled. Ranger Ronald Coffer approached us. Most of the rangers had an attitude, Ronald didn't. "There are three patients, the driver of the pickup and two were in the car. We need your help in getting one out of the car. She's in an awkward position and we'll need the Hurst tool."

I could see a young woman lying in the middle of the road being cared for by Rangers. A man sat beside the road with a towel held to his forehead. Kent, one of PFD's newest EMT went to the man. The driver of the ambulance was Roger Nelson an EMT. He and I were directed to the Toyota sitting sideways in the middle of the road. The small blue Toyota had rolled over one and a half times. It now rested on its passenger side. All the windows were shattered and lay like tiny crystals covering everything with a powdery fine dusting of glass. The patient lay withering and moaning. She was wadded up in the passenger floor board area, under the dash. She was crying in pain. Her eyes were open but they didn't really comprehend. Blood gushed from an ugly wound that formed a perfect "X" dead center of her upper lip. This was wound no plastic surgeon would ever repair satisfactorily.

The car had been stabilized and was no longer in danger of rolling over. The Park Ranger, Ronald Coffer bent down and crawled into the crushed car through the broken back window. He stopped dead. In front of him was a dog. It was of medium size, big enough to be a problem in the cramped spaces of the mashed vehicle. Ronald held his breath. Then he saw the dog was as frightened as he was. The dog was really a puppy and it hung its tail between its legs and hurried to the far corner of the car as far away from the stranger as possible. Ronald crawled on, finally reaching the injured woman.

Outside I was busy hooking up the Hurst tool. The best way into a car lying on its side is through the top. The idea was to cut the roof supports and fold the roof downward exposing the inside of the car. Roger Nelson and I were preparing to cut the roof off and expose the inside of the car for quick removal of the injured girl. Roger was a hyper man and at an emergency scene that behavior intensified. He seldom took a minute to dress for the occasion. I slipped goggles over his head and he reluctantly allowed me to slip the gloves on his hands. I put the hard hat on his head and he was finally ready, whether he wanted it or not. I proceeded to finish connecting up the hydraulic hoses. Although all EMTs with the PFD were trained to operate the Hurst Tool, most had never been allowed to touch it on a real call. If Roger was present, he worked the Hurst Tool. It was always something he would grab and no power on earth could rasp it from his grip. According to the unwritten rule, it was his job and no one else's. He got away with this possessive behavior because at the time he was Rescue Chief of the PFD. I proceeded to finish connecting up the hoses and doing all the behind the scenes work so he could perform for the crowd as the savior of mankind.

It was a hot July morning, around ten o'clock. It was going to be another scorching summer day in Arizona. I jerked the cord and started the motor. It loudly sprang to life. I looked up and saw a large crowd had gathered and appeared to be enjoying the show. I saw Park Service caring for the other woman. They had back boarded her and she now lay beside the road. When we had arrived at the scene to assist Park Service, we had been told they were waiting for the helicopter. Over by PFD ambulance, Kent, the other member of our crew, was loading a man into Rescue-Two with the help of a Park Ranger. I turned my attention back to Roger as he lifted the heavy tool and with the scissors attachment, he cut through the top front roof support as if it were butter. He raised the heavy tool again and cut the center support. He then wrapped the jaws around the back roof support and snipped. Suddenly, gasoline appeared out of nowhere, a steady stream the size of my little finger shot outward from the cut support.

A gas line? Damn. Someone in a moment of brain fade had ran the gas line from the rear tank up through the roof support, across the top of the vehicle and down the opposite front roof support to the motor. At that moment I would have gladly killed the idiot that thought up that one. Gasoline shot out and drenched my leg. I bent down and peered at the cut roof support. The gas line was somewhere down in there, but where wasn't exactly clear. There was a way to stop it, but the needed equipment was on the fire engine back in town. It would take time to get them out here. We could have the girl out by then, if we hurried and our luck held out. The Park Ranger looked up and saw what happened. He saw the gasoline and after a few choice words he announced the victim had an obviously fractured femur and possible fractured wrist. Under the circumstances, the splinting of these injuries would have to wait. It became an *everyone grab a piece of the victim and get the hell out of this bomb"* call.

We bent the roof of the car downward being careful of the sharp edges. I stuck the foot of the backboard into the vehicle near the patient.

13

(Note; a backboard is a flat board about two and a half feet by six and a half feet. It has straps along the sides to strap the patient to the board. It's used to stabilize the head, neck and spine and to move the patient as a unit.) I then stood supporting the top end of the backboard, the part that was the farthest away from the victim. It was propped on part of the front passenger car seat and the folded roof. The board ran parallel with the vehicle as it lay on its passenger side. The ranger and two EMTs prepared to move the whimpering girl out of the vehicle and onto the backboard. The idea was to scoot her up the backboard head first. Her head would come to rest on the end I now held.

Halfway on the board, they stopped, her foot was caught. The gasoline shot out in a steady stream, hit the backboard near my hand and splattered everywhere. I held the board with one hand and with my other I reached out and deflected the steady stream of gasoline off the spot where the girl's head would eventually come to rest. I was soaked in gasoline from the thighs down. I was a human wick dressed in my gasoline soaked cotton jumpsuit. My head swam from the overwhelming fumes. Through the soles of my shoes I could feel the heat of the black asphalt roadway that had been heated by the hot desert sun. All I could think about was the steady river of fuel that flowed down the highway away from the accident to the group of bystanders standing nearby watching. Was one of them smoking? "God, dear God I hope not," I prayed. Here I was standing in the middle of a bomb, waiting for one spark and then whoosh I would be a human torch. I didn't fear death, but I had always hoped to die in my sleep. "Guys, can we hurry this a bit?" I said.

"We see it. Give us a minute," was the tense reply. They were kneeling in gasoline and had soaked up their pant legs too. They also faced death by fire.

My arm ached. The board with the girl half on, half off was getting heavy. She was a big girl. My shoulder was strained and the half crouched position was awkward. Then he appeared, the bystander whose name I will never know. He reached over and replaced my hand with his, holding the spray off the board where the girls head would go. I gripped the board with both hands reliving some of the strain. I smiled. "Thank you." I sincerely meant it. He had bravely stepped in to help. He knew the obvious danger and had chosen to do it anyway. "Look I have to do this, you don't. Can you reach that t-shirt?" I asked. It lay just inside the wreck.

"Yeah," he said as he bent and grabbed it. He too was now becoming soaked with gasoline.

"Wrap it around the roof support. That should cause the spurting stream to flow and drip downward and not spray the girl when we finally get her moved up on the board." The man quickly did as told. The gasoline

14

still ran, but it ran down the cloth now instead of spraying outward. "Thanks. Now get out here," I told him with a grateful look on my face. He smiled and quickly hurried away. I thought "If there's a hero today, it's that man." Due to circumstances beyond my control, in the course of doing my job I found myself in this position and I'm too chicken to turn and run, which is what I wanted to do. That man was the hero. He chose to walk into danger, knowing full well what he risked and knew he didn't have to do it. No one expected it of him. But he did it anyway. He was the true hero.

Then it occurred to me, "What in the world was I doing here?" Why was I doing this? I hate it when my mornings start this way. How I got here didn't matter that much. Why I was here was a question I really couldn't answer at this time. I tried to ignore the now sickening smell of gasoline. I wiped the vision of the fire ball out of my mind. The girl that lay on the board in front of me captured my full attention. She was in her early twenties, slightly overweight. Her sandy blond hair was caked with blood, dust and glass. She was dressed in tan shorts and a brown t-shirt that announced she had visited the Grand Canyon. She was wearing hiking boots. She moaned and cried out. From the looks of her injuries, she would probably never hike again. Walk, yes, but walk for fun? No, never again. I reached out and touched her cheek and spoke soothing words. It managed to get through and she quieted down.

We carried her away from the vehicle. A helicopter hovered nearby and then sat down in a cloud of dust. I shut my eyes as the dust engulfed us. Dust now stuck to my wet jumpsuit and damp arm. The helicopter blades whipped over our heads as we bent over and carried our patient to the helicopter. I hated hot loads. The deadly blades whipped inches above our heads, whoosh, whoosh, and whoosh. We loaded the young woman and backed away. I turned my back and closed my eyes as it took off, whipping up dust and sand. She was heading to Flagstaff Medical Center.

There were really four victims in this accident, the two young women, one young man and the dog. PFD Rescue-Two was a Chevy modular. It had been given to the department by the Arizona Department of Transportation (ADOT) a few years before. I climbed in back and found the male EMT taking care of two patients. An attractive female patient lay on the stretcher, strapped firmly to the backboard in full spinal precautions. She was the woman I had seen lying in the middle of the road earlier. Her eyes were closed and a large knot lay just above her left eye. I noticed a young man was also strapped to a backboard that had been placed on the bench seat. He was about the same age as the female patient. He was a handsome, clean cut, college type young man. The forth

15

patient was the terrified dog was captured by Ronald. Ronald climbed into the front seat and holding the brown dog in his lap, he began to gently try and calm the frightened puppy. It snuggled up to him and welcomed his comforting attention.

"Robin?" the girl asked. She looked up at me with eyes that for the first time really seemed to focus.

"Robin's fine. He's right here." Jumping to conclusions was what I did best. The girl gazed over. The look of hate filled her eyes. The young man turned his head and closed his eyes in shame. "Let me guess, your name's not Robin."

"No," he answered. I wasn't too bright, but then the pieces begin to fit. The pretty girl wasn't traveling with the handsome young man. She was riding with the overweight girl that was now on her way to the Flagstaff Hospital in the helicopter. I silently cursed myself for "assuming." One of the rules in EMS is that we never transport patients from two different vehicles in the same ambulance. But in rural EMS sometimes it can't be helped.

The young man quietly started to talk as the other EMT cared for him. I listened as I cared for the girl that now lay quietly, too quietly. He said he lived up on the hill in Wahweap Trailer Village and as he drove by on the highway below, he looked up and saw his front door standing open. His attention was diverted and he crossed the line on a tight curve and hit the car carrying the two women car head on. He had come out of the accident with a small cut on his hand and a tender elbow. He was wearing his seat belts and his car stayed on its wheels.

Gasoline fumes still clung to me but the overhead exhaust fan was working overtime and the stench was less noticeable. Her vital signs were within acceptable limits. Her main injury appeared to be the blow to the head and her right knee. The knee appeared slightly out of line and could be fractured. Park Service had already splinted it.

We arrived at the hospital and turned the patients over to the ER staff. I took off the gasoline soaked jumpsuit, but the jeans, shoes and socks I was wearing also got soaked so it didn't help that much. I slipped off my jeans and washed them in the sink and removed some of the gasoline. Roger and Ronald also stunk of gasoline fumes but decided to live with it for now. Kent quickly cleaned and restocked the ambulance. We wrote our reports and returned to service.

When I got home, Maurice noticed at once the gasoline smell. "What on earth have you been doing?" I was hyper and launched into an excited rendition of the call. I loved this job! And from a personal point of view, this call had went well, I felt great. I had cheated death. I had won. I didn't die. It was going to be a great day!

16

When it involves tourists, one of the problems with this job is we often do not know how everything turns out. I do know the young man was treated and released. The young pretty girl had a mild concussion. She spent the night in the Page Hospital then transferred out to a higher level of care for consult with an orthopedic doctor about her knee. The other girl had surgery on her fractured femur and plastic surgery on her upper lip. I don't know the final outcome of either of the women.

How did a young mother and housewife find herself wading in gasoline that hot July morning? It was a long complicated road. My grandmother, Alberta Hoover Stacy was a nurse. She had tried to get me to become a nurse. She saw in me something that led her to believe I would be good in the medical field. I regret that I didn't do as she had suggested. I guess my interest in emergency medical started with the popular television program called *Emergency*. How I loved that show. Johnny Gage and Desoto would rush to the scene of an emergency with red lights flashing and the crowd would part and let them through. I loved the ambulance, the drama, the fires, and the excitement. I never missed a show.

But it was the 1960's. Woman didn't do that sort of thing. It was a man's field and I wasn't a man. My life continued on. I did what was expected of me as a woman. I got married and had two sons. I was the housewife that made macramé', joined the women's group at church and of course, the PTA.

My life changed in November of 1976. My husband came home from work with a bid sheet in his hand. He worked for a local power company, Salt River Project. He was currently a Relayman, a good occupation, but it was not the field in which he had received a degree. The job was at the Navajo Generating Station, located six miles outside the town of Page Arizona, around three hundred miles north of Phoenix. Phoenix had been my home since I was two years old. We owned a beautiful home and my family and friends lived there. I didn't want to move.

Seeing his enthusiasm and eagerness, I did what any good wife would do, I helped him type up his job bid and resume. Secretly I hoped he wouldn't get it. My luck had never been very good and he got the bid. In April 1977 we sold my dream house, packed everything we owned in cardboard boxes and moved into a two bedroom trailer in Page. Stephen had just turned five and David's eighth birthday was only a couple months away.

It was a new town, new people, and new situations. I wasn't ready for a small town and it wasn't ready for me. I went in search for something

17

to do with my time. That September an Emergency Medical Technician class was offered. I took it. It wasn't as easy as I expected. I was working full time and had a husband and two small sons, but even with all the demands on my time, I managed to pass the class with a high "B". I had taken the class because we went out on the lake camping. I realized this wasn't Phoenix where an ambulance is only three minutes away. I wanted to know what to do in an emergency. I had no plans on working on an ambulance. I had given up that dream a long time ago.

Near the end of March I received a phone call from Monica Le Garvin. She was an EMT. She asked me if I would be interested in joining the fire department. They were down to eleven EMTs and needed a few more volunteers. During the EMT class she and other EMTs had helped with the skills portion of the class and I liked her and the others I had met, but I told her "No thanks." My husband, who later regretted it I am sure, talked me into giving it a try. He said I had the "book learning" and a little experience would be a good thing. I remembered the TV show; I remembered how I always considered the occupation out of my woman's reach. Now it was an option open to me. I decided to do it just long enough to get experience so I could help my family if needed. Little did my husband or I know that running on an ambulance was addicting.

The next Wednesday night, I went to the fire station. All the Volunteer EMT's were there. They called themselves the P.A.G.E.S. (Page Ambulance Group Emergency Service). They were a group of well-respected EMT's. The group had won the year before the Hon Kachina Award. An award presented each year to an outstanding volunteer or volunteer organization in the State of Arizona. It was a fancy black tie affair at the Biltmore Hotel in Phoenix. It was on the television news and the newspapers. The funny thing about all this is I remember seeing it on television the year before and never imagined I would be joining them the next year. The award today is displayed proudly in a glass case at City Hall. I felt honored to be asked to join this group.

Before anyone could join, there had to be a vote. I was introduced to them. Some of them I had already met, but some were complete strangers. They asked a few questions and then I was escorted into another room. Have you ever heard the term "black balled?" Each person had a white and a black ball. A basket was passed around and each person placed in the basket a ball. All it took was one black ball and the person would not be allowed to join. All the balls were white.

The adventure had begun.

NICE DOGGIE, NICE DOGGIE

I had put it off too long. My driver's license was going to expire if I didn't renew it. To the young bloods reading this, it was before the miracles of doing business on line. Renewing a driver's license required a face-to-face transaction. When on duty, the EMT-Paramedic was not allowed to leave the city limits. The idea was that those on duty had to meet at the fire department, get in the ambulance and go to the scene. It was believed that anything beyond the city limits would take too long a response time.

The Arizona Department of Transportation (ADOT) was located about two miles out of town. I was on duty for the next three days during the day time hours, and the business hours of ADOT. I had tried to find someone to substitute for me, but I couldn't find anyone. It was down to the wire and I had run out of time. I decided to cheat a bit. My plan was to sneak out of town, drive down the hill, across the Glen Canyon Bridge, which spanned the Colorado River and up the next hill to the Driver License Department. It was a small office that shared a building with the State Inspection Station. I was known to those working there and hopefully I could get everything done quickly and sneak back into town between 911 calls. *Oh, the well laid plans of mice and men.*

The Glen Canyon Bridge stands over seven hundred feet above the Colorado River as it leaves the Glen Canyon Dam and continues its journey down the steep walled canyon to the Grand Canyon. It was summer time and the bridge's walkway on each side was full of tourists. They each carried cameras and snapped pictures of the green river and the bright seven-hundred foot high red/orange sandstone cliffs on one side and Glen Canyon Dam on the other. It is a magnificent sight. But for the automobile driver, it was a nightmare. The tourists forget where they are and without warning, spin around and rush across the road to the other side for more pictures. It's like a game of dodge ball and the ball is a three-thousand pound car.

I managed to get across without incident. I drove another mile up a hill and parked. As I got out I took a minute to admire the view. To the north was Lake Powell's Wahweap Bay. And to the East was the original Colorado River Channel as it snakes through the red sandstone landscape. To the south was the dam and bridge. In the distance is the town of Page, mostly sitting on the flat topped Manson Mesa. It was breathtaking. I turned and hurried inside. There was a short line of three people. I took a form and stood in line filling out the paperwork as I slowly advance to the counter. A man came in behind me and then two women. Soon there were six people behind me in line. It was finally my turn. Donald was a friend of mine and smiled when he saw it was me.

"Donald, I'm not supposed to be here, I'm on call. But I have to get my license renewed."

"Ok, let's try and get this done in record time." He looked over the form I had filled out and went to his computer and keyed in my name. He wrinkled his eyebrows. "Sharon, what's your birthday? I told him. "Something's screwed up, they have it the twenty-second not the twenty-first." I assured him it was the twenty-first. "It's just a typo, give me a minute." He went in the back and called the Page police department to verify my birth date.

Now, the PPD dispatcher also knew me. "Donald, why do you need Sharon's birth date?" He explained. She took a deep breath and told him, "Donald, listen carefully. I just dispatched DPS to a one car rollover. Sharon's on the duty roster. He is going to request an ambulance any minute now. She has to get back to town, NOW! I can delay paging until the officer makes the official request, but that won't be long so get her headed to town immediately!"

Donald was very good at what he did, shuffle papers. He wasn't well equipped for emergencies. His body was shot full of adrenaline. His heart speeded up, his breathing increased and he was wired for anything. He slammed the phone down spun around and raced across the room to the counter where I stood. His voice was loud and urgent. "SHARON, GET OUT OF HERE! GET OUT OF HERE! GET BACK TO TOWN, NOW!"

It took only a second to sink in. I grabbed my keys off the counter and spun around, nearly knocking the man behind me down. He and the five people behind him had their mouths open, their eyes were wide with surprise and a confused look was on their faces. I ignored them and rushed out the door. They had no idea what was going on. A woman in line turned to another woman and asked "What do you think she said that made him so mad?"

I spun tires out of the parking lot as I too was full of adrenaline. I hit the road and ignored the speed limit till I got to the bridge. I slowed down, I had too. I got almost across before a man dressed in tacky plaid shorts and a t-shirt with a Grand Canyon logo stretched over a beer belly casually stepped off the sidewalk in front of me and slowly ambled across the roadway to the other side. I stopped and sat there impatiently. I then continued across the bridge and floored it. I was almost up on the mesa by the time the dispatcher paged for the ambulance crew. I owed the dispatcher and Donald one. I got to the station about the same time as the rest of the crew.

Twenty-five minutes before I got the bright idea to sneak out of town on personal business, Dwight decided to drive into Page for groceries. He was forty something, average size and build. Dwight lived in the community of Big Water in Utah. It was about eighteen miles northwest of Page on Highway 89. It was in Utah, but the nearest Utah ambulance was in Kanab, about seventy-five miles to the west so Page handled that stretch of highway with Kanab Fire's approval. Dwight's dog, Wolf, eagerly followed him to the car. Wolf liked nothing better than a ride in the car. He wagged his tail enthusiastically as he bounced about like a one hundred and ten pound puppy. He was a big dog, a German Sheppard and loyal to a fault to Dwight. They quickly were on the highway and heading toward town. Wolf stuck his head out the passenger side window and let the air blow on his face. He was one happy dog.

Dwight saw a white car sitting beside the road about ten miles from Page. He had no warning before they pulled out in front of him. He was going sixty-five miles per hour, the speed limit, when he hit his breaks and the car swerved slightly to the right. The road was narrow and his front wheel hit the sand and dug in. The car began to flip. Dwight and Wolf were not wearing seat belts and both were thrown out of the car as it rolled twice and came to rest on its wheels. Both hit the desert floor hard. The white car continued on, but the car behind Dwight stopped. 911 was called.

The DPS officer arrived and found Wolf standing over the unconscious Dwight. Wolf was showing his teeth and growling at anyone that tried to get near. It was a standoff. DPS had called for the ambulance but now faced an obstacle that might keep Dwight from receiving the care he needed. The officer slowly approached the dog. "Nice doggie, nice doggie." Wolf wasn't buying any of that crap. He barked and snapped at the approaching officer until he backed up. The officer could shoot the dog, but he didn't want too. The dog was protecting his owner. It was understandable and was commendable, but this time it was a serious problem. No one could get near Dwight as he lay face down in the desert.

"Excuse me, officer?" He turned around and found a woman around forty standing behind him. "I am Dwight's neighbor and I know the dog. Maybe I can calm him down?" She wanted to help but deep down she was afraid. The dog was large and angry. It may be a bit confused and/or injured. She wasn't sure if it would be a safe thing for her to do, but she felt she should help if she could.

"Give it a try. I really don't want to shoot him. Here take this," The officer bent down and picked up a piece of rope that lay in the sand. "Try to get him on a leach." The woman walked toward the dog slowly.

"Wolf, it's me. You know me, don't you? Come on boy, let me help Dwight." The dog snarled then stopped. He tipped his head slightly to the right and looked at the woman who was talking so gently to him. He sniffed the air. Then he remembered. She was the nice lady that lived next door. She gave him treats sometimes. The dog remembered that Dwight seemed to like her. The dog sat down and let her approach. She continued to talk in a soothing manner and Wolf calmed down. She tied the thin rope to his collar and led him to the bumper of the car. She tied the rope to the bumper, petted the dog and walked away.

PFD's Rescue-Two arrived on the scene. I got out with the jump kit in my hands. I hurried over to the officer who told me "He hasn't moved." I walked toward the man, not noticing the dog. But, he noticed me. He charged, full speed ahead, teeth exposed and a deep frightening bark. The officer pulled his gun. I hadn't seen the dog lying in the sand under the front of the car. I froze in terror, turning my head toward the frightening sound. Two feet away from me, the rope caught. It jerked his collar and whipped him off his feet. He stood up and lunged out at me. The dog had his hind feet on the ground, his front feet pawing the air in front of him. His teeth snapped as he tugged on the rope that held him to the bumper of the car. The officer didn't lower his gun. He kept it pointed at the dog. "Sorry, should have warned you. The dog's his," indicating the man on the ground.

"I hope that's a strong rope," I commented under my breath as I kneeled beside Dwight. He was unconscious. I did a quick exam as the other EMT's set up a backboard beside him. They too were un-nerved by the monster dog that was two feet away from us, snarling, barking and threatening to eat us alive. We all wondered if the rope was strong enough and how well had the woman tied the knots? An EMT held his head and I applied a collar. We rolled him carefully over onto the backboard. Now that he was on his back I could see Dwight's head had hit one of the many sandstone rocks scattered about the sandy desert. He had a nasty red bump growing by the minute in the center of his forehead. His respirations were normal, but I applied oxygen due to the obvious head injury. The dog continued to paw at the air, snapping his teeth, growling and barking loudly. I prayed the thin rope and knot would hold. I tried to ignore the dog, but it was distracting. I checked Dwight's eyes, they were equal and reactive. He had no blood coming from his head, eyes, nose, or ears. I cut his cowboy shirt and jeans off and carefully checked for injuries. I couldn't find any other obvious injury except his left upper arm was fractured as he was thrown out the driver's side window.

The dog would not stop his violent protest. I looked over my right shoulder and saw the officer standing near us with his gun drawn and pointed at the dog. It was obvious he intended to shoot the dog if the rope gave way. I hoped that didn't happen, but I didn't want to be half eaten by an angry dog, so the officer's intense focus on the situation was comforting. We moved Dwight to the ambulance and loaded him inside. The second the door was shut the dog stopped barking, walked over to the car and laid beside it. I was told a few minutes after we left the scene, the man's best friend showed up and took the dog.

It was about ten minutes to town. During that time we were busy in the back. He was kept on high flow oxygen. His feet moved when I ran my ink pen up the sole of his feet. His pupils were equal and responded to light. His vital signs remained stable during transport. Dwight moaned and moved slightly. I called the hospital on the radio and gave them a head's up. I saw through the back window of the ambulance the ADOT building as we passed it on our way to town. The siren got the tourist's attention and they managed to stay on the sidewalk until the ambulance had crossed the bridge.

We arrived at the hospital on time. As we hit the door we were greeted by a doctor and nurse. I began the report, ". . . an adult male about forty-four years old, unrestrained driver of a mid-size car. It left the road at highway speed and rolled twice. He was thrown out and found prone on sand. I think his forehead hit a sandstone rock. He was completely unconscious until a couple of minutes ago when he moaned and moved his right hand." We lifted the backboard from our stretcher onto the hospital gurney. The nurse switched the oxygen tubing to their supply. "His left upper arm may be fractured, no other obvious injuries found. No known medical history. Vital signs are within normal limits."

The hospital staff took over care and we quickly got the ambulance cleaned and restocked. We then retreated into the chapel to do our paperwork. The driver had to write a simple and short narrative on the accident and fill out the billing slip. I had to recreate the entire incident on paper, what was done, not done, why and by whom. I mentioned the dog briefly and who took him. Arizona law at the time gave a person three years to decide to sue (the ambulance company and/or medic) or not. But if the patient was one year old, the parents could sue any time until the child reaches eighteen years of age. Then the patient has three years. That means the report I write today could reach court twenty-one years in the future so the event and treatment given had to be well documented.

On the way out the door I told the nurse, "When he wakes up and wonders what happened to his dog, tell him the dogs ok and his friend, Edward has him."

When finished at the fire station, I slipped out of town to ADOT. I walked in and Donald smiled. "Did you make it?"

23

"Yeah, I did, but I wouldn't have if you hadn't given me a couple of minute's head start. Thanks, you saved me that time." Donald was efficient and had my driver's license with the correct birth date completed. We finished our business quickly. "Thanks again Donald," I said as I left and he waved. I got in my car and hurried back to town. No one but Donald and the dispatcher knew about this breach in protocol till now. It's nice to have friends that help watch your back, give you a heads up and cover for you when you need it. Oh, by the way, Dwight and his dog were reunited four days later when Dwight was released from the hospital wearing a cast and walking with a slight temporary limp.

I AM WOMAN

Today it is truly different for a woman in Fire, Police and Rescue. It's still a man's world, but if a woman is willing to work hard, she can find a place. Today only eighteen percent of EMT-Paramedics are female. In my Paramedic class, only four women were in the class. In fire the percentage is even less. Some of it may be contributed to the fact fewer woman are interested in this career. It is very physically demanding and at times dangerous. As an EMT-Paramedic I had to lift my half of a two-hundred and fifty pound stretcher. Often the patient was even heavier. As a female it also places additional demands on her child rearing duties as a mother. Duty shifts are twelve to twenty-four hours and it's not easy to find a babysitter for that type of shift. It takes a strong man who is comfortable with his masculinity to accept a wife that chops down doors with an ax, faces down a man with a gun or for him to climb into bed with a women who is considered "high risk" for disease.

In the early days of the battle to achieve equality, many women, such as I, struggled to be accepted in an occupation where women had never served before. To all the young women out there today working in a predominately male field of employment, you may look at your mother and grandmother differently if you really understood how she and others like her struggled so you would have to opportunity, if you so chose, to pursue such a career.

I once stood in the Fire Chief Owens office and witnessed him half-stand and hit his desk with his fist as he yelled, "No woman will ever drive my ambulance!" I became the first female ambulance driver for the Page Fire Department, regardless of what he had yelled at me that day. I also was a member of the first all-female team to respond to a medical emergency for one-thousand square miles of northern Arizona. I am not a radical women libber. I like men, but the female EMT's and I showed everyone women can get the job done just as well.

After three years as a volunteer EMT, Chief Jude Owens moved and his Assistant, Roger Nelson took his job. I was hired as the PFD Asst. Chief/Chief of the Rescue (ambulance) Division. I was the first female to ever hold that position of leadership (or any position of leadership for that matter) in the PFD. I loved working on the ambulance, but when I learned that as Asst. Chief, I had to undergo fire training, I hesitated. I admit I don't like entering a burning building. It just doesn't seem like a bright idea. The department did not have any female fire fighters. I remember the first time I slipped on the turn-outs. The gloves and coat were two sizes too big and the pants were far too long. I was to run an obstacle course. Locally, I would be the first woman to even attempt this feat. I slowly dressed out in full turnouts, mask and the heavy Scott Pack (air tank). I walked awkwardly in the boots two sizes too big, to the starting line. I took a deep breath and on cue I ran to a tunnel built in the middle of the large city garage. I had to get on my knees and crawl through the tunnel as fast as possible. I stood up and found a four foot wall in front of me. I climbed over a four foot wall and fell to the other side. I struggled like a turtle on his back getting up. The turnouts and Scot Pack were restrictive. I felt clumsy dressed in the ill-fitting firefighter gear. I got up and found the dummy. I grabbed it and dragged the one-hundred and fifty pound mannequin across a large room, I lifted him over an obstacle and drug him another ten feet. My breathing increased and I found the mask suffocating but I struggled onward.

I faced the obstacles one after another and managed to negotiate through. We were being timed and I was determined to be the first woman to finish this course, but I was worried about the time limit. I then exited the building and climbed the ladder up onto the flat topped roof and took my ax and chopped a huge log twenty times. The ax felt like it weighed fifty pounds and my arms ached. I had to stop once to regain my breath. Then with new found energy, I climbed down the ladder as the tanks on my back grew heavier and heavier. My hands shook. My legs felt like they were each twenty pounds heavier. My arms and between the shoulder blades throbbed in aching pain from swinging the ax. I was so tired but I couldn't give up now. Then with my last burst of energy, I ran around the building and crossed the finish line out of breath, out of energy and ready to drop. I had finished the course and proved a female was capable of passing the same physical requirements expected of a man. I was thrilled to find I managed to complete it within the allotted time with seconds to spare. I was proud of myself when I discovered some of the men didn't do much better.

During the following years I went to Engineers School and learned how to drive and pump the fire engines. During my time with the Page Fire Department I was more than an EMT-Paramedic with the Rescue Division. I was the first female to achieve the status of leadership and I became the third in charge of the department as "Rescue Chief." Before it was over I became completely cross trained with the Fire Division, including Fire Fighting, Haz Mat (Hazardous Material), Radioactive Monitoring, Rope Rescue, Closed Space Rescue and Incident Command. I also became a member of the Critical Incident Stress Debriefing Team for Northern Arizona, and a member of the Northern Arizona Disaster Preparedness Team. During this busy time I also found time to teach the EMT class for the local community college. I had a full plate and I loved it.

After nine years, I left the Fire Department and returned to school. I became a paramedic. I began working for a private owned ambulance company. I worked two or three straight twenty-four hour shifts on the Navajo Reservation. After a few years I continued to work on the reservation, but when in town, I returned to the Page Fire as a volunteer and later became a reserve paramedic. The department had changed. It wasn't a social group united in a common goal, to serve their community. The department had evolved into a paid, reserve and volunteer organization with *"them and us" attitude*. The full time personnel strutted around like royalty and the volunteers were treated like the red-headed stepchildren. It wasn't fun anymore, but I still wanted to help my community so I rejoined and served at half the paycheck of the full time studs. I became a reserve and tried to make the best of it.

When I returned to PFD a lot of people, with whom I had previously worked, had left. Some new ones didn't know me from my previous involvement with the department. I was now a Paramedic Reserve and I quickly made my place within the evolved department. One summer evening at our weekly drill, the fire and rescue had a joint drill. It involved driving ambulances, fire engines, and the monster airport fire truck.

On obstacle course was laid out at the airport. It snaked around with cones placed to challenge the drivers. The course involved driving in and out of cones, forwards and backwards, parallel parking within a small space, then a long straight run and a "Y" at the end of the run. The driver wasn't told to go left or right until the last minute. Then the wide curve ended in a very tight space with poles bent inward at the top forming a kind of tunnel that is smaller on the top and wider on the bottom. Then it ended with a panic stop. I drove the ambulance and didn't knock down a single cone. Others did as well as I did, but some didn't. Then I asked if I could drive the fire engine through the course. I was given the ok and climbed up into the tall, long red truck. It had been a few years since I had driven a fire engine and many watching me this time didn't even know I had ever driven one.

I started out slow. I snaked my way through the cones, missing a cone by one thin layer of paint. The Fire Captain sitting in the cab with me then told me to do the same thing, but this time in reverse. I put the engine in reverse and slowly I snaked back through the cones. The old timers laughed at the newbie's amazement. I then made a tight turn to my left and came upon a simulated loading dock parking situation with only inches to spare on either side. It wasn't easy. But I have backed travel trailers, boats, RV's towing a vehicle, and of course, ambulances and fire trucks. I jockeyed the long fire truck around and "backed it up to the dock," without losing a cone.

Then I found myself in a speeding fire engine barreling toward a fork in the road. I waited for the Fire Captain to tell me which way to go, but he kept silent. The distance shrunk quickly, I began to get a bit apprehensive. Then he said "Right." I turned my wheel and felt the water in the tank shift. I made the turn and then the road took a wide, long left hand curve. It actually was hard to keep it within the cones. I then straightened it up and headed for the narrow finish. The poles tops were bent inward and could scrape the top of the engine if the driver isn't careful. I must say, this was the hardest part. I approached at a high rate of speed, slowing, but still rather fast. I gripped the wheel and entered the obstacle resembling a tunnel. It was a tight fit. I zipped through and no pole was spun out and tumbled to the ground. All the poles still stood as I slammed on my breaks and came to a stop three inches from the barrier that ended the course.

I still had it! "I don't believe it. How did you do that?" asked the Assistant Fire Chief.

I smiled, "I went through Engineer school and this isn't the first time I have driven an engine."

"Obviously," he said with a smile on his face. It was a lot of fun and I loved it. "Sharon, would you like to drive the airport truck?"

I had never been behind that big a vehicle and jumped at the chance. We went over and climbed up the ladder into the cab. The vehicle was painted a lime green and we all called it the "Monster." It was huge, wide, tall and long. I sat down at the steering wheel. The vehicle was designed to approach an airplane on fire, drive into the flames and extinguish it. Even the tires and underside was designed to tolerate the heat of a direct fire. The chief explained, "We are at times shorthanded and it might come to past that we might need all the firefighters to fight the fire and if the Rescue Division members were cross trained, they could drive this vehicle to knock down the initial fire, allowing firefighters access to the plane and soles on board."

I started the monster and it roared to life with a loud, deep rumble. I shifted it into forward and gently pressed down on the pedal, it slowly moved forward. I drove the truck around the airport, fast at times, slow at others. It was bigger but it handled a lot like my RV. With my right hand I grasped a joy-stick and activated the water spray. It responded immediately. A huge spray erupted and shot out. I then moved the joy-stick around aiming it from nose to tail of the imaginary burning airplane that lay before me. I switched the switch and changed the flow to a direct stream. I also was told how to switch it to foam, but didn't do it then in a cost saving measure. I loved it!

A few months later I was filling in at the PFD for a full timer and was expected to primarily serve as a Paramedic, but if needed I would also assist fire. The department had an attack truck that often went as a first responder vehicle for a fire and some medical calls. I was standing at the rear of the truck trying to remember how to pump water and how to pump foam if necessary. Captain Stewart walked up, "Do you remember how to pump it?"

"At Black Mesa Mine I have a similar truck, but it's older and a little different."

"Show me."

I managed to set it up for pumping water, but I failed to figure out how to switch to foam. The Captain showed me how to switch. I listened carefully because I might have to do this for real five minutes from now. That evening we had a fire drill. Captain Stewart decided to play a little trick on an unsuspecting firefighter. He looked around the firemen and picked one that didn't drive the attack truck that much. "Come up here. Now, show us how to pump foam." He should have known how, but he didn't. He set it up to pump water, but when told to set up to pump foam, he had to admit he didn't remember. From the look on a number of faces, I was sure he wasn't the only one who had forgotten. The Captain then turned to me, "Sharon, show them how."

I knew what the Captain was doing, was going to make the firemen look stupid when a woman who doesn't usually fill in for firefighters, knew how to do it. They had no idea of my experience with the old attack truck and the current one at the mine where I worked part time. I had also had a great review only hours before. I stepped up and flipped the switches as I verbally explained what I was doing.

"Thanks Sharon." He smiled. "Now I want each one of you show me you can turn it on the foam setting." The firemen slowly took turns and finally they all had completed the test. I doubt any of them will forget how to pump foam any time soon.

That night I ran on one unconscious man lying in the park. He had drunk from a bottle of whiskey until he passed out. I was also called to a dumpster fire and tragically, a baby not breathing. At eight o'clock the next morning, I returned home. I changed my "hat" and slipped into my other personality. Maurice's wife and the mother of two had returned home. I unloaded the dishwasher and threw a load of dirty clothes into the washer.

WHO WAS HE? WHO WAS HE RUNNING FROM? WHAT ABOUT THE MONEY?

The man was about thirty-eight years old, in good shape, six foot three inches tall, and about two hundred and twenty pounds. His dark brown hair hung long about his unshaven face. He looked directly at the front desk clerk with piercing blue eyes. The clerk asked no questions when he paid with cash. The man had an air about him that made those around him walk quietly and ask no questions. He avoided small talk. He signed an eligible name. He took the key for room 112 from the intimidated front desk clerk and walked out without a word.

The next morning the maid cleaned all the rooms, saving room 112 till last. She wanted to get home, but couldn't until the man vacated the room. She hated to knock on the door, but it was one o'clock and he should have checked out two hours ago. She walked up to the window and peeked through the gap in the drapes. She gasped, stepped back then turned and ran to the office.

I was busy at home when I heard the radio traffic. The police officer, Jeff Stark, took the call. I found my shoes and keys, I was certain they would be calling me next. Sure enough, three minutes after arriving, the officer called for backup and requested dispatch call F-3 (Fire-Three) to report directly to the scene. I arrived in a couple of minutes. Two police cars now were parked outside the room. The motel was modular in construction. It was one of the less expensive motels in Page. I had gone on some interesting calls at this motel in the past. I walked over to the two officers, Jeff and Anthony. "What do we have?" I asked.

Jeff was slipping on his leather gloves, Anthony was as well. "The maid noticed a trap. There's a crossbow pointing toward the door. I can see a string leading from the bow to the front door. It's cocked and ready to kill the first person through the door."

"Who's inside?"

"Don't know. I couldn't see anyone, but I can hear the shower running."

"How are you going to get in?"

"Anthony's going through the window." I didn't like the idea. This was dangerous. If the guy inside was that paranoid, what would he do if he come out of the shower and found someone in his motel room? I know the officers wanted me here if this went bad. I began to wonder if I should "stage" further away from the door.

The officers moved to the front window. Anthony was the smaller of the two men so he was going to be the one to squeeze through the window. They used a pry bar to open the partially cracked window. Anthony slipped into the room with gun drawn. He moved across the room. At the cross bow, he kneeled down and set the safety. He then cut the string to the door. He let the second officer into the room. They moved toward the bathroom door. The water from the shower could be heard. Anthony slowly opened the door, flung it open, gun aimed and yelled "POLICE!"

I was waiting outside, out of the line of fire. If the guy came bursting through the door, I could easily escape. I then heard Jeff on my radio, "Sharon, come on in." I hurried inside. It was an inexpensive motel room, worn drapes, faded bedspread, small table, two chairs, scuffed dresser, crocked mirror and a cross bow, duct taped to a wobbly chair. "Here, in the bathroom. . . ." Jeff indicated.

I went to the bathroom door. It took no imagination at all to see what had happened. The man lay on the floor. He was naked and very dead. He had obviously showered in the small shower with no tub. He appeared to have stepping out, slipped and his head hit the sink. It was the death blow. I checked no pulse. Lividity (pooled blood, dark purple blotches) had set in so he had been dead for a few hours. There was no evidence of foul play. He was the type of guy you would expect to die in a knife fight, not by slipping in the shower.

I reached over and turned off the water and left the room. Anthony was searching the room. His back was to me when he said "Guys, look at this." Jeff and I crossed the room and stood beside Anthony. He pointed to a black duffel bag lying on the dresser. Anthony had unzipped it then stepped back. It was completely full of money . . . . . a lot of money.

"How much is there?" I asked.

"I don't know but it's mostly big bills. I can't think of a legitimate reason to carry this much cash," Anthony said.

"He was running from someone. That's why he set up the booby trap before he took a shower," theorized Jeff.

"Drug money?"

"Maybe."

Jeff looked in the jeans lying on the bed and withdrew a wallet. "Driver license says he's John Mitchell. Want to bet it's not his real name?"

Anthony walked over and looked at the picture, "It doesn't even look like him."

"Well, if it's ok with you guys, I'm out of here," I said.

"Yeah, thanks for the backup," Jeff said as Anthony went for the camera.

Later it was discovered the mystery man's car was stolen from California. The ID wasn't his. His fingerprints came back no match. There was no central data base in those days. His picture was sent to California police, but they had no idea who he was. No one reported missing a ton of money. We never found out his identity. We never found out from whom he was running. And the money, no one ever claimed it. It's still a mystery, an unsolved cold case

HALLOWEEN WILL NEVER BE THE SAME

It was a dark October night, only a few days away from Halloween. The air was crisp and cool. I sat in the passenger side of the ambulance with Ken Connors driving. He was a new driver and hadn't actually had that much time in the back of the ambulance. He was good, but inexperienced. We were rushing to a one car rollover. There was one reported dead and two injured. The scene was a few miles outside town on highway 98. I always wanted my EMTs to get a good exposure to everything they might encounter on the streets and highways. A dead body was one thing Ken hadn't faced yet. "Ken, when we get there, we will take the two boys and you go over and check the dead body."

He turned and looked at me with surprise. He knew it was

31

protocol for at least two to confirm a death. He had never even seen a dead body before unless you counted his Uncle Tito's funeral. I knew by scanner traffic that Edgar El Terra a local nurse practitioner was at the scene so Ken verifying death was only a legal requirement. To the EMT in the back, I said "Hand me a stethoscope." She did, through the small window that connected the back with the driver's compartment. "Here," I said as I draped it around Ken's neck. "Use this." He nodded. He was a big man, huge in fact. He was always a bit hyper on a call, eager to do his best, and intense. He drove, but his mind was on what he would do when we got there.

The accident was like a hundred others in that area. The woman and her two sons had driven into town off the reservation. The boys, in their mid-teens had gone their way and she went hers when they hit town that day. They met back at the car later that evening, the woman was drunk. The oldest boy offered to drive, but the mother insisted she would. They protested, but she insisted she wasn't drunk and could drive perfectly well. The boys were over forty miles from home and she was their mother. They got in.

She made it about twelve miles before they ran into trouble. Alcohol slows down the nervous system. The eyes of a person that has been drinking are affected by the alcohol. When they drive at night, they experience a type of night blindness. The headlights of an oncoming car cause their eyes to constrict. Then because of the alcohol their eyes don't immediately dilate again. The pupils stay tiny and let only a little light in. For all practical purposes, that person is blind. She didn't see the slight bend in the road and her car sailed out into the desert, burying its front end in the soft sand causing the car to flip end over end.

The two boys were in the back seat. They were suddenly tossed around as glass shattered and metal bent. The sound of their mother's scream was heard as she was thrown out of the vehicle. She landed hard on the desert floor. She would have survived, but the car, still flipping, hunted her down and landed on her then flipped on over onto its wheels. Her two sons got out of the wreck by themselves. They found their mother lying on her back, her head crushed by the car. They fell apart. Luck would have it that Edgar, the nurse practitioner, was passing by and stopped. He was a very competent person, caring, and better than most of the doctors that practice in Page. He took charge.

When the ambulance arrived, I saw the two boys standing with Clare Cooper. She was a Page officer. She knew the boys and was providing the support they needed. We walked them to the ambulance. They weren't hurt. They were bruised here and there, but they didn't 33appear to be injured beyond the band aid stage. Emotionally, was a different matter. The oldest, around sixteen bitterly announced, "I killed my mother."

"You weren't driving, you didn't kill her," the officer said.

"I should have been driving. She was so drunk. I knew that. I should have insisted she let me drive." He buried his face in his hands and cried. The officer put her arm around him and he cried on her shoulder. She gently tried to convince him he was not responsible for his mother's death.

The younger brother around fifteen was also emotionally distraught. But his anger was turned toward his mother. "She never cared enough about us. She always drove drunk with us in the car. All she cared about was getting drunk." He too was crying inconsolable. I cradled him in my arms and let him cry. This treatment isn't in the EMT book and most class rooms don't teach this, but it was the only comfort I could give this boy and it was what he needed.

Outside, in the dark, Ken approached the body that lay on the ground. Edgar was standing beside the woman. He too knew Ken was an untried EMT. He was there if Ken needed him. Ken knelled down beside the woman. Her face was horrible. An eye was bulging out, her cheek bone was depressed inward, her teeth were gone, blood matted her thick black hair and her nose was shoved over to the side and flat. Her head was lopsided and caved in, brain tissue leaked from a crack in the skull and into the sand. She had been partially scalped and bare skull bone was exposed. Ken sat staring at the woman. In his mind he was trying to visualize what she had looked like only a half hour before. He reached out his hand and hesitated and then touched her neck, searching for a pulse everyone, including him, knew wasn't there. He then realized he had looked at a horrible deformed body, actually touched it and lived. He grew braver and took the stethoscope and placed it on the woman's chest. He listened carefully.

Edgar, as tactfully as possible, reached down and flipped the head of the stethoscope around. The way it was made, it was impossible to hear anything the way Ken was using the instrument. Embarrassed, Ken then listened and took them out of his ears and looked up at Edgar. "I don't hear anything. She hasn't got a pulse and isn't breathing."

Edgar and Ken walked back to the ambulance and got a sheet and covered the body. Ken drove us back to town. We took the boys to the hospital to be checked. A Navajo police officer had gone in search for relatives to come get the boys and take them home.

Back at the station, Ken silently wrote the report. He had been affected by the call, we all had. But it was his first time. "Well, Ken, how did it go?" I asked. He laid down his pen and collected his thoughts. He and I talked for a long while. He was doing ok. He was a strong man and although it bothered him, he was doing fine. We all finished the reports and went home.

Halloween came later that week. Ken came to see me the next day. He was upset, nothing he couldn't handle, but upset. He needed to talk. I listened. "You know, Halloween won't ever be the same. I remember opening the door and there stood two little kids. Their masks were horrible. The woman's face flashed before my eyes. Her eye hanging out that way, the blood and brains......." He shifted his great weight in the undersized chair. "I couldn't help but wonder how disrespectful those masks were, how gross they were. How could parents dress two small children up in that hideous way and call it fun?"

"They don't know, Ken. What you saw out there a few days ago, few people see. They know people die and they know bodies can be disfigured, but they haven't actually experienced it. You saw a real woman after she had been killed violently. They may see it in a horror movie, but it's not the same. You know what it is like in the real world, they don't. And they don't want to know." I continued, "To them, it's pretend, fantasy, fiction, television and Hollywood. You know it's actually real, horribly real.

"As long as I live I will never dress my children up like that. I won't let them laugh at violent, horrible death. It isn't something you kid around about. It will be clowns and princesses, from now on."

Ken left. I thought about what he had said. It was true. The bloody movies, the Halloween haunted houses, television, have taken the edge off decapitations, ax murders and other awful ways to die. Children watch Freddy Kruger slice up and disembowel people and they call it entrainment. They spend hours every day playing games where the goal is to kill and dismember as many people as possible.

We encounter the brutal side of life of disemboweled people, decapitation, burnt bodies and dead babies. People do die that way. It isn't pretend. But then, most people live in their own little pretend world and they like it that way. They don't want to get their hands dirty. They don't want to pick up body parts and they don't really know what it feels like to pick up a burnt body and have chucks of flesh flake off the bone into your hand like an over cooked roast. EMTs are exposed to this side of life and it affects them. It will forever change the way they look at ordinary things. They will be different, they can't help it. It goes with the job. Is it bad? I don't know, but it makes your feet become firmly planted on the ground and if you aren't careful, a negative or at least a cynical outlook on life can take hold.

There is good in the world. We can't forget that. And we can't condemn those that don't know what it can really like. We choose this field of work, they didn't. They can live with their limited since of reality, and we can learn to live with ours.

EXCAPED CONVICT ON THE LOOSE

The detention officer was tired. He didn't like transporting prisoners, it was boring. Hunger hit him as he pulled off Highway 89 and drove into Page. There are relatively few places you can walk in with three convicts chained together. Most people would have immediately thought of the take out window, but then the guard was tried and the prisoners were a friendly group that had not given him one bit of trouble. They were all starving and the driver needed a break. He had been at the wheel for hours.

The detention officer pulled into the first hamburger place he could find, RD's Pink Sands. "Look guys, if you behave yourself and not create a big stir, we can all go in here and get something to eat." They all promised to be good little boys. He unchained their ankle chains and their wrist chains. The four men walked into the hamburger place just like ordinary people, well almost. They ordered a variety of tasty treats and sat down to eat.

"Hay, I got to go to the john," said a tall thin man with light red hair.

"In a minute we'll all go." The guard dipped his French fry in ketchup and ate it. The men finished up their meal and together they walked outside and into an outside door marked "Restrooms." The door opened into a dark, short hallway with two doors on the left, one marked *women* and one marked *men*. The bathrooms were tiny and only one person could fit inside at a time. The three men took turns as the guard stood outside. The thin, tall man's turn came and he hurried into the small room. He promptly opened the window and squeezed through the narrow space to freedom.

It didn't take long for the detention officer to see that he had been had. The guard went berserk when he discovered his prisoner was missing. The police were called. They weren't happy either. "Why did you unchain them?" the police asked. The guard had little to say in his defense.

It was around eight o'clock at night and I was at home. My scanner came to life as the Page Police (PPD) suddenly had something to do. They all talked at once in that deep voice that men use when they talk

35

into a microphone. They began to search every dark place in town. We lived in a small town where doors were not locked till bedtime, if at all. I locked my doors anyway since the hamburger place was a short two blocks from my house. I listened as the airways hummed. I jumped when my phone rang.

"Sharon, this is dispatch. We need a transport crew in about half an hour. An Air Evac plane is landing to take a woman in labor to Phoenix."

"Go ahead and page the first out crew," I told her. I knew I couldn't arrange a second crew to handle this non-emergency because most of my people were out of town.

"Sharon, have you been listening to the scanner?" she asked.

"Yeah, what's he in prison for?"

"Rape."

"Who do I have on tonight?"

"Laura, Lilly, and Sally."

"Three women . . . . . ."

"Yeah."

The airport was very dark this time of night. Sometimes it gets a bit lonely and a little spooky waiting for the plane to land. I knew there was little chance the escaped convict would try for a vehicle with a red lights and siren, but you never know. Also, if the crew knew, they could keep a lookout as they handle the transport. "I'm going down to the station and talk to them."

"Good Idea. I'll page." The dispatcher hung up. My husband put down his book as I picked up my keys.

"Need some company?"

"No, I`ll be all right. I won't be long." I walked outside. There was no moon and it was a very dark night. I walked to my car and opened the door. I turned around and saw my husband standing in the door. I waved and got in, locking the doors.

At the station I met the three women getting ready to leave. Lilly was a pretty, slender woman. Her long dark hair was always well groomed. She had a pleasant personality, was well liked and a good EMT. Sally had a house full of children. She was tall and of slender build. She always appeared harried. Laura was "Miss Perfect" and never missed an opportunity to remind you of her perfection. I decided to get to the point. "There is something going on unrelated to this transport that you should know about."

"What?" asked Lilly.

"A group of prisoners were being transported through Page and one of them got away from RD's."

"What did he do?" Laura asked.

"He's a convicted rapist." That got their attention.

"My kids are home . . . . . . alone."

"Mine too." Lilly went to the phone and dialed home. "Lock the doors and don't go outside till I get home." One of the other women called a friend to go get her two children. The other called home and told her husband to lock up and be vigilant.

"I want you to keep an eye out for this man. He's tall and thin, and his hair is slightly red. Even if you see him lying down in the middle of the road, you get police backup before you get near him."

"We will," they assured me.

"And keep your doors locked, just in case." They didn't like it and to tell the truth I didn't either. Bad timing, but it couldn't be helped. I walked back outside and looked around. The fire station was located, at that time, across from a bar, the Windy Mesa. It was not the best area of town after dark. I saw nothing out of the ordinary. I walked to my car, peeked into the back seat and got inside and locked the doors. I listened to the activity on my scanner all the way home. It was interesting.

The women in the ambulance were hyper. They were scared and wished they were safe at home instead of sitting on a dark apron at a deserted airport waiting for a plane to land. It was a moonless night. Shadows moved around and strange sounds heightened their nervousness. They talked among themselves, each feeding the other as they worked themselves up into a hyper state of near panic. In the darkness they saw movement, or did they? What was that sound? They listened to the scanner and knew where the man wasn't, but they didn't know where he was and that scarred them. I couldn't blame them.

Now, Officer Anthony Santiago was driving by the airport and saw the ambulance sitting by the one tiny light. He started to key his microphone but there was traffic. He really should check on them and let them know what's going on. So he turned into the airport gate. He turned off his headlights as he drove up behind the ambulance.

"Well, I don't like it out here. We should have waited."

"He could be anywhere you know . . . ." The women were all talking at once. Silently Anthony walked up to the driver side window and tapped on the glass with his flashlight to get their attention. Lilly's head was only inches from the window. She only knew there was a loud tapping and out of the corner of her eye she could see a dark form of a man. She screamed and moved away, the other women also screamed and the three were just bouncing around inside the ambulance doing laps on the ceiling, running nowhere, but running anyway.

Anthony grabbed the door handle and tried to get inside and that made it worst. He backed away and shined the flashlight on himself. They finally saw it was him and opened the door.

"You scared us to death!" they yelled.

He laughed. "Sorry. I just wanted to make sure you locked you doors and kept a look out for an escaped convict." They explained to him that I had already alerted them to the possible danger. They assured him they would keep a look out and he left.

A sigh of relief was heard as the plane landed. They quickly loaded the two female nurses and their equipment. On the way to the hospital, they told the two nurses about the rapist and the incident with the officer. Now there were five frightened women. The nurses added their horror stories to the already too many running around in the women's minds. They were all wired as they pulled up to the emergency entrance.

The ambulance backed up to the door. The woman started to gather their equipment. Suddenly the side door, which they thought was locked, was violently flung open. The noise and sudden movement caused the women to scream and pull away, knocking over equipment and stepping on each other.

Doctor Birch was a short man, wide and burdened with a deity complex. He often instilled the fear of God into nurses with his brisk and rude attitude, but he didn't expect five women to scream and run as he suddenly opened the ambulance side door. It caught him and the women completely off guard. They screamed and he screamed, adding to the complete hysteria. When the dust settled, everyone was embarrassed. They had to explain why they were so jumpy. He regained his composure and escorted them inside.

The doctor gave the air crew a report. The air crew took a set of vital signs. When they were ready, the patient was loaded into the ambulance with Dr. Birch standing guard. He also insisted on riding to the airport with them. They didn't object. The ambulance now carried five women, one patient and a doctor. It was a crowded little vehicle. They were all shoved up against each other, but no one complained. As they drove to the airport they listened to the police scanner.

Officer De Aquileo was driving by the high school and had noticed movement around some cars. He pulled in and got out. Now De Aquileo is as huge man. His ideal of a good time was to lift weights. When he tried he could be intimidating. He wandered fearlessly over to the place he had seen movement. He walked between two cars and found a tall, thin man with slightly reddish hair crouched in the darkness. "You're under arrest boy," he said in a deep threatening voice.

The man looked up, and from his angle the officer must have looked like King Kong. "Yes sir," he said as he held his wrists out to be

38

handcuffed. When it was announced over the radio that the convict had been arrested, a sigh of relief went out in the crowded ambulance. The patient was loaded on the airplane and the doctor delivered back to the hospital. The women went home and it was over. But everyone, for a change, locked their doors as they went to bed that night.

A DARK SPIRIT

It was a warm fall afternoon in Flagstaff, Arizona. Rachel was eighteen years old. Her black hair hung shoulder length; her dark black eyes were bright with intelligence. Her parents, Mr. and Mrs. Goldstein, were proud of her. They were Jewish and expected excellence. Rachel had not disappointed them. She had been a good daughter through high school and now, as she began her first year at Northern Arizona University, she showed great promise. They had spent the warm afternoon swimming in the backyard swimming pool. Steaks sizzled on the grill. All was right with the world, or so it seemed.

"I'm going to go change out of this wet swimsuit," Rachel said as she started into the house.

"Don't take too long, the steaks are almost done," her mother called out.

"I won't," Rachel, replied, "I'm starved." She hurried into the house. After a while, the steaks were done. Her father removed them from the grill. Her mother called out to Rachel, but got no answer. Mrs. Goldstein got up and went inside to look for her daughter. Rachel was gone. She wasn't in the house. Her mother was confused. She checked the driveway and discovered Rachel's car gone.

She returned to the backyard. "Rachel's gone," she said to her husband.

"What?"

"She's left. Her car is gone." Both parents were confused. Nothing had seemed out of the ordinary. No fights, no obvious problems, nothing to explain her sudden disappeared. The Goldstein's called her cell number, but there was no answer. They called their oldest daughter, but she had not seen Rachel. Rachel's friends had not seen her either. Where did she go? The police would not take a missing person's report since Rachel was an adult and had obviously left of her own accord. The parents waited nervously for their daughter to call.

39

The next morning Rachel's car sat beside the road a few miles east of Kanab, Utah. The small community is about one hundred and forty miles north of Flagstaff and seventy-five miles east of Page, Arizona. Rachel stood beside the car. Highway 89 is a remote two-lane road. In that area, scrub pine dots the rolling hills. Bright red sandstone cliffs stand in the distance to the north. A car passed by and slowed. The middle-aged man and wife inside decided to stop and see if the young lady needed assistance.

They approached her and discovered something was indeed wrong. Rachel stood staring off into the distance with glassed over eyes that saw nothing. She was babbling nonsense. The words came fast, but failed to form sentences. They were a jumbled mess of random words with occasional grunts, groans, and odd sounds. She didn't appear to even see the couple. She just stood, babbling. They called for an ambulance.

In Flagstaff, a couple of hours later, Rachel's parents received a phone call from a doctor at the Kanab Hospital. He explained how Rachel had been found. The parents got in their car and drove to Kanab. The Utah Highway Patrol had not had the car towed. The officer said it appeared that Rachel had driven the car until it had run out of gas. Mr. Goldstein took his five-gallon gas can and poured it into the gas tank. He and his wife then drove to the Kanab hospital. They found Rachel sitting in a wheelchair, staring at the wall. She was quite now. No one knew if that was a good thing or not. Her parents decided to take their daughter back to Flagstaff for additional medical care. The father decided to drive his daughter's car and have his wife follow in the family car. Rachel sat beside her father, staring ahead, saying nothing. This worked for the first seventy-two miles.

On the outskirts of Page, Rachel suddenly "woke up." She turned her head toward her father and yelled, "I want to die and you are going with me!" She grabbed her father, opened her door and with the strength of three men, proceeded to drag her father half-way out the door of the speeding car with her. Mr. Goldstein hung on to the steering wheel as the car swerved all over the road. The father struggled to stop the car and keep his daughter from killing them both. He got the car stopped at the inspection station. There, he continued to struggle with her as she screamed she wanted to die and take him with her. Two truckers and an inspection officer helped the father subdue her. Police and an ambulance were called. The sheriff arrived and cancelled the ambulance. He believed her to be too violent for ambulance transport. The father was scratched, bitten, and bruised, but he refused treatment. The officer handcuffed her and put her in the patrol car. She continued to curse, scream, spit, kick, and struggle. The officer drove her to the hospital with her parents following behind.

At the hospital, Rachel kicked a nurse, spit on the doctor and continued to threaten the life of her father and everyone else. The nurse injected a drug to calm her, but it didn't seem to have an effect. A second dose was given and she calmed down. She lay on her back, staring at the ceiling. Again, she appeared unaware of her surroundings. The hospital called Air Evac to fly her to Flagstaff, but they were told they didn't transport mental patients. A few years before a mental patient had become uncontrollable and attacked the pilot. The plane crashed, killing all on board. Policy was written to make sure this didn't happen again.

Now, I enter the picture. A court order for admittance to a mental facility was obtained and they wanted me to transport her by ground to the Guidance Center in Flagstaff. After hearing about her violent behavior, I agreed to transport her under certain conditions. Everyone agreed to cooperate with my conditions, and the transport was arranged. She would be heavily sedated and restrained to a backboard. I got orders for as much Valium as needed from Medical Control. A large deputy would ride along, just in case.

Rachel lay still in the back of the ambulance. She was restrained to a backboard and drugs had been given to keep her still. Her eyes were closed. I took her vital signs every fifteen minutes and checked her restraints often. An IV of normal saline dripped slowly into her vein. I took a syringe and pull up a dose of Valium. I then taped the syringe to the wall so it would not get lost or roll into some crevice or the floor. At the first sign of movement, I planned on sedating her with Valium. After two hours of peaceful silence, I let my guard down. Suddenly, her eyes opened. She glanced around, tears formed in her eyes. "I tried to kill my father!" she said in disbelief. Her voice became a whisper. "It was a . . . . Dark Spirit." At this point, I don't know exactly how to explain what happened next. Her eyes changed. The eyes are said to be windows to the sole. They turned toward me, black and cold. A chill ran down my spine as I stared into the deep darkness of her eyes. Fear flooded over me. I shoved the syringe of Valium into the IV. Her eyes lingered for, what seemed like a hour, and then turned back to the ceiling. They were again blank, staring at nothing, and then they closed.

"What just happened?" asked the officer.

"I'm not sure."

"That wasn't her . . . . she's possessed," he said in a low voice.

"That's what it looked like," I said, also in a quiet voice. It was as if we didn't want to speak too loud and wake *it* again.

"Is she going to start puking green slim like in the movie?"

41

"I don't know," I answered. "I hope not."

"Damn, that was weird," he said. We continued the rest of the trip in silence, each of us just staring at the girl, not knowing what to expect.

At the Flagstaff Guidance Center, a nurse met us. She was a small, thin woman with a hook nose. Her dull brown hair was tied back into a small bun at the base of her thin neck. She didn't smile. Instead she firmly informed the officer he wasn't welcome inside. "The uniform upsets the guests," she said. The EMT and I wheeled the gurney into the building. It was a depressing place with odd, unpleasant smells. About fifteen people wandered around in a large open area with chairs, couches and a television. They were dressed in t-shirts and jeans and some were wearing PJ's and robes. Most needed their hair combed, and none looked me straight in the eye. About two-thirds appeared to be zombies lost in their own world, the rest appeared to be frightened.

Seeing the leather straps on Rachel's wrists and ankles, the nurse said in a disgusted voice, "We don't restrain our patients here."

"Yes you do. You just use chemical restraints." She had no right to criticize me for restraining a violent patient. Let her ride one-hundred and forty miles with a patient set on killing someone. In the tiny space of an ambulance there just isn't much running room. I for one want to protect the patient and myself and if I have to resort to physical restraints, so be it. She snorted and told us to follow her.

She led us to a steel door with bars on the open window. We rolled the stretcher inside. "Untie her," the nurse demanded. I looked at the EMT and could tell he didn't like this anymore than I did. I told the nurse the patient wasn't to be trusted and was violent. "Nonsense," she said. She bent down, close to Rachel's face. "Rachel?" she said. Much to my surprise, Rachel opened her eyes. She should have been out like a light with the dose of Valium I had given her only fifteen minutes before. But upon reflection, at the Kanab and Page Hospital, one dose had not been enough. "Rachel, I am going to untie you. You won't do anything, will you?" Rachel smiled a humorless smile and slowly shook her head *no*. I had a bad feeling about this. "There, see? Now, let's untie her." The EMT and I untied her quickly, moved her to the bed and rushed out of the room.

We wheeled our stretcher as far away from Rachel's room as we could get. We parked our stretcher along the wall of the open area near the exit. We couldn't leave because the door was locked and "Nurse Ratchet" had the keys and code. Suddenly, a loud scream was heard from the room. I couldn't tell if it was the nurse or Rachel. The door opened and the nurse and two attendants ran out, slamming the heavy door behind them. The nurse rushed to the nursing station yelling, "Give me a cocktail (slang for an IV bag of drugs designed to calm violent patients.)" She glanced up at me, our eyes locked. I know she could see "I told you so," in my expression. A woman dressed in dark blue scrubs handed her a light yellow IV bag. The nurse picked up two syringes and with the two attendants, she re-entered Rachel's room. More screaming, cursing and noise of a scuffle was heard, then silence.

I didn't like this place. It was full of lost souls silently crying for help. I felt an overwhelming wave of depression descend upon me as if it were a blanket. I had to get out of this place. I don't know if it was my cluster phobia or my sense of survival, but I had to get out. My partner appeared to be as uncomfortable as I was. As they all left her room, I motioned to the nurse. She came over to me. "Can we leave now?" She said nothing, but keyed in the magic numbers of the day into the key pad, then inserted an oddly shaped key into the lock and the heavy door opened. We quickly made our escape.

The officer was standing beside the ambulance. "Is she ok?"

"No, she isn't. She's screaming and putting up a fight."

"She doesn't need a doctor, she needs an exorcist," he said.

I agreed. One of the downsides to this job, is we often don't know how things turn out. Rachel's parents were well off and I believe they spared no expense in finding treatment for their daughter. But, I have seen psychiatric episodes before and since. This was unlike anything I have ever seen. I hope she recovered, but I don't think it was a mental illness. I believe she was possessed by what she described as a "Dark Spirit.

LET ME FINISH MY CIGARETTE

"Trailer fire, Space 223 Golden Circle, Lake Powell Mobile Home Village," the dispatcher announced loudly. I was in my PFD car and had just crested the top of the hill on the south access road. I was only about a half mile from the reported fire. I turned around and flipped on my overhead lights. People moved aside as I sped to the location. It was around two o'clock, a bright, clear spring day. I heard over my radio that a police officer was also responding. He and I should arrive at about the same time.

I entered the park and turned my siren off and slowed down. The park had tons of children and they all played in the road. The police officer and I quickly found the trailer. We both pulled up at the same time. The lot next door was vacant and no fence divided the two lots so I parked in front of the vacant lot to allow responding fire trucks easy access to the burning trailer. "F-3, 10-97 (I had arrived), smoke showing, I can see a man inside," I said into my radio. The scene before me was a sight to behold.

I could see a small, thirty foot trailer. It was the type that had a kitchen/dining room in the front of the trailer, a living room in the center and one bedroom and bath in the rear. The front door was wide open. Thick, black smoke boiled from the trailer's door and windows. A black cloud hung near the ceiling (top two feet). It appeared the fire started in the bedroom but now threatened the entire trailer.

I could see a couch directly through the door. An overweight man, about sixty-something, was sitting on the couch. He was dressed in a white t-shirt and a pair of Dockers. He was barefoot and had a nasal cannula in his nose. It was connected to a four foot tall green d-cylinder of oxygen sitting at the end of the couch against the wall. On the other side of that wall was the flaming bedroom. The man's head was just under the boiling black cloud that filled the trailer. He sat in the "good air" portion, but that was getting lower and lower by the minute and the flames were burning through the bedroom door and wall to his right. The flames began licking at the tank and the couch. The man was next, but he just sat there, smoking a cigarette.

I looked at the police officer. We usually didn't run into a burning building with no protective gear, but the man would be on fire if we waited for the fire engine to arrive. I sighed and said "let's go." He silently agreed and we both ran forward. I took a deep breath and bent down and entered the burning trailer. The flames had burst through the bedroom wall and the arm of the couch was now on fire. I could feel the heat radiating into the room. I held my breath but the smoke was thick and burned my eyes. I could see the flames licking at the big green oxygen tank that now sat between the burning bedroom wall and the burning couch. If the tank got hot enough, the air would expand and the tank could explode, blowing chucks of metal outward as shrapnel.

I grabbed the man under one arm and the officer grabbed the other. We turned and drug him across the small living room and with some difficulty managed to get the three of us through the doorway and outside. Unfortunately, I forgot the nasal cannula and as we ran from the flames, the hose tightened and his head whipped backward, almost tearing his head off. He screamed in protest. We stopped, I removed the nasal cannula and we quickly drug the man to safety.

The fire truck arrived, water was put on the fire and it was quickly put out. The bedroom was a complete loss and the couch was partly

44

burned and the green tank was scorched, but the rest of the trailer was saved. I put the man on oxygen. "Why didn't you get out of the trailer?" I asked.

"I have COPD, (chronic obstructive pulmonary disease) and I can't walk." He spoke in a nonchalant tone. He then pulled out a package of cigarettes, removed one and lit up. I took it away from him.

"Oxygen isn't flammable, but it makes everything else burn like crazy. You can't smoke while on oxygen." I wanted to, but didn't add, the cigarettes are what caused him to have COPD in the first place.

"I smoke all the time while on O2."

"Maybe you do, but not in my ambulance." He mumbled but didn't argue the point. I believe if I had been him, I would have crawled on my bloodied hands and knees to escape death by fire, but he apparently felt finishing his cigarette was a higher priority. He never said "thank you" to me or the officer. He came within a couple of minutes of burning to death and all he was concerned about was his next cigarette. I guess this proves the warning printed on the cigarette package is true, "Cigarettes can be dangerous to your health."

FLARES IN THE NIGHT

Some calls start out one way and evolve into something entirely different before they are over. I had been Rescue Chief for a short time, when an out of town call came down. I responded to in town calls as a first responder. I would handle it until the ambulance arrived. I usually didn't go on out of town calls unless on the schedule or obviously needed. This call was a car vs. cow accident near Cedar Ridge. That is about thirty-five miles south of town. There were three people on this call so the ambulance was well manned. I can't explain why but I felt the overwhelming urge to go as a fourth person on this call. Many people don't believe in premonitions but through the years I have grown to listen to that quite still voice. Call it what you may, but it exists and I listened.

Our driver was Patrick Simpson. He was married with children, an attractive man, six foot tall, average weight and brown hair. He worked at the Navajo Generating Station but found time to sign up often for duty with the PFD. Patrick was a great driver. He drove comfortable both feet flat on the floor. He was a fast driver but drove safely. He was the best the department had. He was easy to work with and a good EMT. I rode up front and became the "cow watcher." The road wasn't fenced at the time and the open range could be hazardous to one's health and fenders.

We were within three miles of the accident when we passed another ambulance. They flashed their lights and pulled over. That was strange so we stopped. Patrick and I got out and walked back to them. It was a Navajo Nation Ambulance out of Tuba City. The government operated hospital provided ambulance service but was restricted to providing only care for non-Native Americans. EMS would provide emergency care until a non-Indian agency arrived at the scene. They would transport Anglos only under extreme circumstances. The Navajo EMTs often stretched the rules and assisted Anglos (whites). This ambulance was traveling to Page to pick up a man from the hospital. They had passed the accident and stopped to pick up the woman and girl even though they were white.

We had a decision to make. Take over the two patients or let them continue? Go to the scene or go home? "Is there any reason why we should go on to the scene?" I asked the EMT.

"Well we didn't have any flares and the cow is still in the road but we did leave that man. He was going to direct traffic till the police got there."

"What man?"

". . . . . The driver of the car. This is his wife and daughter."

"Oh ." That changed things. "We have flares. Do you mind taking these people to Page?"

"No, we're heading that way anyway."

"Then we will go on and set out some flares," and check out the man I thought to myself. I felt uncomfortable with them leaving him behind.

We found the cow lying in the road. The man stood in the road with a flashlight. The EMTs went and checked him while Patrick and I located the flares. "Patrick I know I should already know how but I don't. How do you light a flare?"

He laughed. "It's not hard. Here, watch." He took a flare and removed the cap. He struck the flare on the rough cap. Patrick lacked a little in style and instead of striking the flare away from him he struck it on its upward swing. The flare must have been old or damaged because it broke open and tiny crystals flew everywhere. "Damn," he said as he threw it down. I laughed and picked up another one.

We set out lots of flares. Traffic was light and the officer hadn't arrived yet. The Page Fire EMTs came up to me and told me the man suffers from high blood pressure and it was sky high. He hadn't had his medication today and the stress from wrecking his car and sending his wife and daughter to the hospital may have added to the elevated blood pressure. He got in the ambulance with the two female EMT's and Patrick and I took care of traffic.

It was a dark night, early spring. No cars no police, no nothing. We stuck around until the Navajo Police officer arrived. We then left. As we were driving down the road I noticed Patrick swerve a little. He brushed his arm and then his neck and then his forehead and then his neck again. "What's the matter?" I asked.

"I don't know. What's in a flare anyway?" he asked.

"I don't know. Is there a problem?"

"My arm and face are starting to burn. I think I got some of that crap in my eyes." They were starting to water.

"Pull over and stop."

Patrick didn't argue. He stopped in the road (pull offs are rare in the area) and turned on our overheads. We got out and walked to the side door and opened the patient compartment side door. "Patrick got some the flare on him. Give me some water." The patient stared as the EMT handed me the water jug.

I turned to Patrick. "Take off your shirt." It was cool that night, maybe forty degrees, maybe not quite. Patrick did as told and while standing in the desert I drowned him in water. He shifted in discomfort but allowed me to wash off his face, neck chest and arms.

"My eyes still sting," he said.

"Get in the back." He did and they wrapped a blanket around him. "Take the saline solution and drip it in his eyes and just let it run out. Keep it dripping till be get to the hospital." (Trick of the trade: A oxygen nasal cannula is used.) The tube end is connected to the IV bag. The nasal prongs are placed over the bridge of the nose and the elastic band is slipped over the patient's head. Water drips through the tube, through the nasal prongs and into the eyes.)

I got behind the wheel and started to drive. Now I know why I felt I needed to go on this call. Out of the three EMTS only Patrick knew how to drive the ambulance. I called on the EMSCOM radio, but we were in a dead spot and got no answer. I was hoping to patch through to a hospital and find out if we were doing all we could do. Patrick's eyesight could be at stake. To be completely honest, I didn't know for sure if the normal saline flush was the correct treatment. Normal Saline has the same chemical composition as tears. It was just a guess, but Patrick, who was also an EMT had agreed. It was probably the right thing to do.

One of the EMT's got out the Hazardous Materials (Haz Mat) book but flares weren't listed. I hurried. As we got within ten miles of the hospital I called dispatch. "We are ten miles out and have two patients. Call the hospital and ask them what we should do for a patient that has the chemical found in flares in his eyes."

The dispatcher did as told and came back and said to use sterile water. We didn't have sterile water. "Patrick" I yelled through the window. "The doctor says to use sterile water. We don't have sterile water only normal saline. It's your eyes what do you think we should do?"

"I don't know."

"Stop for a second." (Stop the eye flush.) They did.

"It's starting to burn again."

"OK if it feels good let's do it."

"Ok with me," said Patrick. We continued normal saline drip in his eyes. I didn't know what a stir my radio transition caused in town. Apparently the EMTs were very good at adding one and one and getting two. They knew Patrick was driving going out and suddenly I'm driving coming back. They had heard the Navajo Ambulance on the radio earlier and knew they were transporting two and left one victim at the scene. They all came to the same conclusion. Patrick was our second victim and he had flare chemicals in his eyes. When I pulled up at the hospital back entrance there was a large greeting party everyone was there except the fire chief. We took our two patients inside.

The nurse asked me "Is this industrial?" Well I was Patrick's boss wasn't I? This was new for me, a boss decisions.

"Yeah" I said as I assisted Patrick to the small exam room. I rubbed my arm absent mindedly as I watched the doctor and Patrick. Later the Fire Chief Nelson arrived. He was mad. I had failed to call him. (Wow the whole town knew and we had been at the hospital a whole eight minutes and I hadn't called.) Then he got even madder when he found out I had declared this an industrial injury.

"What else can it possibly be? He was hurt while on active duty." I never took well to being yelled at especially when I hadn't done anything wrong.

"He works for Salt River (Navajo Generation Station) let their insurance pick this up."

"His eyesight could be damaged. This could be nothing or something really big. It's our responsibility not SRP." The Fire Chief huffed off to check on Patrick. The doctor said he had ordered sterile water but since we didn't have it normal saline was just water with normal salt content of tears so we had done the right thing. We all stayed while the doctor brought the man's blood pressure down with medications. The doctor called Phoenix trauma center and found out how to best treat Patrick's eyes. They were burned but not badly and he was given some ointment and told to wear sunglasses for the next couple of days. I walked him to his car with his wife, absent mindedly rubbing my neck.

We went back to the station and cleaned the ambulance. "It was a good thing you came with us. Neither of us knows how to drive the ambulance and it's really dark tonight," said one of the EMTs.

Luck? No. I had known, with a certainly, that I would be needed. How, I don't know, but again that little voice had paid off. I drove home. When I got home I begin to tell my husband all about the call. During my narration I was rubbing my arm and neck without noticing, but my husband noticed. "Sharon, you better take a shower. You got that stuff on you too."

"No I didn't."

"You're scratching. Now go take a shower." I then noticed my arms did itch and my neck stung. I took a shower. The next day one arm and the side of my neck were red and felt as if I were sunburned. I hadn't noticed at the time but I too had some of the chemical on me when the flare exploded.

I made a list of all EMTs with the department that were not trained as drivers. I began a training program designed to train all PFD EMTS to drive the ambulance. Patrick's eyes healed quickly. That was the first time I had had to deal with *one of our own* injured. It was different very different. Unfortunately, it would not be the last time.

FLASHFLOOD

Maud and Henry had finally retired. They were ready to do what they wanted to do for a change. They bought a motor home, a big one. It was a few years old, but nearly new. Henry spent hours upon hours mapping out their route, what to see, where to camp, and every detail. Maud began nesting. She filled the RV with dishes, pots and pans, food, clothing, DVD's, cameras, everything they could possibly need for the next three months.

It was a bright, beautiful day when they pulled out of their driveway in Mesa, Arizona. Maud had never been behind the wheel of the huge RV and Henry had only driven it from the dealership to home and once to his friend's house about five miles away. But, both were excited and looking forward to three months of freedom. No alarm clocks, no idiot boss, no crisis with the children, no boring day after day routine of work and no play, just the two of them on an adventure to see what was beyond the hill and around the curve. An old Chinese proverb says, "Be careful what you wish for." Little did they know, life and death excitement laid waiting for them two-hundred and twenty miles to the north.

Their first day had been tense. Driving a big RV through traffic had demanded all the skill and luck poor old Henry could muster. But he made it, unscratched through their journey across Mesa, Phoenix, and the long, slow uphill trip out of the Valley of the Sun. They reached Flagstaff and pulled into the Wal-Mart parking lot, found a spot near the edge, next to the other RV's and settled in for the night.

The next morning, bright and early, Maud and Henry continued their journey. Maud played with her new digital camera as they headed for Monument Valley. She wanted to be ready for a picture taking frenzy. She completely ignored the dark angry clouds to the west. Highway 89 heading north of Flagstaff is an old narrow, bumpy, two lane road. It had no emergency parking, just a foot of extra pavement beyond the solid white line that marked the outer edge of the road. Henry struggled keeping the big motor home between the solid white line and the dotted center line. Confidence lacking, but spirit willing, they continued on their journey.

As they were closing in on the Tuba City turnoff, Maud announced she needed to go to the bathroom. Henry was annoyed. There was no place to pull off. She decided to walk back to the bathroom while they were moving. She staggered to the back and finished her business, awkwardly, but successfully. She staggered back up front in time to see the turn off to Highway 160. Before she could get back into the seat and buckle up, Henry made his tight right hand turn. That's when life became exciting.

I was on duty in Tuba City, in the middle of my seventy-two hour shift. I stood in a dirt field beside the road, cash in hand. Tony and I were preparing to purchase our lunch, barbequed mutton and fry bread (food of the gods!). The elderly Navajo woman had slaughtered the sheep herself and now stood beside her grill, slowly turning the thin strips of mutton. Her grand-daughter was preparing to drop the fry bread dough into the hot lard bubbling in the cast iron skillet. Our pager sounded "962, (auto accident with at least one person injured) at the junction of 160 and 89." The elderly woman smiled, she was use to our quick departures. "We'll be back," Tony, the EMT Driver said as we turned to leave. There were five more people waiting in line behind us so the food she was cooking wouldn't be wasted. We hurried to our ambulance and took off, code-three, lights and sirens blaring.

"Looks like rain," I said. Tony agreed. We were driving west, toward the large black angry cloud that now covered the entire western sky. There was a lot of water on the way. I could see it coming over the

50

mountain of rock and heading toward us. Flashes of lightening lit the dark sky.

We quickly covered the thirteen miles. As we pulled up to the crash, I looked it over. It was quite a sight to behold. Maud was lying on her back. Two Navajo Firefighters were securing her down to a backboard. A cervical collar was on her neck. She did not look amused. Henry was what I found interesting. The highway is elevated at this point because of a deep, well-worn wash (gully) that flowed with runoff from the infrequent, but intense desert rains. One large drainage pipe ran under the pavement to divert the water under instead of over the highway. Henry had swung too wide on the turn and went off on the opposite side. The motor home had tipped over and rolled once down a steep hill about fifteen feet. It now rested on the bed of the sandy wash. The RV was on its wheels. Henry was still strapped in the driver's seat. His hands were still on the wheel, and a dazed disbelieving look was on his face.

The odd thing about this is the motor home had disintegrated. It had broken apart as it rolled over and went down the hill. The only thing left intact was the floor, wheels, undercarriage, the motor, the toilet, the seat Henry sat on and the steering wheel. Everything else was scattered down the hill and in the wash. The desert floor was littered with clothing, cooking utensils, a toilet seat, can food, papers, and tiny chunks of insulation, wooden 2 by 2's and what was once the walls and roof of the motor home.

I walked over to Jim, the Navajo EMT. He looked up and smiled. "Sharon, she was standing up when the RV rolled. She got tossed around a lot. She was sitting over there (he pointed about twenty feet away from us) when we got here. chief complaint is her right shoulder." I made a mental note of the information. The men picked up the board and carried her to the ambulance and loaded her inside. As they loaded her into the ambulance, I told Jim, "That cloud is heading our way. It's close. That wash fills up fast so you might need to get that man out of there now."

"I know. Keep an eye out. Let us know when you see water in the wash."

"I will," I answered as I watched him hurry down the hill to help the others.

The back door to my ambulance was open and I could see the rescue efforts. They were gently moving Henry from behind the wheel and onto a backboard. A Navajo police officer walked up. He introduced himself to the woman and asked a couple of easy questions. "Could you please get my purse? It's white, my ID and papers are inside," she asked him. Navajo's are taught to show great respect to their elders. She was old enough to be his grandmother; he could not deny her request. He said he would and hurried down the hill, looking for her purse. It started to sprinkle.

I turned my attention to my patient. She was sixty-five years old, about five foot, four inches tall, and around one hundred and thirty pounds. She was well groomed and handling the situation better than most. I palpated her shoulder and believed it to be intact, but badly bruised. She had good movement and neuro's were intact. On further examination, she had minor neck pain and pain to her lower back. When the RV rolled it must have been like being inside a blender. It's amazing she wasn't injured that bad. I started an IV, hooked her up to the cardiac monitor and ran a base line strip. She was very stable and I expected the x-rays would be negative. She would probably be able to leave the hospital in a few hours.

The rain increased. I could see the men struggle with rescuing Henry. He would let out a loud verbal protest occasionally if they moved him the wrong way or too fast. They were taking their time and they didn't have time. The rain became a cloud burst as only the desert can have. It was like standing under a raging waterfall. I saw the police officer wandering around the muddy floor of the wash still in search of her purse. I was high and dry, but everyone outside the ambulance was soaked to the bone and probably would have drowned if they had dared to look up. Lighting flashed. The men hurried. This time Henry didn't complain.

Then I saw it, a wall of water. It was about four foot high, rolling and churning down the wash heading toward the accident scene. I jumped outside and screamed "Get out, the water's coming! Get out NOW!" Instantly every man in the wash understood they were all in immediate danger of drowning. No man can stand in rushing four foot deep flood water. Without a word, each man sprung to action. Henry was unceremoniously tossed on the backboard and handed down from the RV to waiting hands on the ground. No straps held him to the board, it was scoop and run.

I looked up the wash; the water was almost to the road, they had a minute and not a second more to get out of the wash. The water looked like churning chocolate milk. Small boulders and bushes rolled in the churning water. "Hurry! HURRY!" I screamed, and they did. Six men surrounded the backboard and rushed up the steep and slippery hill. Henry hung on for dear life. Torrents of rain fell down on them as a stiff wind blew in their face. One man fell to his knees but quickly got up, they were not about to abandon Henry, but they also had no intentions of being in the wash when the water hit. Again, a fireman stumbled, but they charged on and upward, reaching the road with a handful of seconds to spare. Two men fell to their knees, gasping for breath. Jim and the others

52

took a minute and checked Henry. He was hanging in there, scared but very happy he had not died that day.

The officer found her purse, scooped it out of the mud and took off running as fast as he could through the rain, wind and mud toward the road. I wasn't sure he was going to make it. Everyone held their breath, watching him sprint for his very life swinging a white purse flapping in his right hand. The water went under the road and exploded on the other side with great violence. The officer hit the base of the hill and started clawing his way up the muddy, slippery incline with a speed and determination that only fear of death can inspire. The water filled his boots with muddy water, but he reached the safety of the asphalt. He rolled over on his back, gasping for breath and almost drowned in the effort as the rain poured down on him, washing the mud from his clothing.

The firefighters carried Henry to the ambulance and loaded him on the bench seat. I strapped him in securely. "Are you ok?" I asked as I covered him with a warm blanket.

He looked up at me, gratitude in his eyes. "I'm ok, tell them thank you for me." He closed his eyes. I looked at the men standing at the back door, I smiled, and they smiled. They had cheated death again, and the feeling was wonderful! They had saved the man's life and managed to keep theirs. It was a good day.

The woman reached over and took her husband's hand. "Henry?"

He opened his eyes, "You ok Maud?"

"I'm ok Henry."

"It's all gone," he said.

"I know," she answered. "We're alive, that's all that matters."

I looked up and saw the flood wash all their belongings downstream. We drove off to the hospital. I went to work on Henry. His head had been hit, perhaps by the windshield or some other portion of the RV as it rolled and fell apart around him. He had serious back pain, his left hand was cut and bleeding, he had a headache and a knot on his forehead that was the size of a golf ball and getting larger by the minute. His left eye was swelling shut and the ribs on his left side were painful when touched. He wasn't going to die, but he was going to be in the world of hurt the next morning.

I got the necessary medical history and vivid details of the accident as we speeded down the road. They were both freezing and I covered them with blankets and used heating pack to warm their numb fingers and toes. We pulled up at the hospital with the rain still pouring down with a vengeance. Lighting flashed here and there. We unloaded them and hurried into the emergency department. We took them to the larger room so both of them could be together. Doctor Fisher was waiting for us. I started to give her a verbal report. She then began asking questions. "Was the windshield starred?" She asked as she began examining her patient.

"The windshield was gone," I answered. I had described the scene, but apparently it didn't sink in.

"How much intrusion?" (Meaning how far was the side of the vehicle pushed into the passenger compartment). She asked a couple of other questions that made it very clear she didn't understand what these two people had just gone through.

"The RV was a large one, it left the roadway, rolled down a fifteen foot hill and landed on its wheels. It fell into tiny pieces on the roll over. The floor, bottom frame, tires, driver's seat, steering wheel and motor is all that is left." The doctor stopped examining the woman and looked up at me. I had got her attention. I continued "the walls, ceiling, plumbing, chairs, everything was scattered over the desert in tiny pieces. The flash flood then washed all the debris down the wash. It's probably in Lake Powell by now."

The doctor looked down at Henry's face. "It's all gone," he said with a touch of disbelief in his voice. He was still trying to digest what had happened.

"Ok. . ." Dr. Fisher said, almost to herself. She returned to her examination of the patients with a renewed knowledge of just how horrendous this accident had been. We left the ER and went outside and opened the back doors of the ambulance. Mud lay three inches deep on the floor. The bench seat and stretcher was dripping muddy water and mud. It was an unbelievable mess and took both of us to get it clean again. I then sat down and wrote my report. When I finished I checked back in. Henry had a mild concussion and cracked ribs. He got a few stitches and would probably walk funny for a few weeks, but other than that, he was doing great. Maud's shoulder had sustained a hard blow in the rollover but with a sling and a few pain pills she would get through the next few weeks. They had called their son in Phoenix and he was on the way up to get them.

I drove by the accident site later that day and the flood water had receded. Mud and tiny pools of water was all that remained. The frame of the RV was still there but everything that had been inside and the wreckage debris had been washed away. The tow truck was pulling what was left of the RV up the hill. By the time their son turned onto Highway 160, there was nothing left to even hint of his parent's accident.

IT'S IN GOD'S HANDS

Religious freedom is one our priceless rights as Americans. Today it's become convoluted to freedom *from* religion, but early in my career, it was still freedom *of* religion. Early in the evening the pager went off. It was a report of an ill man at a local address. We drove up in the ambulance, got out and walked to the door and rang the bell. A woman, around fifty-eight years of age opened the door. She was an attractive woman, well dressed with a gentle dignified manner. I will call them Mr. & Mrs. Black and their son will be called Junior. Mrs. Black seemed surprised to see us. After some discussion, it appeared a neighbor had visited her and was concerned about Mr. Black, who was ill. The neighbor had called the ambulance without telling the family. It sounded odd, but odd people walk the streets of every community. I asked if I could come in and check her husband. She said it was ok.

Mr. Black was lying on the couch in the living room. Junior, around thirty-two years of age, was sitting in a chair nearby reading from the Bible. Mr. Black was obviously ill. His face was flush with fever and he was very weak. He smiled as I approached. "Thank you for your concern, but I am alright," he said.

"You don't look alright," I commented. He appeared to have an infection, possibly septic. "Have you been ill long?"

". . . . . . . For three or four days now. The fever just won't go away." He appeared to be experiencing serious abdominal pain.

His wife interjected, "He can't keep anything down."

After some questions, which he politely answered, I decided this man probably had appendicitis. I believed it may have burst and he was now in serious danger of dying. I told him what I suspected.

"Yes, you are probably right, but I don't want to go to the hospital," he said.

"Sir, I don't think you understand. This is probably a treatable problem, but if you wait much longer you will die." I decided to not pull my punches.

"Perhaps," said his son. Mrs. Black looked down with a hint of a tear in her eye and shook her head as well.

"Do you want your father to die?" I asked Junior.

"No, of course not. But it's in God's hands and His will be done."

Now I understood this family. I am a Christian and strongly believe that nothing I do can add one minute to someone's life unless God so wills it. I also believe He uses me and others like me to add to the quality of a person's life. I usually keep my beliefs to myself and outwardly remain neutral at the scene of an emergency call. But this time I couldn't

55

resist commenting. "Have you considered that God may sometimes use doctors and EMTs to do his work?"

In a polite voice, the father spoke, "God works wonders. He can heal me if it's in His plan. If it isn't, He will take me home to be with Him."

"Of course, you can refuse my help and transport to the hospital, but many religious people choose to do everything they can do to stay alive so they can do God's work. If God decides to take you, he can do it in the hospital ER. You appear to be giving up and choosing to die."

"No, I am not making a choice to die. We have put this in God's hands. He will either heal me or not. If I go to the hospital I will be saying I don't believe in God's ability to heal me. Whatever happens is His will."

I turned to his family, "You all understand that he is dying, don't you?" They all shook their heads. "You understand that with medical treatment he would probably live?" They were polite, but firm, they refused transport and any medical treatment. I tried to convince them one last time and was politely told that "God's will be done." I had the man sign a refusal (his wife and son as well) and we left. He died less than 24 hours later of a massive infection. His appendix had burst and he had developed peritonitis, a deadly infection. His wife cried at the loss of her husband and his son mourned the loss of his father, but they were people of deep faith and accepted God's will.

JINGLE BELLS, JINGLE BELLS, JINGLE ALL THE WAY

I grew up in the desert and love the rain. But snow was an entirely different thing. I hate snow. I was on call that night and we expected snow. My husband put the snow chains on his pickup in anticipation of needing them the next morning to get to work. He suggested I take his truck if I got a call during the night. I didn't like driving his pickup. My legs were too short and climbing into it was a struggle. It was stick and the clutch was stiff and required a lot of force to push to the floor. I knew how to drive a shift but I didn't like shifting gears. But, when it snowed, it was a good vehicle to drive. I went to bed hoping it would be quite and I would not have to drive on the snow covered streets. But that was not to be.

I was snuggled in my warm bed completely unaware of what was happening across town. Connie and Carl had been at the local tavern celebrating his job promotion. They were not drunk, but the drinks they had didn't help with the delicate balancing act required to walk up the icy steps leading to their front door. Connie slipped and Carl reached for her. They both began a strange sort of dance, slipping, sliding, swaying and staggering this way and that. Their arms flung out attempting to find something to steady themselves. Connie managed to grab the hand railing and cling to it in an awkward half standing, half kneeling position. Carl wasn't as lucky. He finally completely lost contact with the icy stairs and fell backward to the snow covered ground. He was in the perfect position to make snow angels, but I doubt that thought crossed his mind.

The pager woke me up around one-fifteen in the morning. The timing of the call was just after the local bars closed so whatever the emergency was, it probably involved a person with a few beers on board. I got dressed in winter attire, including snow boots, gloves and layers of warm clothing. I opened the front door and a blast of cold air hit me like a slap in the face. The front yard was solid white. The road in front of my house was covered in around four inches of newly fallen snow. Not a tire mark marred the smooth surface of the snow.

Earlier I had placed a sheet on the front windshield of the truck. I whipped it off and presto, a clean and clear windshield. As I climbed into the truck I noticed my husband standing in the doorway smiling. He was singing *Jingle Bells*. That man was walking a fine line. I grumbled and he laughed again and waved as I slipped and slid around the corner.

Page was deserted. Most of the streets had no tire tracks visible. Everyone was snug in their bed, fast asleep. I slowly made my way to the fire station. The crew assembled and we took off to a local address. The ambulance slipped once and caused me to gasp as we slid around a corner, barely missing a car parked on the street. We arrived at the locationt. As we approached the house I noticed the imprint Carl had left in the snow. We knocked on the door and Connie answered and invited us inside.

Carl sat in a recliner. "I'm ok." He looked ok, but sometimes it was hard to tell. He let me check him over and cooperated. I couldn't find anything wrong with him. I offered to take him to the hospital, but he refused. He signed the refusal forms and we left.

At the station I climbed back into my husband's truck and took off toward my house. The streets were quiet and completely deserted. It had begun to snow again. I took a different route and approached my house from the bottom of Date Street. Date ran in front of my house. It was a quiet residential street. My home was near the top of the street. It sloped gently downward for a long block. As I neared my house I heard something. It was children laughing and singing. I peered through the foggy windshield just as something dark slid past my vehicle on my left. I was surprised and couldn't identify the object.

As I got closer to home, I saw my husband standing in the drive way. He was bent over a form sitting on a plastic bag. It was my youngest son. My husband shoved him and he slid forward, down the driveway, hung a tight left onto Date Street and sailed down the street pasting my vehicle. I could hear him singing *Jingle Bells* as he passed. My oldest son appeared from behind me and ran to my husband, sat down on the trash bag and my husband shoved him forward. My husband then got on a plastic trash bag and followed his oldest son down the driveway, sliding into a tight left turn and down Date Street. I parked near the curb in front of my house. I got out and the sound of children laughing and singing drifted through the night air. It was a beautiful sound, like music. "It's the small things in life that count," such as the sound of children's laughter or the enjoyment of the spontaneous moment.

I remembered back when I was six years old and had just moved to Prescott Arizona. My father woke me up in the middle of the night. He took me outside for my first introduction to snow. My backyard glittered in the moon light. It was a winter wonderland and I marveled at its beauty. We had a snowball fight and my giggling woke my mother. She threw a fit that I would catch the death of a cold. But my father ignored her protests. When we grew tired, he scooped up a large handful of new snow and we went inside. He added sugar and can milk to the snow and we sat at the kitchen table and ate snow ice cream. I had forgotten that joyful childhood memory. I reconsidered my opinion of snow. Anything that can bring that much pleasure to a child in the wee hours of the morning had to be a good thing.

RACING THE GRIM REAPER

Joe's life was coming to an end. He had lived a selfish life, doing exactly what he wanted to do without any regard to how it might affect those around him. He drank too much, lied, cheated, and stole. He seldom worked and lived off others. He never appreciated the help family and friends gave him. He often borrowed money with no intentions of every repaying the debt. He had worn out his welcome and moved far away from his family and the few friends he had left. Years passed by. He didn't change, he just used different people.

Joe's lifestyle finally caught up with him at age forty-two. His liver finally died from years of abuse. His skin and eyeballs turned yellow. He couldn't keep food down and became thin as a stick. He was so weak, he couldn't stand. Physically he became a withered shell of the man he had once been. He knew it was over and he looked back on his life and saw he had wasted it. He saw the pain he had caused those who loved him, and he wanted to tell them how sorry he was and beg their forgiveness. He wanted most of all to hug his mother and tell her how much he loved her and how sorry he was for the pain he had caused her. He didn't want to die alone.

I was called to the Kayenta Clinic to transport him by ground ambulance to the hospital in Shiprock. His family had been notified and over fifty of them, were waiting for him at the Shiprock Hospital. Even after all he had done, they still loved him. I was told he had only hours to live. It was possible he wouldn't make it to Shiprock, two hours away. I walked over to Joe as he lay still in the bed of the emergency room. Tubes and wires lay everywhere in a tangled mess. Six IV bags hung on two poles at his bedside. The drugs dripped silently and slowly into his veins. They were the only thing keeping him alive. The heart monitor beeped quietly. I looked over his vital signs, they were scary. He opened his eyes and looked at me. His eyes were filled with sadness. I introduced myself and told him I was going to transport him to Shiprock.

Joe looked me in the eyes and placed his hand on my arm. "Please . . . . . I have to tell them, I'm sorry . . . . I have to tell them goodbye . . . . please. . . . my mother . . . ." His voice trailed off.

"I'll get you there," I promised. Little did I know how difficult it was going to be to keep that promise.

I went over to the doctor. She explained his dire medical condition. "He's dying. We can't do anything. He just wants to say goodbye to his family."

"Why don't you fly him?"

"There aren't any planes available, and there's a snow storm between here and there." The doctor went on, "He's a *no code*. Don't work him if he codes on you." I didn't want to think about that because I wanted more than anything at that moment to help this man. I wanted to grant him his one last wish. I then spoke with the nurse that had been caring for him. She wasn't encouraging. I took note of the many drugs he had been given prior to my arrival and the many drugs he was getting continuously by IV. I got orders for pain meds and a few other drugs needed to keep him alive, at least for a few more hours.

It was going to be a cold trip, even with the heater. I took a blanket and lay it on the stretcher. We loaded him on the stretcher and brought up the blanket and wrapped him like a baby. I then covered him with another blanket. Packaging him for transport was no small task with all the wires and tubes. As we opened the door, a cold wind hit us. I glanced over my shoulder; the eastern sky was dark gray. The snow clouds were between us and Shiprock. I wondered if the snow would slow us up. He didn't have time to spare. Two people walked out with us, holding IV bags, our cardiac monitor, and his bag of personal belongings. Finally, he was loaded in the ambulance.

I sat on the bench seat. I hung the IV bags from hooks in the ceiling. I took his oxygen tubing off the small cylinder on the stretcher and connected it to the wall unit. We pulled out of the parking lot, code three, lights and sirens. I leaned forward and sat the cardiac monitor on the shelf located on the front wall of the patient compartment.
Suddenly the monitor began that long loud scream of flat line. I turned and looked at him. He was looking at me with wide eyes filled with terror. "Are you ok?" I asked as I moved back beside him.

"I don't know," he said with fear and confusion in his voice.

I began moving the blanket aside to expose his chest. "Hang in there, I don't think it's a big deal" I told him. I don't think he believed me. I located the EKG leads and found one had been disconnected. I plugged it back in and the monitor began to beep in a regular rhythm. He closed his eyes and sighed.

It was a long trip. In the back of an ambulance people open up and say things to me, a total stranger, they would never say out loud to someone they knew. He would sleep for a while, and then wake up. He began to talk quietly, telling me his life story. He told how as a boy, he use to run and play in the desert around his home. He spoke lovingly of his traditional Navajo parents. He spoke fondly of his brothers and sisters, nieces and nephews. He told me about the son he didn't know, and his wasted life of self- indulgence. He told of the few triumphs of his life and his many mistakes. He was proud of his military service and ashamed of his drug and alcohol abuse.

Snow began to fall. The large flakes collected on the windshield. The driver turned on the wipers. The wind rocked the ambulance gently. I looked out the back window and saw the desert was now coated in a light dusting of snow. The road turned white. The truck in front of us left tire tracks in the snow for us to follow. The snow continued for a while then stopped. We continued onward.

Joe's vital signs were becoming strange. The blood pressure was going down. His heart rate was also going slower and slower. I cranked up one IV and turned down two more. I gave him a dose of medication, turned up his oxygen and crossed my fingers. We were a little over half

60

way there. Joe improved, slightly. It was cold outside, really cold. We continued on. Have you ever heard of the "middle of nowhere?" Well, we were there. As far as you could see, there wasn't a living soul. Occasionally a small hogan could be seen in the distance. Smoke curled skyward from unseen homes hiding behind barren hills. The ambulance slowed as a herd of sheep crossed the road. We speeded up and then it happened. A strange sound was heard and the driver slowed up and began checking gauges.

"What's wrong?" I asked.

"I don't know," he answered. We slowed down and coasted to the side of the road. Troy turned off the lights and sirens.

"NO! NOT NOW!" I screamed silently to myself. My heart dropped into the pit of my stomach. Troy, the EMT Driver, got out. He opened the hood and poked around. I sat, silently praying it was something small. It's strange, but almost immediately, without the heater, the ambulance became cool, then cold.

Troy got back in. "Man it's cold out there," he said, rubbing his hands together.

"How bad is it?" I asked.

"Bad. I don't have the tools to fix it."

My mind raced. Now what do we do? Troy and Joe were looking at me for the answer.   I didn't have one. I considered my options. I had a few. Our portable radios wouldn't work out here, but my EMSCOM Radio might. I keyed the radio. "Kayenta ER, this is 1545" I waited. Time ticked by, time Joe didn't have to spare. No one answered. I decided to try another approach. "1190 (Flagstaff Medical Center) this is 1545" I held my breath. They answered. "1545, this is 1190." They heard me!

"1190, we picked up a patient from Kayenta a little over an hour or so ago. We have experienced a vehicle problem. We are stranded beside the road about ten miles west of Teec Nos Pos. Will you call Kayenta Clinic and let them know. We need an ambulance to come out and get this patient. He is in critical condition and needs transport as soon as possible to Shiprock. Are there any helicopters in the area?"

"No, I'm afraid there are no helicopters available. I'll give Kayenta a call. Do you need anything else?"

"Yes, call Shiprock and let them know about our situation and tell them we will be a little late." She said she would. The ambulance grew silent. Joe woke up. He looked around. "We have car trouble. Another ambulance is on its way to get you." He looked disappointed. He closed his eyes, resigned to the possibility he may not live long enough to see his family one last time. The thought occurred to me as well. I checked his vital signs, and found they were starting down, again. I corrected the flow of IV meds and paid closer attention to the cardiac monitor. His pulse began to slow. We were almost out of time. I felt so bad for him. I felt as if I had let him down.

The temperature continued to drop. I noticed Joe was getting cold. I was out of blankets so I took my coat off and tucked it around him. "Thanks" he said. "My feet are really cold too." I lifted the bench seat and searched for another blanket. I only found some towels. I laid them across his lower body. I took out heat packs and struck them, activating the heat. I laid them up against his feet. I gave him one to hold. He smiled up at me.

"Don't give up yet," I told him. He nodded and drifted off to sleep again. I checked his vital signs. They were erratic; the pulse was slow, then fast, then very slow, then ok. It made me nervous. His blood pressure just stayed low. I raised his feet, it helped a little. "Where was that ambulance?" I wondered. I was getting cold. I was wearing a shirt and sweatshirt, but it wasn't enough. I began to be very uncomfortable. Joe needed the hot packs and coat more than I did. Troy complained of the cold as well. Snow began to fall again.

Then my prayers were answered. I saw an ambulance pull behind our ambulance and back up. That would make loading the patient easier. The EMT opened our back door and got in. The ambulance was from Teec Nos Pos. They were both basic EMTs. EMT-B's are great in an emergency, but this man needed an intensive care unit, not basic care. I couldn't just give him to them. I quickly made a decision. "He needs to get to Shiprock as soon as possible. Let's get him in your ambulance and I will go with you." One EMT and Troy unloaded Joe while the other EMT and I stripped my ambulance of anything ALS. I know their ambulance has basic supplies, but I need Advance Life Support stuff too. I grabbed my drug box, monitor, an extra oxygen tank, and some other odds and ends and loaded it into their ambulance.

We were all moving on fast forward because it was freezing outside and Joe had run out of time. Troy chose to stay with our ambulance. The Navajo EMT was good. I put her to work. Joe needed some attention. He was covered with more blankets and hot packs. I adjusted meds and gave him another dose of drugs. His vital signs improved but not as well as they had previously. That wasn't a good sign. I radioed Shiprock Hospital and told them we were en route again. I gave them an update on the patient and our estimated time of arrival.

The traffic became heavier as we approached the city. The ambulance was flashing code lights and weaved in and out as some cars pulled over and some did not. I held on as the ambulance swayed this way and that. Joe opened his eyes. "Are we almost there?" he asked weakly.

"Yes, we are in Shiprock. The hospital is only a couple of miles away. Hang in there Joe, your family is all waiting you. I called and gave them a head's up."

He smiled. "Thank you. Thanks for everything." He now had hope.

Suddenly the ambulance swerved hard to the left. A pickup had pulled out in front of us. I lunged forward, but managed to catch myself. "Damn it!" yelled the Ambulance driver. The Teec Nos Pos EMT in the back with me fell off the seat and landed on her knee and become wedged between the foot of the stretcher and the back door. The driver was good and he had managed to miss the pickup. "Are you guys ok?" the ambulance driver asked.

"Yeah," I answered as I reached for the Navajo EMT and pulled her back up on the seat. She wasn't hurt. This type of accident is fairly common and she shrugged it off.

"Joe, are you ok?"

"Yeah, what happened?"

"Some ding-bat pulled out in front of us. I guess the bright flashing lights blinded him."

Joe actually laughed a weak little laugh. "Joe, I can see the hospital." Wonderful! I don't know who was happier, Joe or me. We pulled up and unloaded him. We wheeled him into the ER. We were met by a doctor. He was smiling.

"So, you finally made it. How is he?" he asked.

"He's hanging in there. He's anxious to see his family."

"They are all in the room at the end of the hall." We wheeled him into the room. It was full of people, young and old. They rushed around him. Everyone wanted to touch him. He was showered with kisses. Tears flowed from everyone in the room, even the EMT's and I had tears forming in our eyes. We got Joe all tucked in bed and left.

Joe got his last wish. He got to say goodbye.

THE GERMAN TOURISTS AND THE NATIVE AMERICAN

Lars Vandenburghe, Hans Schultz and Clas Beenkerslauze were three college students on their first trip to America. They were a long way from Germany. Their cameras had almost overheated and burst into flames from overuse since they landed in Las Vegas, Nevada. Las Vegas was a wonderland for the young men. They then set out on their adventure in a rented car. They had seen Canyon of Fire, the Virgin River Valley

Gorge, Zion National Park, and Lake Powell. The Southwest is an area of magnificent scenery beyond imagination. They were excited and having a wonderful vacation.

It was early evening and as they drove by the Lake Powell turnoff and the Glen Canyon Bridge. They planned on coming back in the morning for a tour of the dam and a boat tour on the lake. They were hungry and as they reached the top of Manson Mesa, they found themselves on the main street of town, Lake Powell Boulevard (previously known as Seventh Street). It was a beautiful summer evening and tourists and locals alike were walking up and down the sidewalks, wandering here and there enjoying the evening now that the sun had gone down. Motels, fast food, and restaurants lined the street. They looked back and forth trying to decide where to eat.

Arnold loved alcohol. He had spent his day enjoying the one thing in his life that made him happy, whiskey. He noticed a couple of friends sitting on the benches near the sidewalk across the street from Taco Bell. He stepped into the road to walk over. He didn't look, he never did. He just concentrated on not falling down as he staggered across what local police and EMS called "the crossing."

Lars was distracted by the movie marquee. When Lars turned his attention back to the road he let out a short scream. Arnold had stepped in front of the car. He stomped on the breaks but it was too late. Arnold never saw the car. The car was traveling at about twenty-five miles per hour when it hit him. He felt the impact on his right side, mostly his thigh and knee area. He was launched forward and then landed on the hard pavement. He didn't move. His buddies ran into the road to help. People gathered around him while others dialed 911.

I arrived at the scene before the ambulance. I walked over with jump kit in one hand and oxygen bottle in the other. I was met by a very excited group of Germans. They were all talking at once with heavy accents. "Follow me," I said, "talk to me as we walk." They walked beside me and I listened as I walked toward Arnold. I kneeled down and recognized him. This wasn't the first time he had walked in front of a car. I began my initial examination. He had pain in his right leg, but it didn't look fractured. He had bumped his head but there was no lump to be found and no blood. He was slow to answer my questions and didn't seem to understand what had happened to him. Was his confusion the alcohol or a head injury? It was hard to tell.

I looked up and saw the ambulance arrive. The crew hurried over and I told them what I knew and backed off. I decided to check out the driver of the vehicle. Sometimes they are injured as well, or have a medical condition that needs attention or maybe drunk. I walked over to the tall blond man I later learned was named "Lars."

"My name's Sharon. I'm with the Page Fire Department. Are you injured?"

"No. What about him? (indicating the injured pedestrian)." He sounded worried.

"He's injured but I think he will be ok."

Lars was hyped up. He had never been in an auto accident before and he was looking around at the flashing lights and talked a bit fast. He told of their adventure so far. I listened and was convinced he did not appear to be drinking or impaired by drugs. He was acting normally for the situation. He then mentioned a problem they had been having. After they crossed the Arizona border, they had been looking for an Indian. "Are there any Indians around here? We want so much to see one." he asked. He and his friends had the idea that many European tourists have about Native Americans. They see them in John Wayne movies and believe they still live in teepees and wear buckskin loin cloths with a feather in their hair. They have no clue that with the occasional exception and the traditional elderly, Native Americans dress like everyone else, eat pizza, watch direct TV and live in a regular house.

I smiled. "See all those bystanders?" A crowd of around sixty or so people had gathered in the street watching the EMS crew care for Arnold.

"Yes," he said.

"Well, about half are Indians and the man you hit is a Navajo Indian."

Lars became excited. He yelled at his friend standing about twenty-five feet away. "Hans......! Hans! We struck a Native American!!!!!" Hans quickly pulled his camera out of his pocket and ran over and began snapping pictures of Arnold as he lay on the pavement with the EMS crew around him. Clas ran for the car and got his camera and started snapping pictures of the crowd and Lars posed beside his dented fender. They had at last found an "Indian."

Arnold spent a few hours in the ER and was found to be only bruised and banged up a bit. There is no law against public intoxication in the state of Arizona so he only got a ticket for crossing in mid-block and not using "due caution." Since witnesses said Arnold walked right out in front of the car and there was no way they could have avoided the accident, Lars got a ticket for "failure to honk his horn before striking a pedestrian." I kid you not. In Page it is standard procedure to ticket both parties involved in such an accident and this was the only thing the Police could find. Lars and his friends continued their trip across America with memory cards full of pictures of Native Americans.

DOING BATTLE WITH
THE MONSTER CALLED "FIRE"

I hope this doesn't sound wrong, but I enjoy fires. There is something exuberating about doing battle with this monster called "Fire". It bellows and roars, hungrily devouring anything in its path. While working for the Page Fire Department I had a front row seat and the view was spectacular. My main function at a fire was multi-level. As first responder, I would give status reports to responding units. Move the public out of the hazard zone and prepare for arriving units. I was fire command until the fire chief arrived. I would then take medical control. I had complete power to pull any firefighter off duty if I felt his medical condition warranted it. I commanded the EMTs, and did a lot of crowd control. I also worked the crowd to find out if anyone knew what happened. Where are the owners? I acted as a behind the scene "safety officer." I was cross trained as a firefighter, engineer and Incident Command.

My enjoyment of fires diminished when my husband joined the fire department as a volunteer firefighter. I didn't think it would bother me, but it did. On calls I could successfully block out my personal life and concentrate on the emergency, but that was impossible when the man in turnouts entering the burning building is the man you love. I began to experience a strange disturbing fear for his safety. This fire was to drive it home hard.

To stand by and watch Maurice disappear into the burning structure was very hard to do. I couldn't go up and kiss him and tell him good luck. We both had a job to do. Good-bye's and good lucks were a luxury that we couldn't afford. I wanted to yell, "Be careful!" But I never did. I couldn't forget he was working the fire and I usually knew where he was and what his assignment was at any given time. I would like to believe I didn't let my concern show. I think I kept it from interfering with my job. I may not be the best judge of that, but I think my concerns were not obvious to the casual observer.

Maurice was a reckless sort. He took risks. Oh, yes, he was a good firefighter and wore his protective gear and played by the rules, but the unknown factors of a fire gave it a danger unlike any others. I knew he was a good firefighter. I had seen him train and he was very good. But deep down I knew even good firefighters get hurt and sometimes die. And the one thing that frightened me the most was that somehow he always seemed to be in the most dangerous place at just the most exciting time.

During our years with the fire department, three fires stick out in my mind as the most disturbing in relationship to Maurice's firefighting.

The biggest was the Corn's Fire. It was "the Big One," the big fire all small communities dread. It's the test of their training and resources. I have devoted a chapter to that fire near the end of this book. The other two weren't as big, but they are etched forever on my memory.

The first fire was early in Maurice's career. He had fought a few fires, but not a full structure fire. My husband was an eager volunteer firefighter. He worked hard and mastered the skills to fight a fire. I trusted his skills and judgment and didn't expect to experience any emotional issues with his new interest in firefighting.

The trailer was located in Lake Powell Mobil Home Village, Vermillion Trailer Park to old timers. It sat down the hill, off the mesa. It was very late at night and there was no moon. I remember being woke up by my pager announcing the fire. Maurice and I sprung out of bed and ran around bumping into each other, getting dressed. I rushed to my car and headed to the fire. He got in his truck and hurried to the fire station.

I started down the hill and at once I could see the fire. It was big. Half of the long trailer was blazing brightly in the darkness. Thick smoke rose in the still night air. I keyed my radio. "F-3 . . . . Page."

"F-3, go ahead," answered the dispatcher.

"The trailer's fully involved." I laid the radio down and hurried to the park. I drove into it and found the roads full of people. They were flowing out of their trailers. The police officer's sirens and the excitement had awakened them all. They were dressed in strange attire, whatever they could throw on. I had to slow, children clothed in pajamas ran into the street followed by their parents. All eyes were on the bright orange glow a few blocks away.

I pulled up and began working with the police to move people back. The fire was hot and growing larger. We needed room for the responding fire and medical vehicles to park. I checked around and found the people who lived in the burning trailer were out of town and the trailer was unoccupied. The fire trucks soon arrived and the ambulance was on the way. I got preoccupied with radio traffic with the ambulance. I had picked out where I wanted them to park and I warned them about the large number of pedestrians.

I still remember with frightening clarity the scene that confronted me when I turned around. The area took on a strange ire orange glow. The blackness of night was illuminated by the flames that leaped and danced out every window and door. I could feel the heat on my cheeks even though I was an acceptable distance away. I knew my husband was on Engine two. I searched and found it. I then listened and discovered two firefighters from that truck were attempting to extinguish the burning car that sat parked beside the trailer. The gas tank had not yet blown, but the car was burning with a fury.

I moved to get a better view. I then saw Maurice. He and Don Parks stood between the burning trailer and the burning car. The flames licked out at them from both directions. They held the hose pointing toward the car. Maurice reached out with gloved hand and opened the door. Flames jumped out, engulfing his arm. The turnouts kept his flesh from roasting, but through the gloves his hand had been burned, but he didn't know that yet. They turned the hose inside of the car. The flames died with a loud protesting hiss. They could feel the hot breath of the monster breathing down their necks. Their body dripped in sweat under the heavy turnouts. Flames licked at their back, so they turned the water back on the trailer fire. Huge bursts of orange/yellow flame would lick out like the tongue of a fire breathing dragon and completely engulf the two men, hiding them from my view for what seemed like hours but in reality were only a fraction of a minute.

I watched the scene with a hypnotic stare. Two tall trees had caught fire and stood like giant torches, with flames reaching into the night sky, lighting the area with an unreal glow. The fire in the car again sprang to life and licked out at the men's back causing them to turn around and try to drown the hungry flames

BOOM! I jumped at the sound of the first tire exploding. Maurice and Don didn't even appear to notice the explosion. Another tire went and I again cringed. I didn't worry about tires blowing, but a drive shaft, a shock absorber or a gas tank could seriously injure or kill anyone within fifty feet of the exploding mass. The men were only inches away, too damn close. With their attention diverted, the trailer fire saw its chance and reached out to engulfed them again. I held my breath. Then the flames were forced back as the men turned and resumed their fight. The power lines caught fire and the insulation on the phone, electric and cable wires burned dark orange and sparks shot out like the fourth of July.

The ambulance arrived. I tore myself away from thoughts of widowhood and concentrated on getting medical control set up. The ambulance crew and I set up a rehab station. Tired firefighters would come over and sit down. We would give the exhausted firefighters Gatorade to drink and take their vital signs. I was surprised to discover early into my career that the young men, age nineteen or twenty or so took over twice as long to recover and return to duty than the man in his late forty's. Why? I don't know for sure, but I believe it's because the older more experienced men pace themselves while the young ones burst forth in one hundred and ten percent of pure raw energy, therefore they burn out quicker and are much more worn out when they arrive at rehab. We would monitor the men until their vital signs had stabilized and they were rehydrated. I was busy and forgot about my husband for a while.

The fire had too good a foot hold by the time water was applied and all they were able to save was the neighboring trailers. When it was all over and the last tired firefighter was taken care of, the overhaul was over, and the investigation completed, I finally allowed myself to become the wife of Maurice Holbert again. I looked around for him and found him loading hose. Maurice smiled as I walked up. His face glowed with excitement. "Now that was some fire!"

"Sure was, and what in the world were you doing standing in the middle of it?"

He laughed. "You know me, the cautious type." Nothing could have been farther from the truth. Fires were a lot more fun before my husband had joined the fire department.

THE STUN GUN

With backup being an uncertainty in rural EMS, I quickly decided a basic knowledge of self-defense wasn't enough. In the back of an ambulance, there isn't much running room and when I responded ahead of the ambulance for PFD the possibility of walking into a dangerous situation was a real possibility. I purchased a stun gun and a small canister of pepper spray. I carried them just in case. One night I was glad I had them.

It was around midnight. I was asleep in bed when the sound of the pager tore through the peaceful silence. As I got up, my husband mumbled and rolled over trying to ignore me as I slipped on my jumpsuit. I hurried down the hall to the front door. I grabbed the keys as I slipped on my shoes and hurried out the door. I stopped and stood for a moment, looking around. The neighborhood was silent. No movement except the two coyotes that were digging through my neighbor's trash. I had been receiving a few hang-up phone calls recently. The last one wasn't a hang-up. I heard a man's voice say "Do you want to die?" It takes a lot to intimidate me. I had received such threats before and they didn't scare me, they make me mad. But I wasn't stupid, I took the threat seriously. Perhaps I should have, but I hadn't told my husband about the new threat. He was working a lot of overtime and had his own problems.

I went to my car, peeked in and again looked over my shoulder. I had my hand on my stun gun as I opened the door and got in. All a person had to do to get me out of my house in the middle of the night was to call

911 and request an ambulance. I knew I was a sitting duck right now and later when I returned home. I wasn't scared, but I was vigilant. I responded to Ken's Old West, a restaurant/bar across town. I pulled into the parking lot beside the police car. I walked up to a man sitting on the curb of the parking lot. He looked up at me. "I'm ok," he said.

"He got into an altercation with another man and got a split lip. He came outside and passed out. A buddy found him over there on the sidewalk." He pointed to a spot about five feet away.

I kneeled down and introduced myself. "What happened?"

"Nothing, I'm ok." His voice was quiet and unthreatening.

I was trying to decide if he was drunk or if it could be something else. "How much have you had to drink this evening?"

"I don't know two or three beers. I'm ok. I don't need an ambulance."

"Do you have a headache or blurred vision?" He shook his head "no."

"You should be checked out at the hospital."

"No. I'm ok. I just want to go home."

"Is there someone I could call to come pick you up?"

"My wife . . . . maybe?" He gave me her number and I called her. She seemed mad but said she would be down in a few minutes.

I told the officer his wife was on the way. Just then a call came in for the officer. The dispatcher's voice had the slight edge of urgency. "We have a request for backup, domestic violence situation. Officer is on the scene of a man with a shove and a woman with a rake circling around their front yard threatening a physical confrontation. The officer on the scene says they ignore him and won't put the weapons down."

"I got to go," the officer said.

"Go on, I think this is under control. I'll just wait for his wife."

"Thanks," he said and hurried off. Page only had two officers on duty at this time of night and it sounded as if the other officer might need help. I watched as the officer spun out of the graveled parking lot. I turned around and saw the patient had stood up.

He looked like a different man. His expression was no longer friendly. "So, he left you . . . . . What are you going to do now, bitch?"

His behavior surprised me. I hadn't done anything to provoke him. My hand slipped into my jacket pocket and my fingers went around my stun gun. "Sit down Mr. Jones. Your wife should be here anytime." I worked at keeping my voice calm and reasonable.

"I don't like being told what to do by a dumb woman." His voice was low and threatening. Only four feet or so separated us. I was alone with him in the deserted parking lot. I keyed my radio so what I was

70

saying could be heard by dispatch and the two officers, "Mr. Jones, your threats are beginning to make me uncomfortable. Just sit down before this gets out of hand."

"No way you *&%$#%^&^*& bitch." His hands formed fists at his side. He took a step toward me.

I took out my stun gun and pushed the button. A bright flash of blue lightening lit the night as the loud zap accented my point. He stopped dead in his tracks. I raised my voice and tried to sound confident and strong. "Sit down and shut up or I will fry you." I meant it.

He stood in a moment of indecision. He stepped back and sat down on the curb. Just then a police car slid into the graveled parking lot. He leaped out. He was mad. "What the hell is going on?" he asked as he stomped toward us.

Mr. Jones sat still. His face had assumed his unthreatening facade. "Nothing's wrong," he said in a calm, reasonable manner.

"The hell it isn't. I heard you cuss her out over the radio." The man now realized he was in trouble. Just about that time his wife drove up. She appeared to have a calming effect on her husband. When she found out how he had been behaving, she begged us to just let her take him home.

"He's a mean drunk. He hasn't had a drink in three months. We're working on the problem with counseling. Madam, I'm sorry he threatened you," she said to me. "Please let me just take him home."

The officer looked at me. "It's up to you, Sharon."

I didn't like being threatened, but this wasn't the first time it had happened and it wouldn't be the last. "I'll let it drop this time. But if this happens again I will press charges." His wife thanked us and took her husband home.

"Thanks for coming to my rescue," I said to the officer.

"No problem," he said. His radio came to life. "I gotta go." He hurried to his car to investigate strange sounds in an elderly woman's back yard.

I drove home and as I neared my house, I looked around. Nothing stirred. I pulled into my driveway. I didn't get out at once. I looked around and saw no movement in the shadows. I pulled the stun gun out of my pocket and grasped it in my hand. I got out and hurried into my house. I stepped over Sheppard, our dog, who lay asleep in the hallway. I entered my bedroom. My husband was snoring. I took off my jumpsuit and climbed back in bed. I quickly forgot the drunken man and drifted off to dreamland.

THE DUMBEST SKIER ON THE LAKE

Over the years I have heard some fantastic stories. Some are hard to believe, but true. Other times, after one or two sentences, it's clear where it's going. Didn't they see it coming? No. They set themselves up and are genuinely surprised when something goes wrong. This is one of those cases. I am willing to bet, early into this story you will see where it's headed.

Chris was in his early twenties, full of recklessness masquerading as bravery. He was a show off, performing for a boat load of pretty giggling girls. He considered himself a hot shot skier. He was being towed by a ski boat at a high rate of speed. He wove back and forth, jumping waves, and lovin' every minute of attention. Then he got the bright idea to take it up a notch and ski with no hands. He took the handle of the ski rope, a triangle of rope with a wooden handle on the base of the triangle that the skier was supposed to hold. He took the triangle of rope and slipped it over his head, extended his arms, and continued skiing. Can you see where this is headed? He didn't.

Something went wrong with the boats speed, or the water, or perhaps he shifted his weight, somehow he went down, hard. With the rope around his neck, he began being dragged face up through the water with the wooden handle under his neck. It was a tossup, was he going to be choked or drown? The driver was a bit slow to react and after some hesitation the boat slowed down and stopped. The skier sank like a rock.

Two guys and a girl jumped overboard and reached him. He didn't drift downward in the water far because he was still being hung by the ski rope. They untangled him and brought him to the surface. He gagged, coughed, and complained of sharp pain in his neck and throat. They called on the marine radio and turned toward the boat launch at Wahweap. National Park Service EMTs responded and called for a Page Fire Paramedic. This patient could need advanced airway management. I was on call, and responded in the PFD ambulance code-three.

We arrived just as they had finished back boarding the patient. He looked scared. He was loaded into our ambulance and I told the driver to move it out, code-three. The man's voice was harsh and raspy. This indicated a possible crushed larynx (voice box). He also complained of server pain in his neck, back and both sides. It probably was just bruising, but it could be a broken neck. He had good movement in his extremities, but it was getting harder for him to breath. His throat was swelling shut. This is common in strangulation or hangings.

Vital signs were good, except his oxygen saturation was low. I put him on high flow oxygen and notified by cell phone the hospital. I chose

72

my words carefully, not wanting to add to this man's worries. Paramedics, EMTs and ER staff at times talk in "code." I told them mechanism of injury and how I found him. I told them "he's on a backboard with high flow oxygen. I am preparing for advanced airway management if necessary". They filled in the blanks. I took the Cricothyroidotomy kit out, opened it and looked up. The EMT's face drained of color. He now understood where this was headed and he didn't want to be involved but couldn't get out of it.

If this man's throat swelled shut from the traumatic neck injury, he wouldn't be able to move air. As a paramedic I could not intubate a conscious patient. If he went unconscious and I tried to intubate in the normal manner, I would probably not be able to get the tube past the crushed and swollen larynx. If I did manage to do so there was a good chance I would do more damage. If he lost his airway, I had no choice but to cut an incision in his throat, below the larynx. I would then cut through the membrane in the patient's neck into the trachea (windpipe) then insert a tube. This would bypass his airway obstruction and provide a breathing passage, allowing air into the lungs. This emergency surgery is seldom necessary but in this case it would keep him alive until surgery could repair the damage and time would shrink the swelling. I didn't want to do the procedure, but I prepared my equipment and hoped we could make it to the ER before his throat slammed shut.

The EMT driving the ambulance was driving very fast and I didn't object. I held on for dear life and watched the EMT in the back near the panic point. The siren blared as we topped the mesa and soon we were at the hospital back door. Chris still had an airway, barely. His respiration was labored and very noisy. He struggled for every breath. He could talk in one word sentences, but his voice was raspy and deep. Due to lack of oxygen, he was becoming confused and slightly combative.

We unloaded him and rushed him into the ER. The doc and staff stood by. They had already called for the helicopter which arrived quickly. The anesthesiologist from the hospital also arrived. He decided to do a Rapid Sequence Intubation. This procedure involves giving the patient a sedative and then Succinylcholine (or similar type drug). It paralyzes the conscious patient so they can be intubated. Ventilation is done by using a bag valve mask (BVM) to force oxygen down the tube to the lungs. The anesthesiologist along with the specialized helicopter crew and ER staff intubated the patient. With the TV camera attached to the ET tube the doc carefully guided the tube through the maze of crushed bones and twisted tissue into the patient's lungs. They then began to bag him since he couldn't move his chest muscles to breath due to the drugs. His eyes were open, but he couldn't move. The great thing about Succinylcholine is he won't remember anything.

I went outside and put up my cricothyroidotomy kit. "Man, you freaked me out when you opened that thing," the EMT said. I laughed and pretended it was no big deal, but deep down, it was a big deal and I was glad we didn't have to cut him. The patient was flown to Flagstaff Medical Center and underwent surgery. The air crew checked on him off and on and reported he made a complete recovery. He holds the record, as far as I am concerned, as the dumbest skier I have ever met.

A CASE OF DOMESTIC VIOLENCE

I could write and entire book on Domestic Violence calls. Often it involves alcohol and/or drugs but not necessarily. It's a complex topic. In this book there are seven stories on this subject. Disagreements are part of life and at times emotions may run high, voices may rise a bit, but most adults control the impulse to strike out. I could never understand why a person would allow another to bust their lip, shove them down, kick them, break their bones and then allow them back in their bed. I know what the text books say and it makes a strange kind of sense, but no matter how many calls I went on, no matter how many times I saw the text book proven right, I still can't say I understand.

That morning I was in the office working on pre-plans for a new hotel when Tom Harkin stopped by. Tom was about five foot eight inches tall, of slender build. He spoke softly, moved slowly and was always ten minutes late for any non-emergency situation. Even on emergencies, he always arrived last even though he lived near the station. I don't remember how, but the topic of domestic violence came up. "I just think this entire domestic violence thing is exaggerated. A husband would never really hurt his wife. Sure, they yell, shove, and maybe slap sometimes. I know it isn't' right, but it's just not that serious an abuse." Tom Harkin refused to believe women were often beaten and sometimes killed by their husbands. I know he and his wife would never resort to blows and his range of experience was limited, his world view small. In a few hours, he was to be introduced to the real word.

The pagers sounded around nine o'clock in the morning. "We have a report of an injured woman at space two in Seiko Trailer Park." Sarcastically, *Seiko Enchanted Gardens* was what many people called it. It was a small trailer park off Vista Avenue. Vista was a short street filled with small business. The streets inside the trailer park were dirt and the trailers were all old, mostly small single wide trailers in desperate need of repair. Many good people lived there because they were poor. But mingled among the normal people were druggie's, thieves, alcoholics, and common criminals. We went on a lot of calls to this park. Tom Harkin and I drove to the address. It was a small twenty-eight foot trailer. An older woman (the patient's mother) opened the door for us to enter. Tom and I walked into the trailer. Our patient was perhaps nineteen years old and lay on the couch. Her mother gave us the details. "I came over to check on her and found her like this, that bastard beat her last night."

"Her husband?" I took a wild guess.

"Yes," she answered.

I looked at the woman. Both eyes were puffy blue and had swelled shut. Her nose was leaning to the side and covered in dried blood. Her face was puffy and her lips were encrusted in blood and hugely swollen. She had teeth missing. On her chest I found triangle shaped bruises, the tips of her husband's cowboy boots had left their marks as he kicked her about her chest and abdomen. She could hardly breath, couldn't open her eyes and everything hurt. We put on a c-collar and gently placed her on a backboard.

"Where is the husband?" I asked, almost as an afterthought.

"The bastard is in the bedroom, sleeping," the mother said.

"Oh, crap," I thought. The scene wasn't safe. The monster that had attacked this helpless woman was sleeping only feet away. "Let's get her out of here." We hurried outside with the woman. I called the police on the radio as we drove to the hospital. They found the husband passed out on the bed in the back bedroom. He was arrested. At the hospital, after it was all over, Tom came up to me.

"Sharon, I remember our conservation. I was so wrong. I now see it really happens." Tom joined a local support group that helped battered women. He had finally become aware that not all men respect women. I also joined the local group and I was made aware of something I had never considered. A man who worked in the group spoke to me concerning a comment I had made. It was derogatory toward men who beat their wives. He softly said, "Sharon, do you really think the men who do this are happy? Do you really think they like hitting the woman they love? They are not happy, I know, I use to beat my wife. I got help and now I try to offer help to other men."

He was right. I now saw the other side. The men needed help too. I volunteered for a while as the organization helped victims of domestic abuse. But as I became more involved, I discovered the organization also spent a lot of time and money encouraging abortions. They didn't even discuss the option of adoption or keeping the baby. I had a moral dilemma. I had dedicated my career to saving lives. I couldn't morally advocate stopping a beating heart. I finally decided to withdraw from the group.

AFTER CURFEW

Bobby had pushed his father too far this time. The past year Bobby had changed from a good kid to a troubled teen. He was fifteen and thought he knew everything. It would be years before his hormones leveled out and he matured enough to realize his father was smarter than he had thought. A wise man once said, "Raising a teenager is like being pecked to death by chickens." I completely agree. This is the time that tries a parent and will years later define how good a parent they were. Robert loved his son and was struggling to be a good parent.

"That's it. I'm tired of you coming in after curfew. If you aren't in by ten, I'm locking the door." I know Robert was desperate, but he didn't foresee the problem this would cause.

I remember another call where a man had told his daughter the same thing. In Page it was and still is common to not lock your door. She staggered home drunk and found the door locked. She took off all her clothes and lay down on the patio. It was January and she almost froze to death. In her drunken mind she was getting back at her father by freezing to death. She didn't die. A neighbor called for an ambulance. And she actually did get back at him because he was arrested for child abuse.

Robert meant well, but by Saturday night he would see the error of his ways. Bobby stomped to his room, and slammed the door behind him. Saturday night arrived and Bobby's friends pulled up front and honked. Robert didn't approve of Bobby's new friends. As Bobby ran out the door Robert yelled "Be home by eleven."

"Whatever," Bobby mumbled as he turned and left. Robert sighed. The evening progressed until the clock struck eleven. Bobby wasn't back yet. Robert locked the doors and he and his wife went to bed.

Around two in the morning Bobby stumbled out of his friend's car. Bobby was drunk, very drunk. He had some difficulty climbing the stairs to the front door but after a couple of tries he made the top of the steps and stumbled to the door. He tried to open it. "Damn it" he said out loud as he realized his father had really locked the door. He kicked the door and stumbled back down the stairs. He made his way to the back door and found it locked as well. Now Bobby was mad. It was cool that night and he wanted inside. He noticed the large window in the dining room. He walked up and drew his right arm back and hit the glass hard, shattering it. Bobby climbed through the broken window. He then staggered down the hall to his bedroom. He fell face first onto the bed and passed out.

Robert sat up in bed. He heard something. He listened and heard some odd noises at the other end of the house. He got up to investigate. When he entered the dining room he noticed glass all over the floor. Then he saw the blood, a lot of blood. Whoever broke the window had been cut. A burglar? No, he realized it was probably Bobby. Robert picked his way through the glass that covered the floor and began to follow the blood trail. It disturbed him. There was so much blood, everywhere, even smeared on the wall. The blood trail led him to Bobby's room. He opened the door and turned on the light.

Bobby lay face down on the bed. "Bobby?" Robert said. Bobby didn't move. "Was he breathing?" Robert wondered. He kneeled on the bed and tried to wake his son. When his knee hit the bed he felt squishy cold moisture. He rolled Bobby over and saw his son lay in a pool of blood. He searched his son body and found a one and a half inch slice in Bobby's right wrist. Robert jumped up and ran to the phone and called 911. He yelled for his wife, waking his daughter in the process. He rushed back down the hall and grabbed a t-shirt lying on the floor and tried to stop the blood coming from his son's wrist. It didn't work, the blood kept flowing. He pressed harder. After what seemed like an hour he heard the ambulance crew enter the home.

I came through the front door first and Bobby's mother motioned down the hall. I noted the blood trail. It indicated heavy bleeding. I entered the room and Robert looked up. He was covered in his son's blood and the look of sheer panic was in his eyes. "I can't get it to stop." He got up to let me in.

I quickly could see Bobby had cut his radial artery. The pulsing bright red blood squirted from a cut about one inch up his arm from where the hand connects to the forearm. He was completely unconscious and I was certain it wasn't just the alcohol. I wished I was a paramedic but at that time I was an EMT. Robert told me what happened as I worked on his son. I placed a stack of gauze bandages over the wound just above the wrist. I then took the blood pressure cuff and applied it over the bandage. I pumped it up until the needle stopped moving. I then let out a little air and splinted the arm.

While I was doing this the other crew members got the stretcher set up and put oxygen on Bobby. He was in serious shape due to sever blood loss. I backed out of the room and told the rest of the crew to load him on the stretcher and get him in the ambulance. I went outside to the ambulance and called the Page Hospital ER. At that time in history the doctor on call wasn't physically at the hospital. He had to be called at home and respond to the hospital when needed. I wanted a doctor waiting at the back door when we pulled in. The only chance Bobby had to see his sixteenth birthday was surgery. The crew opened the back door of the ambulance and loaded our patient. The bleeding was under control, but not completely stopped. It had slowed down to a small trickle.

In five minutes we pulled up at the ER door. I was pleased to see the ER staff waiting for us. I jumped out and we got the stretcher out. "Where's the doc?" I asked.

"He's scrubbing up. They are almost ready for him in surgery." We wheeled Bobby into the hospital and at a run we rushed through the ER to surgery. "What's that?" the nurse asked.

"BP cuff . . . . . . It was the only way I could control the bleeding."

"Good call."

I stopped at the door to surgery and watched Bobby disappear from sight. He was still wearing the BP cuff on his arm. His parents and sister arrived. I showed them to the chapel where families waited. Many of our patients were Navajo and when a person is taken to the hospital the whole family follows. Navajo's have big families and so Page Hospital had to use the chapel as a waiting room most of the time.

I completed my paperwork and the ambulance was cleaned. It was a mess with blood soiling the usual white interior. Bobby was still in surgery when we left the hospital. The next morning I got another ambulance call and while at the hospital I met his father in the hallway. "How is Bobby?" I asked.

"He's going to live. He came so close to bleeding to death. Thank you for saving his life."

"I'm glad I could help. But you're the one who saved his life. You put pressure on the wound and slowed the bleeding before I arrived." We shook hands and I left. Bobby and Robert had another chance. I hope they came to some understanding and hopefully this brought them closer together.

TWO-CAR HEAD-ON

Mary and her sister Beth were returning from a family reunion in Salt Lake City, Utah. They had spent the night at a hotel in Page. They got on the road around nine in the morning and hoped to reach their apartment in Mesa, Arizona by mid-afternoon. Both sisters were of slender build and pretty. It was August 2003 and Beth was eager to return to classes as Arizona State University in a couple of weeks. Her older sister Mary was in a hurry to get home to her husband. She was three months pregnant and looked forward to motherhood. The small white car they drove was older and had been given to them by their father when they went off to college. Mary was driving around sixty-five miles per hour as Beth sat in the passenger seat studying a map.

Ed was thirty-six years old. He had spent most of the night drinking with his two friends, Sonia and Ned. They had drunk a cheap wine and Ever Clear until they passed out. The morning sun woke them and they decided to head into Page and get more liquor. Ed was still impaired by the alcohol he had consumed only hours before but it didn't keep him from driving around five miles over the speed limit. His old compact car was a rusty blue with each and every fender dented. The back driver side window wouldn't roll up but it didn't concern Ed.

Mary saw the blue car wander over the center line once as it approached her. She moved to the edge of the roadway hoping to give the car a little extra maneuvering room. Suddenly it crossed the line and she barely had time to scream before it hit her car head on. The front of Mary's car caved in and buckled. The dashboard folded in and down. Glass broke and the sound of screaming and scraping metal filled the car. Then there was silence.

PFD Attack-One and Rescue-One arrived about the same time. The attack truck was manned by J.C. Harper a Fire Captain/Paramedic and a firefighter whose name I have completely forgotten. Rescue-One was manned by Jessie Blake an EMT and Kasie Lane a Paramedic. Captain J.C. Harper took incident command. He did a quick triage of all five patients.

At a scene where there are multiple patients and multiple vehicles it can get confusing. Sometimes a medic and ambulance crew is assigned one patient and they do their job without knowing what is happening elsewhere. At other times incident command has to reassign rescue workers to fit the incident as it evolves. This is one of those times. There were five patients. I never saw one, and had a part in evaluating, care and/or treatment of four others but only transported one. There were two ambulances with one doing two trips and a helicopter that also did two trips. The scene was orderly, but to put it down on paper was a challenge. Here we go, I hope it makes sense

Captain Harper called for a second ambulance, a helicopter and additional manpower. He decided the three in the blue car appeared the least injured. He moved to the white can and found Mary was trapped behind the wheel and Beth screaming in pain. Captain Harper and a firefighter began sitting up the Hurst tool. Out of the five, Mary appeared to be the most seriously injured. They were going to pop the door of the white car providing access to Mary who was in and out of consciousness. Captain Harper decided she would be the first to be flown by the helicopter.

Beth was easy to get too so EMT Jessie Blake and Paramedic Kasie Lane extricated her from the front passenger seat. She appeared to have fractured her right ankle. I pulled up in Rescue-Three. My ambulance was smaller so we traded ambulances and they rushed her to the Page Hospital with orders to do a quick turnaround and come back for another patient as soon as possible. Page was twelve miles away on a narrow highway with summer traffic and two miles of six percent downhill grade. It would take them awhile to return.

Captain Harper and the firefighter started the Hurst tool about the same time the helicopter lifted off from Page. Harper was determined to have access by the time it arrived on scene. I was assigned the blue car with three patients. I had gotten lucky and was able to bring two firefighter/EMTs with me on the ambulance. I quickly looked over the three people in the blue car. The woman was screaming and the man in the back passenger seat was singing and the driver was now unconscious, so the driver came out first. We slid Ed out onto a backboard and lowered it to the ground. I hear the helicopter land. I cut his shirt off and checked his chest and abdomen and pelvis. He had the most severe seatbelt injuries I have ever seen. Where the belt crossed over his left shoulder and across his chest was bright red were it had rubbed the skin raw. His respirations were rapid and shallow. Where it went across his lap, was also raw. He was wearing the belt too high and he popped his bladder. I believed his abdomen was slightly ridged, indicating a possible abdomen bleed. He appeared seriously injured. I left him with the basics and told them to strap him down and I would be back when they had him packaged. If I had not cut the shirt, most of his injuries would have gone undiscovered at the scene.

The female front seat passenger was still screaming and the rear passenger was still singing so I hurried over to Captain Harper. The RN and Medic from the helicopter were starting an IV on Mary, preparing to transport her. "J.C. I think the driver of the blue car is critical."

Before he could answer, Senda Monroe the RN turned to her partner Paramedic Bigalow and said "Jack, go check him out and see if we should take him first." Jack and I hurried back to the blue car. The EMTs had strapped him to the backboard and a baseline set of vitals. His heart rate was up and his blood pressure was down. Jack listened to breath sounds and palpated the abdomen.

"It's rigid. He's bleeding into the abdomen." He turned and hurried to report his finding.   Now my radio sounded, it was J.C. "Sharon, have the EMTs get the driver loaded on the helicopter and you check out the other two patients. When the EMTs get back give them the two patients in the blue car and you get over here."

The EMT's lifted Ed, driver of the blue car and hurried to the helicopter meeting the flight crew at the door. I popped the driver's seat forward and climbed into the back seat. Ned had stopped singing. He had layed down in the seat and appeared to be sleeping. I woke him up. He had blood around his face and mouth, but was able to answer questions. His speech was slurred and he was slow to answer. He moved all extremities and didn't appear to have any obvious injuries except for small cuts from the broken windows and a few red spots that would become bright blue bruises in a few hours. Then I noticed something on his neck, almost hidden by the collar of his shirt. It was a very deep two inch slash in his neck, missing his carotid by only an inch. There was very little blood. I almost missed the deep wound. He was lucky. He had come very close to dying from a slit throat. The inside of the car was covered in beer bottles and the smell of beer was overwhelming. Ned had been taking a drink of beer at the time of the accident and the neck of the bottle broke off his front teeth, but he didn't swallow the bits of teeth or broken glass and his airway was open and clear. He would drop off to sleep unless disturbed. I considered him stable for the moment. I took a piece of paper and wrote simple vital signs (pulse, respiration rate and capillary refill) the injuries I had found as well as his name. I taped it to his sleeve for whoever eventually got him as a patient.

I then went to the woman in the passenger seat. Sonia was now moaning but still conscious. She was unrestrained and I was told she was found lying in the driver's lap by first arriving bystanders. I don't know how she ended up sitting in the passenger seat where we found her. Her left arm was her main complaint. I was certain her left arm was fractured and possibly her left shoulder. She screamed if you got near her neck which caused me great concern. I slipped a c-collar on her with a fireman holding c-spine. I was preparing to start an IV when Captain Harper radioed me to take over care of the driver of the white car. The helicopter was going to do a quick turn-a-round and return for her. I told him I just getting ready to start an IV on the female passenger of the blue car. He said he would come over and do it. We then traded patients. Why? I don't know but in the middle of an emergency, you don't ask questions, you just follow orders.

I went to the white car and for the first time saw the patient. She was young, small, and injured very badly. At the time of the crash, she must have stomped on the break and on impact, her right femur broke. It was obviously bent inward. The IV sat on the dash. I knew the helicopter was coming back soon, so I decided my priority was to get her out of the vehicle and packaged. Then I heard over the radio that the helicopter had another call to go up lake for a wake boarder with a deep laceration to his arm. His arm was numb and he was fourteen years old. I began to worry if they were coming back for the driver or not.

Mary was conscious so I talked her as I decided how to get her out of the car. I also looked over the notes left on the dash by the nurse and noted that Mary was three months pregnant. The flight crew had taken vital signs and given her four milligrams of morphine for pain. Together, the EMTs and I decided how to extricate her from the car. I explained to her what we were going to do. "Mary, we will be as gentle as possible, but this is going to hurt." I believed the truth helped a patient prepare themselves for what was to come. I told her she could scream, but we would do the move quickly and not stop even if she yelled. She said to "do it" and we did. We carefully removed her with her screaming loudly. I supported her right leg and outside we were going to temporarily prop her femur on a pillow.

We considered a hare traction splint. I told them to get it ready, but to not put it on till I found out if she could fly with the splint on. I found DPS Sergeant Baker and he said the helicopter was coming back for a quick load and go of Mary then they were leaving to handle the emergency on the lake. He quickly contacted the helicopter and found out she couldn't be transported with the hare traction splint.

I returned to find Hank, an EMT and the new firefighter had Mary securely strapped to the backboard with her head secured. She lay still as the last of the morphine did its work. We cut her pants and found the right femur obviously fractured as I had suspected but I was surprised to find the most horrible tib/fib fracture I have ever seen. The tib/fibs are two bones that rest between the knee and ankle. The bones of the right lower leg extended out of a horrible open wound on her shin. The firefighter gagged when he saw the raw bone protruding through the skin. It made the hare traction a non-issue even if the helicopter could have flown with it on. I then cut her ankle high topped leather shoe and sock. Her left ankle was fractured and left knee was lacerated.

I sent a firefighter to get a dressing to cover the bone ends. He brought it and with shaking hands he dampened the dressing and applied it to the bone ends. I used a flat splint to support the right lower leg fracture. The femur (thigh) remained propped on pillows. I wrapped another pillow around her left ankle to support the fracture. She continued to have a pulse distal (below) to the fractures so that was good. I had EMT Hank, take another set of vital signs. I held off giving her more morphine because she was doing ok if she lay still. But the helicopter would be landing soon and I wanted her morphine to be at its strongest for the move and hospital arrival.

The helicopter soon landed and I gave them her vital signs and suggested it was time for more morphine. I then informed them of the new injuries we had found. If we had not cut the pants, we would have not seen it. They flew off with her, taking her to Page Hospital, where she was stabilized and flown to Flagstaff later for orthopedic surgery. It was a repairable injury, but complicated by her early pregnancy.

The new firefighter who had applied the dressing to the tib/fib fracture went over to edge of the scene, sat down and became sick to his stomach. He had never seen such a thing before and it upset him. Later, when we heard about it, we tried to comfort him by explaining that his action was normal. He had nothing to be ashamed of and shouldn't worry about it.

Jessie and Kasie returned from transporting Mary. They took the back seat male passenger to the hospital. Ned was injured but nothing life threatening. I heard him break into song as they loaded him into the ambulance. Kasie later told me the note I had taped to his shirt was extremely helpful. I transported the female passenger in the blue car. Sonia was stable but her arm was badly injured with fractures in two places. It was awkward to splint. Her neck was not broken but it was badly strained and I am sure she had neck pain for months after the accident. She was also flown to Flagstaff Medical Center for Orthopedic surgery and rehab.

After completing tons of paperwork, extensive cleaning and restocking of the ambulances I returned home. It wasn't even lunch time yet.

Beth's fractured ankle was casted and she was released the next day. She couldn't drive because of the cast so EMT Jessie Blake and his wife were driving to Phoenix anyway, so they drove Beth to the hospital where her sister was in intensive care. The two girl's family had flown into Phoenix that morning. Mary lived and her baby was fine. Beth returned to college on crutches. No one died, but three of the victims had to undergo extensive surgery, a long hospital stay and months of rehab just because a drunken man got behind the wheel.

IF YOU STOP CPR, I'LL KILL YOU

Mr. Carnell was a huge man with a booming voice. I came in contact with his family three times. The first time his trailer caught fire, then his daughter died and finally when his son died. Needless to say, the only time I saw Mr. Carnell was at the worst possible times of his life.

The fire wasn't that big. The only thing that makes it stick out in my memory was the owner, Mr. Carnell. When PFD arrived he was standing out front screaming, waving his arms about and yelling in a booming voice that his trailer was on fire as if we couldn't see the plumb of smoke drifting high in the sky. I moved him back away from the front door so the firefighters could gain access. The trailer was smoke filled. I moved to the door of the cabana attached to the front of the trailer. Firefighters were running in and out. I noticed a red gas can sitting by the doorway, with its top open. A fireman in full turnouts can't see where he's walking and one was storming right for it. I pictured the open gas can kicked into the cabana and igniting in a blazing path of fire. I bent down and grabbed it and jerked it from the fireman's path. Not exactly hero stuff, but it made the call memorable.

Now, Mr. Carnell was a very excitable man. He saw I had an oxygen bottle and suddenly he started coughing and gasping. I gave him oxygen and suddenly he improved and was fine. It was either all in his head or he was faking. I don't know which. Across the street his daughter and son were standing beside their small, worn out mother. She was old beyond her years, a quiet, simple woman. I had a feeling he did all the talking in this family.

The source of the fire was the water heater. The fire was extinguished without serious damage to the home. The heater, one washroom wall and small section of the ceiling were charred. The rest of the home had been saved.

Later he sent his insurance company a bill for a new water heater and repair of the washroom. He also insisted on replacement cost of new drapes, new carpet and furniture because of smoke damage. In reality, he had furniture that had seen better days and a simple shampoo would have done the job on the couch. The two chairs were vinyl. The carpet needed cleaning anyway and the drapes were washable. The insurance company complained. Mr. Carnell complained and the fire department was in the middle because we estimated the damage confined to the hot water heater, a small portion of the washroom and only the cleaning costs to the furniture drapes and carpet. The insurance company won.

The second time I met Mr. Carnell was when his daughter died. She had Parkinson's Disease. She was only in her late twenties but she

84

slowly lost control of her body and finally was found dead in a trailer where she lived, a few doors from her family. At this time, Page didn't have a mortician so the ambulance would go pick up bodies and take them to a refrigerated building by the hospital. Now, I have been on many dead body pickups but this one was very different. Mr. Carnell's wife had passed away suddenly the previous year in the Flagstaff Hospital. So he had become a single parent with a seriously ill daughter. He loved his daughter and he helped her. That morning he had gone to check on his daughter and found her dead. She had died peaceably in her sleep. There was no evidence of foul play. When we arrived, Mr. Carnell unexpectedly left. He went home to get his son. A few minutes later I heard his loud voice yelling outside. I looked up and saw him approaching, literally dragging his older teenage son down the street to the trailer and into it. He said, "See, I want you to face this. This is what it does and it will do this to you too."

I stared at him in disbelief. His young son had just been diagnosed with the same disease a short time before. He had very few symptoms but as he looked at his dead sister you could see terror written on his face. He was looking at his own death and not too far off. I felt sorry for him. He turned and ran.

Detective Stark took out a camera to photograph the body before we moved her. She lay peacefully on her back on a sofa bed. She was wearing pajamas. Stark took a couple of pictures. Mr. Carnell was screaming and sobbing and wailing. He rushed to his daughter and picked her up and cradled her in his arms. He looked up, "You can't take her picture this way. Wait a minute." He rushed off and returned with a tank top and shorts. We humored him and let him dress her and comb her hair. It was an understandably painful situation for this man and we wanted to help ease his pain if possible.

Stark then took another picture. Then Mr. Carnell got up and returned with another top and changed it. Then he combed her hair again, this time with bangs. Stark took another picture. We then took her to the morgue. I saw Stark and told him I bet his pictures of the body are the only ones on file at the PD where the body changed clothes and hairdo's three times for the pictures. I know it isn't funny, and the comment wasn't meant that way. But someday, someone is going to wonder what happened that day and no one will remember.

The third time I met Mr. Carnell was years later. It was not near as tame this time. I responded to a call of a man choking. When I got there, almost the same time as the ambulance, I rushed inside. Mr. Carnell was kneeling on the floor performing CPR on his son, the same son that he had dragged to see his dead sister, years before. The boy was now a man, but the disease had twisted his skeleton thin body into a small contorted shell

85

in which he lay trapped. Mr. Carnell had been feeding the boy and the boy choked. The boy and the father fought sometimes because the boy would "choke" on purpose and spit up on his father. The father thought it was one of those times and ignored the boy. By the time he realized the boy wasn't kidding, the boy went unconscious and his heart stopped. Doing CPR on such a patient would almost seem obscene, but it had been started and we couldn't stop it legally since we were EMT-B's. So we continued.

He was loaded on a backboard with great difficulty since he was permanently curled up in a semi-fetal position. The ambulance crew continued CPR. It was driver Tom Harkins, Lead Tech. Dona Arch and Tech. Shawna Kemp. Shawna was the same age and had gone to school with her patient. It hit her hard to see him that way and to be forced to do that to him. She felt guilty of prolonging his torture. But she did as she was told.

While the crew worked at getting him out of the tiny room and into the ambulance, I tried to keep Mr. Carnell out of their way. He cried on my shoulder and sobbed and talked a thousand miles a second. He insisted he killed his son. I don't know if he was talking about the heredity factor or the food he fed the boy. But either way, the man was hurting. He appeared a little theatrical and one police officer questioned his behavior as maybe suspicious, but I told him that was just Mr. Carnell.

As the ambulance pulled away, I left and drove to the hospital. I walked into the ER in time to hear Dr. Birch yell at my crew, "Stop it! Doing CPR on him is a waste of time. He's dead! Why on earth did you start it anyway?"

Doctor Birch had a near terminal case of Deity Complex. He was five foot nine inches of total inflated ego. I was very protective of my EMTs. I stepped in, "CPR was being performed when they arrived. They can't legally stop," I explained to this irritating man.

He looked up and in a sarcastic voice said "Well, stop it now." Just then Mr. Carnell burst through the ER doors, bellowing "WHERE'S JERRY!" He then saw me and moved toward me. The room was on the corner where two hallways met. I stood in one of two doorways leading to the ER room. He took one look and bellowed, "Don't you dare stop CPR!" My crew had a decision to make and they made it. They continued CPR.

"Mr. Carnell, Jerry is dead," said the doctor in a condescending tone.

"No he isn't, not if you don't stop CPR." Now I understood, as long as CPR was being done, Jerry's blood flowed through his body and Jerry wasn't "dead". And as long as Jerry was "alive," in his own mind, Mr. Carnell hadn't killed his son. I had great sympathy for Mr. Carnell. I couldn't begin to understand the pain he must be feeling. He had accepted

my comfort at the house so I tried to comfort him again. "Mr. Carnell......"
I reached and gently touched his shoulder. His arm shot out and caught
my shoulder and drove me violently into the door frame. Pain shot
through my shoulder and arm. I knew I was going to feel that in the
morning.

"Don't you dare stop CPR! Don't you stop! You hear me?" he
yelled ignoring me and stepping two steps toward a now frightened
doctor. My EMTs faces showed fear, but no indecision, they continued
CPR.

I moved out into the hallway, six feet away and keyed my radio.
"Could you send an officer to the hospital, we need assistance." Only once
before had I called for police back up at the hospital (see *There Must Be A
Full Moon*). That time my radio broadcast had been screamed into the
radio and my fear and panic blared in loud volume for all to hear. I had
vowed that if I ever called again, I would be calm and clear. I had even
rehearsed what I would say. This time my voice was clam and my request
clear and concise.

Behind me Mr. Carnell was becoming more agitated. "I'll kill you;
I'll kill you all if you stop CPR! You hear me? Come on Jerry, fight! Fight!"

But unknown to me, Mr. Carnell's screaming and threats were
broadcast loud and clear over my radio. Every officer within thirty miles
heard my request and his bellowing threats in the background. I was
surprised when every law enforcement officer in the area rushed to the
rescue. Before it was over two city police and a detective, two DPS officers,
one sheriff, two park rangers and a Navajo police officer came.

The first through the door were PPD Anthony Santiago and Brody
Smyth. Both men are good police officers but physically the two of them
barely made one Mr. Carnell. Anthony knew the man and tried reason. It
didn't work. Mr. Carnell struck out at him just like he had me, but this
time he met with resistance. "I'll kill you, you M . . . . F . . . . !" he
screamed as he lunged at Officer Smyth. The two officers grabbed him.
Detective Prim rushed through the door. He is a big man and together
they tried to subdue the now violent Mr. Carnell.

The EMTs stopped CPR and Dr. Birch kept the door to his back
staring out the other door at the fighting men. I got out of their way and
stood watching. I had seen the officers take a man down before. They did
it very well. They usually run them into a wall and then slam dunk them to
the concert. This time, they did it differently. They didn't want to hurt
him, but he was out of control and had threatened to kill. He was big
enough to do that with his bare hands. They walked a slender line of
subduing him without hurting him and not letting him hurt anyone else.
They ran him into the wall, but not that hard and they took him to the

floor, but they lowered him carefully. He lay on the floor still fighting them. He was screaming, "Don't kick me. Stop kicking me!"

I didn't see them kick him so I move around and looked down at the officer's feet. They weren't kicking him, not even accidentally. About that time Dr. Kilmer picked around the corner. He too had heard the part about kicking and came to investigate. He looked at the four struggling men and then up at me. "I don't see them kicking him."

"I don't either," I answered. He shrugged his shoulders and walked away. I stood by rubbing my shoulder and watching the struggle men on the floor. The cavalry started arriving. Each stormed in ready to do battle. Mr. Carnell was finally subdued and cuffed.

They lifted him up and walked him outside with a police escort of six officers. I followed. They talked to him. He was still very mad and threatening. "If you'll just calm down, we will release you, Mr. Carnell," Detective Prim said in a compassionate voice. Mr. Carnell took a long time to calm down. They finally uncuffed him and lead him in to view his dead son. He was again very loud, theatrical and emotional. But the doctor and the other EMTs were long gone. Tears replaced death threats.

"Do you want to press charges?" Prim asked me.

"No, he didn't hurt anyone."

"He shoved you and you're rubbing your shoulder."

"Well, yeah, he did, but I'm all right and I won't press charges."

"He threatened to kill you, the EMT's and the Doctor . . . . " his voice trailed off. He knew none of us would press charges. Unfortunately, Mr. Carnell didn't see it that way. Later he filed a complaint of police brutality against the two officers who had arrived first. My crew and I had to give very lengthy depositions and undergo over a hour each of questioning during the investigation that followed. The doctors and nurses were also questioned. All the stories were pretty much the same. The one thing that lost him his case was his tape recorded threats to kill us all if CPR was stopped on his son. The transmission I made requesting help was taped as part of all radio traffic and his voice came in loud and clear in the background.

The decision was that "no unnecessary force was used against Mr. Carnell," and that they had actually bent the rules in dealing with him by being as gentle as possible and then letting him go, considering his serious threats and actions. Mr. Carnell's immediate family was now deceased. He moved out of town a few months later. I don't know where he moved. I never saw him again. I am hopeful his luck improved and he found peace.

THE TSUNAMI

The wind had been blowing at over sixty-five miles per hour for two days. The record was one-hundred miles per hour set a few years before. We had just returned from a reported 962 (motor vehicle accident with at least one person injured) thirteen miles south of town. It had been a nerve wrecking trip. The ambulance is a high profile vehicle and the wind did it's best to blow the vehicle over on its side. It almost succeeded a couple of times, but the driver of the ambulance, Roger, managed to keep it shinny side up. We arrived on the scene just in time to be cancelled by the DPS officer. The vehicle had left the roadway, but had managed to get back on the road and had driven off into the sunset before the police arrived. The return trip back to Page was scary as the rig was rocked back and forth by the wind. We were pulling into the fire station when dispatch called on the radio to report a request for an ambulance at a local address. It involved a man, whose wife couldn't wake him from a nap. She was panic stricken. The driver did a "U" turn and off we went. Roger parked the ambulance in front of a small house. We took a minute loading up with our jump kit, and other equipment. Roger rushed in ahead of the crew, running down the hall and into the bedroom. The man lay on his back, his arms resting at his side. He was dressed in pajamas. His eyes were closed and he was very quiet. Roger rapidly rushed across the room to the man and kneeled on the edge of the king size bed. It was then we all realized it was a water bed. He sunk down when his two-hundred and seventy-five pounds of junk food pressed on the edge, displacing gallons of water. The victim was caught in the tidal wave and lifted straight up two feet above the bed in mid-air. He still maintained the prone position and appeared to be sleeping in mid-air like a magician's assistant.

The man came back down with force creating another tsunami wave that crossed the bed and caught Roger, propelling him up in the air, still in the keeling position. With the look of surprise on his face, he came back down and the man was again air born. The wife stood with mouth gaping open in shock as the crew burst out laughing. The carnival side show came to an end when Roger managed to stand up and let the poor unconscious man settle down on his restless bed of water.

Trying to regain some shred of dignity, Roger cleared his throat and took out a stethoscope. The crew struggled to regain composure, for the woman's sake, not our partner. The rest of the call was routine. The man's vital signs were within normal range. His condition turned out to not be serious. I can't remember with any degree of certainty why he couldn't be awakened, but I think he had taken an extra sleeping pill. What does remain clear in my memory was the waterbed. There's something about watching a man who takes himself so seriously bouncing around on a king size water bed with another man.

SHOW AND TELL

The last Basic EMT Class I taught was for Coconino Community College in Page. The Page Campus is nice with a pretty block building with furnished classrooms. The academics (full time instructors) live in a cloistered environment. Everything's nice and neat and people are always polite and say please and thank you. I found them interesting and completely out of touch with the real world. One example involved Northern Arizona University (NAU, a four year college) that had space in the Page CCC building. It was noticed that there was a high dropout rate in first year students on the main campus in Flagstaff and the classes held at Page. Guess what they did to address the problem? They changed the school's logo. During my career my title has changed from "teacher to instructor to educator, to learning facilitator." I find it amusing that my title changed so many times but the job remained the same. I love teaching regardless of what you call it. It is such a fantastic feeling to see your students go from awkward, clumsy, unsure people to EMT's that have the confidence to step in and handle an emergency and do it well. Many of my past students are working as EMT-Basics. Some are now paramedics and registered nurses. Two went on to be Physician's Assistants. It was my honor to have a small part in their educational process.

Before CCC came to Page, Yavapai Community College offered classes in Page but didn't have a campus. The Basic EMT Class it was held at the Page Fire Department. Setting up a classroom involved moving Rescue-Two outside and using the bay as a classroom. Oil drippings were soaking in a type of "kitty litter "that crunched as we walked on it. The students sat at old folding tables on scratched and dinged metal folding chairs. In the summer everyone would sweat even if the fan was on and in the winter they would wear coats in class. It was primitive, but it was all we had and we made it work.

One evening I was teaching the class. There were around sixteen people in class, most were awake. Unexpectedly, a man in his sixties walked into the bay. Everyone turned around. He looked at me and said, "I'm having a heart attack."

For a brief moment I stood there absorbing the information. I then looked at my class and said, "Student's, he's having a heart attack.

You know what to do. We studied that last week. Do it." They all stood up at once and began to move rapidly. I smiled as I saw they each automatically took a task and began caring for the man. One student helped him sit down; two ran for oxygen and a mask. Another started taking his blood pressure while still another took his pulse as a third student counted his respirations. One student began to question him referring to the class notes he held in his hand. Another student stood at his elbow writing it all down. There wasn't enough of the patient to go around and some students stood and watched, offering suggestions here and there. I walked from the room into my office. I called dispatch. "Page the first out ambulance crew and have them report to Station One for a possible heart attack." She paged and I went back in to check on the students.

They had documented all his vital signs with the time taken. He was on high flow O2 by non-rebreather mask. His medical history had been written down and the drugs he took documented. They were hovering around him as a student took a second set of vital signs. He looked better. Oxygen works wonders for a heart attack.

The on call crew burst into the bay and was met by one of my students. "He walked in and said he was having a heart attack. His name is Drake; he's sixty-four years old and had a heart attack one year ago." A student hurried up and gave them the paper with vital signs on it. Quickly the crew stepped in and took over. One EMT opened the bay door and removed the stretcher from the ambulance and wheeled it into the classroom next to where Drake sat. The students backed off and watched as they loaded him on the stretcher in a sitting position and loaded him in the ambulance. Off the ambulance went code-three to the hospital.

I walked over and closed the bay door. "Let's take a break and then we can talk about what just happened." The entire class was excited. They had just experienced their first emergency and didn't even have to leave the classroom. After a very short break they sat down. One student after another told the same story from their point of view. Each person proudly told what part they had played in the drama. I let them talk. I then answered questions. When everyone had had a chance to talk and all questions had been answered, it was my turn. "In EMS you never know what you will be doing in the next five minutes. It's spontaneous and unplanned. Tonight you were presented with your first emergency. I want to say how proud I am of all of you. You did exactly what you should have done. No certified EMT could have done better."

They were all smiling and quite proud of themselves. They should be. The patient lived for many years after that and many of the students went on to work in EMS. They had found a confidence I could have never given them. They were pleasantly surprised to discover they knew what needed to be done and did it. This turned into the best classroom learning experience in my entire teaching career.

This isn't the end of the story. Five months later our patient, Drake Miller exited an insurance office and again experienced what he had become to recognize as the beginning of a heart attack. Should he drive himself to the hospital? Should he return back inside and have his insurance agent call an ambulance? Before he could come to a decision he saw the Page Fire Department Attack Truck heading his direction. The truck was designed to arrive first to a fire. That day Mitch was driving the truck. He was a great firefighter and a good fire engineer, but he had never been interested in becoming an EMT. He was heading west on North Navajo (don't ask). He saw a man in his sixties run into the road waving his arms and yelling for the truck to stop. Mitch slammed on the brakes and came to a stop two inches from the man's chest. He reached for the door handle to get out but Drake hurried to the passenger door, opened it and jumped in.

Mitch looked over at the stranger who had just got in his truck. "I'm having a heart attack. Take me to the hospital," announced Drake. Drake buckled his seat belt. Mitch sat there with a stunned look on his face. It was against the rules for a non-employee to ride in a city owned vehicle. They were one and a half blocks from the hospital. If the man was indeed having a heart attack, Mitch was reasonably sure he should call for an ambulance. But it might be faster to just do what the man asked and drive him to the hospital. But then what if the man dropped dead in his truck? For a minute Mitch was racked with indecision, Finally he reached a decision. He reached up and lit the code lights, turned on the siren and stomped on the gas. He reported over the radio he was en-route code-three with a man having a heart attack, ETA (estimated time of arrival) one minute. I was sitting at my desk at the fire department when he sped past the station with siren blaring loudly. What in the world is going on? I though. I got up and went to my car and headed to the hospital.

I saw the red attack truck do a tight right into the ER driveway and skid to a halt. I watched as Mitch exploded from the driver's side door and ran screaming into the ER "Man with a heart attack in the parking lot!" Due to his short transport time the dispatcher had not been able to warn the ER of the unorthodox "incoming" patient. I parked behind the attack truck and jumped out. I ran forward and met Drake climbing out the passenger door. He didn't look that bad, but with his history I decided to take his word for it; heart attack it was. The ER Tech joined me and we escorted Drake into the ER Department with Mitch running circles around us. The doctor and RN were setting up the crash cart. They turned and saw us as we entered the hospital. Drake was known to the staff. He had been having serious cardiac issues. We assisted him to the gurney and connected him up to the EKG monitor. I slipped an oxygen mask on him and cranked it up. I backed off and left the room. The ER staff appeared to have it in hand. I found Mitch in the parking lot frantically sucking on his cigarette.

"What happened?" I asked. As Rescue Chief I had to find out why he chose to ignore department protocols.

"He just ran out in the road, damn it, I almost hit him!" Mitch was still high on adrenaline.
"He told me to drive him to the hospital because he was having a heart attack. Shit, I could see the hospital; I just thought it would be faster." Mitch took a deep draw on his cancer stick. He was coming down and his hand shook.

As a supervisor I couldn't say it out loud, but sometimes the rules have to be bent a little. Common sense dictates t was a lot faster to just transport the man the one and a half blocks. Its possible Mitch may have saved Drake's life by getting him to the hospital so quickly. "Look, no was harm done. But the department policy says you are to call an ambulance." I hesitated, then continued, "With that said . . . . . off the record. . . . . . good job." Drake had an internal automatic cardiac defibulator implanted in his chest. He hated the thing but it kept him alive for many more years.

MVA, SNOW, ICE, AND THEN THE INTERRVIEW

Snow fell, covering the world in a layer of white. Fog and clouds obscured the hills. Ice covered the road causing vehicles to slide back and forth, fish-tail, and do donuts while traveling backwards or sideways down the steep hill from the top of Black Mesa. I lay on my stomach on the snow covered black dirt at the side of the roadway. I could feel the cold damp earth seep through my clothing. I reached deep within the overturned car through the broken back window, groping for the woman that lay moaning in the twisted metal. My forearm hit sharp metal, cutting a thin, line that began to bleed. A car slid past, sideways, a few feet from me. I tried to ignore it and concentrate on removing the injured woman.

Perhaps I should back up a bit. In January 2003, the private ambulance company I worked for in Tuba City began hinting they may be forced to pull out of Tuba because their contract with the hospital may not be renewed. There were no problems with the company's service but because of the Navajo Preference Policy, they may have no choice. A Navajo man with no business experience had sent in a bid for the contract. He was a questionable choice but he was a Native American. The company for which I worked employed mostly Native Americans but that didn't seem to count. The hospital made it clear they preferred the company I worked for and asked the Navajo Government to make an exception, but they refused to bend the rules. In the world today, discrimination is allowed if the person you are discriminating against is white, so the Anglo owner of the company lost the contract. I lost my job because of the color of my employer's skin.

The Navajo who got the contract asked me to work for him but I knew him and I didn't want to work him because we had worked together on an ambulance in the past and didn't play well together. I stayed busy by working part-time for Page Fire and I taught an EMT class for Coconino Community College. I wasn't working full time when I ran into an old friend in the Tuba City ER. Vicky Del La Cruz. She was my administrative assistant (and EMT student) when I was Rescue Chief at the Fire Department. We were good friends. She was an attractive woman, a Navajo, thin build with long black hair. She was well organized and highly skilled as a paramedic. After she left the fire department I saw her off and on through the years. She worked as a flight medic for a local helicopter service and Navajo Nation EMS.

Vicky currently was working full time for Peabody Western Black Mesa and Kayenta Mines as an independent contract medic. The mines had a clinic and ambulance that served the workers and locals leasing the land to the mine. It was a great job, paying around sixty percent more than I was being paid in Tuba City. Vicky and a RN alternated weeks of duty at the mine, working seven days on, seven days off. She wanted me to substitute for them when they were sick, on vacation, or at work related conferences. It would be about a total of five weeks a year. I would be a contract paramedic. A contract medic is an independent medic offering their services as a small businessman. I would provide my own insurance and other required legal requirements. I jumped at it. I would provide clinic care for employees and their families. I would have considerable leeway. I also provided ambulance for the employees and their families and there was a small attack truck for small fires. Mileage wasn't a factor since it was under a hundred miles southeast from Page around the same distance I was driving at that time to Tuba. When I told my husband about the job he commented, "Great. I never expected to be sleeping with a coalminer."

A few days after Vicky approached me with the part-time job at the mines, Lynn Brown called me. She worked for Navajo EMS. We had worked together in the past and she heard I was looking for a job. She was an average sized woman with a massive head of long black hair that she wore in tight curls. I don't know how she did it but she always had neatly groomed hair and perfect makeup even at three in the morning. Her shoes were polished and her uniform was neatly ironed. Lynn was a hard person to like. As most people who consider themselves "perfect", she lacked tact and believed her way was the only way. She made enemies easily. I learned to ignore her cutting remarks which she saw as being honest and straightforward while those that disagreed with her were stupid, rude and confrontational. She's the only paramedic I know that was threatened by a Hopi Ranger with arrest if she didn't back away, take her ambulance and leave the scene of an accident (without the patient). She and I got along reasonably well. I learned a long time ago, confronting someone like her was a waste of time because she would never change and I would create an enemy.

Lynn had heard I was looking for a job. She said the Kayenta Clinic needed medics to work in the ER and for long range transports. I had worked out of the clinic a few years ago with a private owned ambulance company and was familiar with some of the clinic staff and how they did things. The pay was very good and a bit more than Peabody paid. It was also full time, two 24 hour shifts, back to back a week. Kayenta didn't provide quarters so I would have to park my RV or rent a motel room. I was certain I could do both jobs, but was it want I wanted? I can't explain it, but I began to have a strange negative feeling about this job. I wasn't certain if I should pursue it or not.

On paper it was a good opportunity and I was looking for full time employment. There was no logical reason why I shouldn't consider this job. I scheduled an interview at Kayenta Clinic for the same day of my eight hour orientation at the mine. The town was only twenty-four miles away from the turnoff to the mine so I decided to kill two birds with one stone. I then turned my concentration to jumping through the many hoops required for both jobs. I got my own insurance since I was going to be an independent Paramedic Contractor (at the mine and the K-town Clinic). I became familiar with my new Medical Control's protocols. I became New Mexico Paramedic Certified (a requirement for both jobs). For the mine job I went through a three day safety/orientation class. I also reviewed rope rescue and fire suppression. There were a lot of loose strings but I got them all tied together and was ready to go one day before I was to start work.

I also had the interview scheduled at the clinic after I had completed orientation at the mine. It was going to be a long day. I left Page at six o'clock that morning (March 18) even though it was only eighty miles away and I had allotted myself two hours to make the trip. I started early due to the weather. It was raining in Page, but it turned to snow at Inscription House on Highway 98. The wet roads froze and then the snow covered the icy road making it slick. The snow became thicker and the ground was covered in a white blanket. The tops of the mountains were hidden by thick clouds. I hit the junction of Highway 160 and 98. I turned east on 160. It was just twelve miles to the Black Mesa turnoff. Then there was another eight miles up the hill to the Peabody Clinic on State Route 41. Highway 41 was paved, but narrow. It winded its way up the steep hill to the top of Black Mesa (a flat topped mountain.) It was a beautiful, peaceful area with scrub pines and grassy hills. It is considered a joint use area and both Navajo and Hopi share the top of Black Mesa.

I left highway 160 at the Black Mesa Trading Post. It is well over six-thousand feet and the snow increased, visibility dropped. I reached the bottom of "THE Hill." It climbed up the north side of Black Mesa. It was very steep and curved up the side of the mountain like a snake. A light fog was in the air. Snow was falling and the road was covered with a thick sheet of ice and several inches of snow. No snow plow or gravel truck had tackled the hill yet (it was early). It was slick as snot and dangerous.

I was driving my new Chevy Impala and headed up the hill behind two pickups. We were going about twelve miles per hour. To my left, I saw a pickup sideways in a narrow area between the roadway and guard rail. He had spun out there and was now digging out. A car went past me heading downhill fishtailing followed by a large pickup with brakes locked and still traveling forward. I was getting nervous.

About three-fourths of the way up the steep hill, a truck in front spun sideways and stopped. The pickup in front of me and I (plus those behind me) managed to get stopped. The pickup spun its tires. The rear tires whipped back and forth and regained forward motion. The next pickup did the same. I sat and watched them fishtail up the hill, just missing a van sliding down the hill with tires locked and a driver with a terrified look on his face. I lifted my foot off the break and slowly depressed the gas pedal. My car slid backwards. My tires spun, but I didn't move forward. I braked to a stop. I tried again, and again. Each time, I would slide backwards. I now sat slightly to the center of the road, partially sideways. Vehicles behind me worried me most. They began to drive around me. Visibility was very poor and the vehicles coming up the hill had very little time to adjust their path to miss me. They couldn't stop or they might be stuck by those behind them. I was scared. One truck went around me on the right, taking half the lane and half on snow covered dirt at the side of the road. I checked it out.

There was about three foot of dirt then a shallow drainage ditch, then the side of a rock cliff. If I could maneuver over to the dirt and get one wheel in it, I might get traction. But, to do it was to risk sliding into the ditch. I wouldn't die, but my new car would require a tow truck and body work. I took a deep breath, turned my wheel to maneuver the tail of my car toward the side of the road and took my foot off the break. I slid backward. In three short attempts, I managed to slide off the road into the snow and black dirt. I then put it in drive and after a few seconds of panic, I moved forward. Slowly I went up the hill, sliding slightly back and forth. I gained the top. I was thrilled. I continued to drive on ice, snow with poor visibility, but no more steep hills.

Just minutes after I had gained the top of the hill, a small white car started down the steep incline. The driver was a twenty-six year of age Navajo man and the woman was a twenty-two year old Navajo female. They both were dressed in Peabody Security uniforms. They were just getting off work. The car began to slide sideways. The woman screamed, the man gripped the wheel, and struggled for control. It crossed in front of a pickup heading uphill, struck the snow covered dirt, flipped over onto its top and slid along the rough bolder lined ditch to a stop. The sound of screams and crushing metal stopped. The unrestrained people lay in the overturned car's roof, the space was crushed down, and limited movement. Snow silently fell, covering the underside of the car, now exposed to the elements.

I drove up to the Administration Building. The clinic was inside the building. Vicky had arrived in the ambulance just before me. We walked into the clinic together. The phone was ringing. ". . . One car rollover, on the hill . . . . multiple patients."

"Wonderful" I thought to myself. I didn't want to go back to that hill. We jumped into the ambulance and headed back. The ambulance had four-wheel drive, but on ice that isn't that much help. The rig was very heavy, which helped but didn't guarantee safety. Ice covered the roadway. Vicky drove slowly, lights flashing red/white/blue with siren blaring. Cars tried to pull off the road, but most had problems due to the mud and snow.

We started down the hill. Through the fog, a line of cars and brake lights became visible. We moved to the wrong side of the road and slid alongside the overturned vehicle. The placement of the ambulance provided some protection from sliding vehicles, but one could still get us.

97

Was this scene safe? No, but it was about as good as it could get under the circumstances.

The driver was out of the car and pacing around, very upset. I led him to the ambulance and put him inside and told him to sit there and we would go get the woman out of the car. He climbed inside and took some deep breaths. He had scrapes and scratches, and was wet and dirty, but looked reasonable uninjured. I grabbed a backboard with straps and hurried back to the car. The woman was lying on the roof of the upside down car. Her feet were pointing toward the front dash and her head toward the shattered rear window. Security guards (five or so) showed up. One who was a first responder got on the cliff side and I crawled under the trunk on the road side. We positioned the backboard. Our plan was to slid the woman head first out through the broken back window and slid her onto the backboard. We wanted to do it quickly because of our dangerous location. I felt the cold moisture soak into my clothing. I struggled to position my body around the antenna that protruded from the trunk downward to the dirt. The falling snow began to cling to my long hair, soaking it. We reached in and grabbed a hold of the woman. My arm scrapped against a piece of twisted metal and my forearm was cut. Blood seeped from the wound. I ignored it. The patient moaned and answered questions with one to two word sentences. I slipped a c-collar around her neck and told her to not turn her head. We began scooting her out head first. It wasn't easy. Vicky climbed into the vehicle through the driver's window and untangled the woman's feet that were trapped by the car's head rest. I heard a bystander scream and I looked up in time to see a pickup slide sideways past us followed by a blue car, also sideways.

The woman was soon extricated and secured to the backboard. I shivered as we carried her to the ambulance. I was soaking wet and chilled. Quickly we got her on the stretcher and inside the warm ambulance. I grabbed a 4x4 gauze dressing and taped it over the wound on my forearm. Vicky and I set about getting the patients checked out. She took the woman and I took the man. Someone had cancelled the Kayenta ambulance. Vicky asked that it continue and meet us at the trading post. The Kayenta ambulance was a basic unit and would take the man so I kept him a "basic" patient by not starting an IV. I got him on a backboard with c-collar, vital signs, etc.

Convinced our patients were ready for transport, Vicky climbed into the front to drive and I was in the back. I hung on as she started down the slippery hill. The drop off beyond the guardrail was several hundred feet down, and of course, the ditch and cliff on our left. I couldn't believe I was back on that steep hill where I was stuck only a few minutes before.

The patients were nervous too. They had just slid off on the ice and now they were tied to a backboard, helpless and traveling down the same hill.

Vicky had security stop traffic coming up the hill so we would have the whole road to ourselves. I set up to start an IV on the female patient. Before I made the stick, I looked up and saw a UPS truck in the middle of the roadway, slightly cocked to the right as it slid slowly down the hill. Vicky moved to the left and passed it. I started the IV. To help warm her up, I wrapped the IV tubing around a heat pack. As the fluid flowed through the tubing it would be warmed by the heating pack. We gained speed, but to hit the brakes would guarantee a slide. We continued down the hill. We reached the bottom. All four of us in the ambulance sighed with relief. We pulled into the trading post parking lot to await the Kayenta ambulance. The female patient was an Advanced Life Support (ALS) patient so we planned on keeping her in our ambulance. She had a number of complaints that might be serious or maybe not. It was a good plan to prepare for the worst and be pleasantly surprised.

The Kayenta ambulance soon appeared and we transferred the male patient to their care. They quickly left, heading to Kayenta. As Vicky maneuvered the ambulance back on the highway, I turned my attention to the female patient. I got vital signs every five minutes. She complained of right shoulder pain, clavicle pain and mid-sternum pain on inspiration so I put her on high flow oxygen and the EKG. I found all her vital signs within normal limits and her EKG was normal sinus rhythm. The oxygen made it easier for her to breath and she relaxed a little.

We pulled out onto Highway 160 and headed east toward Kayenta. It was twenty miles away, twenty miles of low visibility and a solid sheet of ice. I checked the IV of normal saline and took another set of vital signs. It was slow going. I called Kayenta Clinic on EMSCOM Radio. I identified myself as Peabody Ambulance, Paramedic Holbert. I didn't know it then, but several people in the clinic ER recognized me from the time I worked out of there years ago. Vicky was a good driver, so we arrived safely around a half hour later.

We wheeled our patient into the ER. I was met by three people saying "Welcome back, Sharon." I smiled and greeted them. We took the woman into a curtained area. The doctor was Dr. Heinz, a doctor I had previously worked with in Tuba and Kayenta. She was very pregnant and waddled up to receive a report. The patient didn't look too bad right now, but with pain on taking a deep breath, she could develop serious problems. In the next bed was the male patient. Nurses were working over him. The man's wife arrived and the female patient's parents arrived. Later I found out the man was treated and released, the female was taken to Tuba City Hospital (75 miles away) and admitted for further monitoring.

I took a deep breath; it was time to start the paperwork. I washed my hands and looked down. My navy blue uniform was covered in mud and soaking wet. Thick black mud covered my boots and I think I was a bit taller for the caked mud on the bottoms. My uniform pants were wet and mud clung to the fabric from the hem up to my thighs and belly. My sleeves and the front of my jacket were wet and mud covered. My mud caked hair hung dripping wet from the snow about my red face (red from exposure to cold). I shivered from the chill I was just beginning to notice. I heard my name called. There was Lynn. She was working that day at Kayenta and was dragging a short woman, obviously from India. "Sharon, this is Dr. Actshaw." I looked down into the face of the doctor I had called a couple of times in an attempt to set up a meeting about employment at the clinic.

My mind raced about. I stood in front of the doctor, dripping wet and covered in mud. My face was smeared with mud and my hands were filthy. Black dirt encrusted my finger nails and my right ear. I could not have looked worse. In the past, I have always gone out of my way to dress well for interviews. I smiled, "I am happy to meet you at last, Doctor. I am dressed to impress." She smiled and chuckled.

We talked briefly about the job. I was pretty well hired if my paperwork is found to be in order. Vicky wasn't that happy, but let me take the time necessary to get things in order. I left with phone and fax numbers to send my paperwork. I would be a contract paramedic and purchase orders must be completed and a contract signed. I was set to work at the Peabody mines Monday and made arrangements to drop by the clinic before noon and drop off the paperwork. My schedule was going to be tight for a couple of weeks or so since I now had three jobs instead of one, but you must grab opportunities when they present themselves. If you don't, they pass you by. I won't have the Tuba job much longer, and Peabody was an erratic part time job, so I needed Kayenta. But, that uncomfortable feeling lingered. It didn't seem right somehow.

I struggled with the feeling that I shouldn't take this job. I can't explain it, but the feeling increased as it became time for me to put my name down on the schedule. Finally, I sent a fax and followed up with a phone call stating that I had a "family situation that made it impossible for me to follow through" and I would have to "decline their generous offer." The doctor was too polite to ask for details of my "family situation." After backing out of the job offer I felt relieved. I didn't know why, but it had been the right decision, I was certain.

Over the next four months the company, for which I worked, pulled out of Tuba City. I filled in at Peabody a total of six days. I continued to teach the EMT class for Coconino Community College and increased my activity as a reserve for the Page fire Department. I didn't regret turning down the Kayenta Clinic job.

The Kayenta Clinic is staffed by a dedicated group of people. They are very busy and work hard. On long range transports they followed New Mexico rules that requires only one trained person on an ambulance. They took it to the limits, and allowed a desk clerk to drive the ambulance one day. The clerk had never driven an ambulance before, she had no training, and she turned on the red lights and sirens and took off toward Tuba City Hospital, seventy-five miles away. In the passenger seat was an off duty RN. In the back rode a paramedic and a very stable patient with a fractured wrist.

On the main street of Tuba, the desk clerk sailed along at sixty-five miles per hour in a thirty mile per hour zone. She struck a man crossing the street. He flew up in the air and landed with a sickening thud on the pavement. She slammed on the breaks (after hitting him) and violently threw the paramedic forward and fractured his arm in two places. In a car sitting at the stop sign was an off duty paramedic and EMT. They witnessed the accident. They got out and ran to the man lying in the street. The medic felt for a pulse, there wasn't one. "Start CPR," he said. He and the EMT started CPR. They were shocked when the ambulance drove off leaving them in the middle of the roadway with no equipment and a man in full code arrest.

The Kayenta ambulance delivered the patient with the fractured wrist to the hospital (about three blocks away) and the paramedic went in to be treated. The Navajo Police arrived at the scene of the accident and called for an ambulance. The officer was very angry and when another officer arrived at the scene, the first officer drove to the hospital. He entered the ER spitting fire and ready to kick ass and take names. He said the Kayenta ambulance had struck and probably killed a man then left the scene of the accident. He arrested the driver in the middle of the busy ER. After treatment the entire Kayenta crew ended up at Navajo Police headquarters. They were eventually released, but they all were in deep legal trouble. The paramedic allowed the inexperienced driver to drive code-three. The off duty RN was the highest ranking person on board and had allowed the driver to exceed the speed limit by thirty-five miles per hour on a busy city street with pedestrians everywhere. She also told the driver to leave the accident so the medic could be treated at the hospital.

It was hushed up. Since it occurred on the reservation and all involved were Navajo's, the rules were different. The Navajo legal system handled the case. There was enough blame to go around and punishment was passed out to all involved. Kayenta stopped transporting people and took bids for the service and the same company I had worked for in Tuba City got the contract. By Sept. 2004 I was back working in Kayenta for that company. Now, looking back, I see I did the right thing to turn down the job. It only lasted four months and I could have been on that ambulance. It is often best to follow gut feelings. My decision to not take the job was one of my better decisions. On a lighter note, this job interview goes down in my personal history as the most strange.

Note: November 22, 2004. I had just began working for a private ambulance company who had taken over the long range transports and backup 911 duties for Kayenta. I was at the Kayenta Clinic preparing to pick up a patient. A short woman from India stood behind the nursing station. She looked at me as I walk up, "I know you, don't I?" she asked.
"Yes" I explained, "I was going to work for you doing transports and I had to drop out due to family problems."
She smiled, "So you're back working now?"
"Yes, I am."
"Good," she said. I guess this proves arriving at an interview dripping wet and covered with mud makes an impression!

IF YOU HAD BEEN THERE,
THIS WOULDN'T HAVE HAPPENED

I was awakened by the pager sitting on my nightstand. "We have a report of an unknown medical at . . ." I was really tired. I usually rolled as first responding EMT, but not tonight. I lay in bed and as soon as I heard F-2, Timmy Alto, Assistant Fire Chief, go on the air, I rolled back over and went back to sleep. I didn't know it then, but I would regret that decision.
The call was to a small two bedroom apartment on Eighth Avenue. The family that lived there had called because their nineteen year old daughter had "gone crazy." The EMTs, Susan Elders, Tex Manning, Timmy Alto and Officer Anthony Santiago found the woman standing in the kitchen screaming and beating on the cabinets with her fists. She was a young adult Navajo female. Her name was Shoshone. She wore her black hair long, was of tiny build, and very pretty. She was crying and screaming. The crew could not really understand the problem. Why was

she so mad? The rest of the family that lived there was her mother, father, younger sister and a couple of brothers. They all said they had no idea why she was behaving this way. She lived in Phoenix and had come for a short visit and went off the deep end for no apparent reason.

There are some basic survival rules in dealing with unstable people. Never back anyone into a corner. Also, never back an angry person toward weapons. And never underestimate an emotionally disturbed person. They broke all three rules. EMT Susan talked with Shoshone as she slowly backed away, into the corner of the kitchen, next to the dishes that were drying. "We just want to help."

"You can't help."

"Yes I can."

"No one listens," (sob) "No one believes me." Her voice was laced with pain. She looked at Susan. "Just go away! Leave me alone! I don't need your help . . . . I don't need anyone!" Without warning, she reached over and picked up a steak knife that was lying on the counter and with the other arm grabbed Susan around the throat. Susan was in trouble. The small woman suddenly had a weapon and a hostage. The officer and the two male EMTs realized they had blown it and Susan just might be the one to pay for their sloppy inattention. Shoshone held the knife to the EMT's throat. "I'll kill her. I swear I will kill her if you come any closer!" The girl shoved Susan forward and they began to slowly work their way to the front door. They slowly entered the living room and began to move across the room. Outwardly Susan tried to appear calm, but inside she was terrified. Her eyes were wide when she saw what the men were planning on doing. The men started to slowly circle the girl. They moved as one and on an unspoken command they grabbed her. The officer took the arm with the weapon and jerked it away from Susan's throat. Tex took her other arm. Timmy grabbed her knees as Susan bolted away. They took Shoshone down to the floor hard and handcuffed her as she lay crying on the floor.

Shoshone was loaded in the ambulance and taken to the hospital. En route she calmed down. She started to softly talk. "I hate them both."

"Who?" Susan asked.

"My parents." She sat quietly for a minute and then continued. "I was only nine when he started coming into my room at night, ... he. . . . .touched me."

"Who?"

"My father. He made me . . . . you know. By the time I was thirteen he forced me into . . . intercourse." Her voice trailed off. She fell quiet, lost in dark memories.

Susan just sat there. This small young woman had threaded to kill Susan a short time ago and now Susan felt only sorrow for the poor tortured young woman. "Did you tell anyone?"

"I told my mother, but she said she didn't believe me. She knew what he was doing and did nothing. He had a good job and provided for the family and she sacrificed me so she could dress well and my two useless brothers could watch Direct TV." Anger dripped from her voice. "At seventeen, I packed up and left. No one seemed to care. I moved to Phoenix and lived with my best friend's family. I made a life that didn't include them. I went to school and became a Certified Nursing Assistant. I have a good job. I thought I had put it all behind me. I came up to Page for my cousin's wedding. That's when I found out that bastard was abusing my little sister. That %$*@!^&! I just lost it. I'm sorry if I hurt you."

"I'm ok, don't worry about it." Susan now understood why the girl went berserk. Years of pent up rage exploded that night in frustration and anger that now her younger sister faced the same abuse and again no one cared. The ambulance pulled over to the side of the road. Susan got out and Officer Santiago, who had been following behind in a patrol car pulled over and got out. Susan told him the girl's story.

"That son-of-a-bitch just sat there and pretended to not know why his daughter was so upset." He took a deep breath the continued. "Look, take her to the police station. I'll call a detective. At the station Officer Santiago and the EMTs sat and listened, as well as a detective that had been woke up to come down to the station. It was a disgusting story of incest and dirty secrets exposed. After enough evidence was taken, they called D.E.S. (Arizona child protection). The officer s escorted the Child Protection worker to the home where the younger sister, Sheena, was removed.

It was now early morning. I heard unusual radio traffic and went to the fire station to see what had happened. I wasn't ready for what I found. Susan turned on me and verbally assaulted me. She got in my face and yelled. "If you had been there, this wouldn't have happened!" She was very angry. No one was watching her back and she had almost been killed. Assistant Fire Chief Timmy Alto was totally useless and everyone knew it. I hesitated. I thought about what she had said. She was right. I would have never allowed it to escalate into a hostage situation. "I'm sorry. Timmy was on call, not me."

She screamed, "He's a waste of skin, you know that. He almost got me killed. You better come the next time it sounds dangerous or I will quit. I will not enter another situation with him to protect my back." I felt bad, but there was little I could do. Timmy was F-2 and I was F-3 and could do nothing to change that. The Fire Chief was a control freak. He liked

Timmy because he did whatever he wanted and gave him no grief. He was a puppet. This issue would rear its ugly head again and again until eventually Timmy finally would have to resign.

Was there a happy ending? No, there never is a happy ending in something like this. The best you can hope for is that the abuse ends and the healing begins. Susan refused to press charges of assault but went to the Fire Chief and complained loudly about Timmy. It accomplished nothing. The father stood trial for the molestation and rape of his older daughter and molestation of the younger daughter. He was found guilty and sentenced to prison. The mother and brothers were angry at the two girls. The father had had a good paying job, but now he was in prison and was unable to support the family. The boys had to go out and get jobs and the mother assumed the martyr persona.

Shoshone got legal custody of her younger sister and took her back to Phoenix. I was told by the DES worker that the two girls had been scheduled for counseling. I hope they were able to regain some measure of self-esteem and find a way to let go of the anger inside. I would like to think they were able to heal.

I personally made a point of going to any call that could go bad. I felt guilty for what had happened to Susan. I made certain it never happened again while I was Rescue Chief.

THE SQUARE DANCING EMT

The life of a volunteer EMT can be challenging. They wander about their life knowing at any moment the pager could go off and they will be expected to drop whatever they are doing and report for duty. In the early years, the Page Ambulance EMT Volunteers signed up for two or three person ambulance crews. Shifts were 12 hours long (6 am to 6 pm and 6 pm to 6 am). The ones that were not on the schedule would listen to their personal scanner or if they were and EMT and a Fire Fighter, they would have a radio. If a "full call out" was paged, everyone available was expected to respond. Most of the employers in the community allowed those at work to leave. It was considered part of the "community spirit." Unfortunately, today that isn't the case. With a full time staff scheduling is simpler, but motivation comes down to money. Most volunteers have deserted the fire department due to the working environment and lack of continuing educational opportunities.

Let's get back to the good old days. Monica was a volunteer EMT. She took her duty seriously but she also enjoyed her Tuesday Square Dancing Group. She never missed a meeting, well . . . . . almost never. While Monica was dosey-doeing I was throwing in a load of clothes into the washer. My husband was taking a shower and my two sons were in their tree house. "Beeeeeeeeeeeeeeeeeeeeeeeep" sounded the pager. I quickly added detergent and turned on the washer. I got to the front door I slipped on my shoes, picked up my jump suit and reached for my car keys. They weren't there. I usually left them on a table next to the door. I looked around the floor, thinking they may have slipped off the table. I didn't see them. Now it's only a theory, but I have always though there was a black hole in my home. Sometimes items would slip into that hole and completely disappear only to reappear a few hours or days later in exactly where I had looked previously. Now my keys had slipped into that black hole.

I spun around in circles in pure panic. I then saw my purse. I unzipped it and dug around looking for my keys. I found nothing. I tossed the purse down and hurried to the desk and ripped the drawer open. I usually kept the extra set of keys in the drawer, but not this time. I panicked. I was almost a fanatic about keeping my keys and shoes handy, but this time I blew it. I ran into the bedroom. My husband was out of the shower and dressing. "I can't find my keys!" I screamed. He was a volunteer EMT and Fire Fighter so he completely understood my panic. He grabbed his car keys lying on the nightstand and tossed them to me, "Here, take my truck."

I caught the keys. "Thanks" I said and rushed from the room. As I climbed into his pickup I heard the driver of the ambulance announce on my scanner that "Rescue-One was "10-8," (in service). I was running late. We had ten minutes to arrive at Station One but usually five minutes or so was the normal response time. I wasn't certain how long it took for me to find car keys, but I was sure it was more than five minutes I speeded to the station down Date Street and skidded onto Elm and turned east on North Navajo. Now it was a straight shot to the station. As I approached the Fire Station sitting on the corner of Lake Powell Boulevard (known in those days as Seventh Avenue) and North Navajo Drive, I noticed the traffic light at the intersection I saw the light flashing green. Most of the volunteers lived on the west side of town and the dispatcher would flip the switch and give us a green light at the intersection.

Rescue-One was still waiting. I sighed a sigh of relief as I pulled up, thrilled that they had waited for me. I ran to the ambulance and was surprised to find only the driver, Doug Alton. I jumped into the passenger seat and buckled up. "Where's Monica?" I asked.

"I don't know. I was beginning to believe I had imagined the page out." He contacted dispatch over the radio and found out they had not heard anything from Monica and it had been ten minutes since the page. "We can't wait any longer," he said. I had only been a member of the department for a year or so at that time and Doug was an old timer.

"Then let's go." I hung on as Doug turned on the code lights and pulled out on the street. I was looking for traffic when I saw her. About two-hundred feet on the other side of the intersection ran Monica. She was running down the middle of North Navajo dressed in her square dancing attire. It was a blue dress with lots of cotton lace, ruffles and can-can's. For those of you that are too young to remember can-cans, they are a many layered net and lace slip that when worn under a skirt will gives lots of volume and holds the skirt outward. She carried her stethoscope in one hand and her jump suit in the other. She was waving her arms, screaming and trying to get our attention. "There she is!"

Doug pulled over and waited until Monica opened the back door and jumped in the back. Doug got back on the road. Monica was out of breath, "I'm sorry, I . . . . . had trouble. . . . getting out . . . . (gasp) of the . . . . parking lot (her car was blocked by another car) and then . . . . I ran out of gas (gasp) back there," (a long block and a half away).

Monica began to slip off the many layered can-cans so she could dress in the jump suit. Doug went around a corner and Monica lost her footing and fell to the ambulance floor. "Sorry," said Doug. "Are you ok Monica?"

She didn't answer Doug. She was a small woman and slid partway under the stretcher. The can-cans were shoved up and now she resembled a giant blue flower with her face in the middle. I laughed, I couldn't help it. Monica went crazy "#@!(&*^$%&@%$&!!!!!" I watched through the small window from the cab to patient compartment as she struggled to push the can-cans away and regain her feet. She got up and slipped off the can-cans and skirt. She then sat on the bench seat and put her feet in the jump suit just as Doug hit the brakes and swung right. I was laughing so hard I had forgotten to check traffic. A car pulled out in front of the ambulance without warning and Doug had no choice but to go to evasive maneuvers.

Again Monica slipped off the bench seat and sat flat on the floor. This time she addressed Doug. "What is %$#@^*&*%$@ matter with you . . . . . you . . . . . %$#@%&*&%$!@!!!!." She was mad. She tried to stand, but her feet were hung up in her jumpsuit and she lay on her back with her feet in the air kicking off the jump suit. She ignored the fact that she was now dressed in pink panties and a square dancing ruffle and lace covered blue blouse. She continued to curse as she got up and finally slipped on the jumpsuit and zipped it up. She tried to smooth her rumpled hair in place and put on her shoes.

We pulled up at the house and were met by a police officer. "They aren't here. They got tired of waiting. They took her to the hospital in their own car." We knew we had taken too long even though we were still within expected official response time. We walked back to the ambulance. Doug looked over at Monica. Her hair was sticking out in every direction. She was usually so well groomed it looked odd to see her so disheveled. "Are you . . . ." Doug couldn't even get the words out without bursting into laughter. I joined him. Monica wasn't laughing. We rode back to the station in silence. At the station, Doug begged forgiveness and Monica finally accepted his apology. Doug went back to work.

I went over to Monica, "Seriously, are you hurt?"

"I don't know. I don't think so." She and I looked around for injuries. She had a number of red spots that would be blue by tomorrow morning. She had bumped and tumbled about but there didn't appear to be any serious injuries. She admitted to being very sore the next couple of days and blue marks all over her body, but she continued to "run on the ambulance" without any time off. Monica eventually saw the humor in the incident.

IT'S A MATTER OF TIMING

Johnny was fourteen years old. He lived with his parents and two brothers in a double wide trailer in Page. "Time for bed," his father announced as he tossed another log into the cast iron fireplace that stood in the living room. Johnny and his brothers complained a little, but they were good boys and knew school came early and their father insisted they go to bed at a reasonable hour. The family had purchased the used trailer last year and now Johnny and the other boys each had their own bedroom. Johnny's was a small room, but it was all his. He got ready for bed and soon was sound asleep.

While the family slept the fireplace warmed the trailer. It was mid-October and the evening had a chill to it. The fireplace had been put in the trailer four years previously. The wall behind the fireplace was thin. The heat from the fireplace dried out the wood over the years and tonight the wall reached the point of no return. The bone dry wood two-by-twos began to smolder. As the family slept the small smoldering fire grew larger, then larger still. Soon it ate through the pretty wallpaper of yellow sunflowers and began to lick at the ceiling and anything else the flames could find to eat.

Around midnight, Johnny woke up. He didn't know what had awakened him, but he was wide awake. He looked around and noticed a faint glow under his door. He stood up and found the top half of the room was full of black smoke. He took in a lung full and started to cough. He opened the door and looked down the hall and saw the flames as they devoured the living room. He spun to the left and beat on his parent's door and staggered down the hall and beat on his two brother's bedroom door yelling "FIRE!"

Officer De Aquileo was on patrol in the area. He was a huge man and lifted weights every day. He was good looking and knew it. He had a thing about germs and wore leather gloves while on duty and tried to not get dirty. I liked him but he was a bit neurotic for a police officer. A neighbor had called in the fire and the dispatcher hit the key and paged a full call out for the Fire Department. Officer De Aquileo spun his car around and headed to the fire. He pulled up at the address, leaped out and hurried to the burning trailer. This time of night meant people were probably sleeping inside. He took his huge mag light and at the rear half of the trailer he began to pound on the siding and yell "FIRE! WAKE UP, FIRE!" He pounded down the side and the rear of the trailer and up the other side.

Johnny's family, one by one sat up in bed. They had heard Johnny pound on the door but were in deep sleep and were confused about what was happening. Then they heard the officer beating on the side of the trailer and his loud yell of "FIRE" got their attention. They leaped up and ran for their doors. Flinging them open the father, mother and two sons ran halfway down the hallway to the laundry room and out the back door. The father assumed Johnny was in front of them and already out of the trailer.

Johnny had breathed in a lot of smoke and he was confused. The lack of oxygen had left him dull and unable to make quick decisions. Johnny thought he was heading for the back door but found himself back in his bedroom. He stood in the middle of the room, trying to collect his thoughts. They were all jumbled up and didn't make sense. He knew the trailer was on fire and he realized he was in real trouble, but didn't know what to do. Just then he heard pounding on the outside wall of his bedroom and a light through the window. He coughed and concentrated on what he saw. He realized it was a window and he knew it was his only hope. He was unsteady on his feet, his eyes stung, he felt dizzy and couldn't breathe. The flames were crawling through his open bedroom door and he was about to pass out. In one final burst of glory he ran at the window as fast as he could.

Officer De Aquileo had looped back around and was beating on the trailer trying to wake anyone inside. He was a powerful man and didn't realize that in the excitement of the moment he was beating giant dents and holes in the trailer. It looked as if someone had beaten the trailer with a bowling ball instead of a mag light. He reached Johnny's window and pounded the side and yelled. The trailer sat about four feet off the ground and the officer couldn't see inside the window. He didn't expect what happened next.

Johnny exploded out the window. Glass and shreds of wood blew outward. De Aquileo looked up and saw the hundred and ten pound fourteen year old burst outside and fly through the air toward him. Johnny's head hit De Aquileo's forehead, his arms went around the officer's neck and the officers arms went under Johnny's arms and Johnny's knee went into the officer's groin. They both fell backwards. De Aquileo landed on the lawn and Johnny on top of him.

I arrived in time to see Officer De Aquileo running from the now fully engulfed trailer with Johnny in his arms. Blood covered both of them from head to toe. The flames illuminated the area and it was a spectacular sight. I jumped out of my car and ran with my jump kit toward them. De Aquileo laid Johnny in the road where the next door neighbor's car usually parked. In the distance the sound of the ambulance's siren could be hear.

"Whose blood is that?" I asked.

"I think it's the kids," he said as he began to inspect his own body looking for injuries. I was checking Johnny over as his family found us. The mother stood nearby crying, her two older sons tried to comfort her. The boy's father kneeled down beside his injured son. His hand gently stroked his young son's face. Tears were in his eyes as he said, "He's a hero. He saved our lives." I took out dressings and roller bandages and began to bandage Johnny's arms. They had been sliced to pieces as he dove through the window. I got the bleeding slowed down. The ambulance arrived and took him to the hospital.

"Are you hurt?" I asked the officer?

"No, just a few small cuts, nothing big. My head hurts but I think I'm ok." He looked down "But my uniform is ruined." I laughed. He was always Mr. Clean, groomed to perfection. He now looked as if he had been sacking wildcats.

"You sure you're ok?"

"I'm sure." He then began to tell me about his surprise when the boy came sailing out the window into his arms. Later, at the hospital the rest of the story was discovered and everyone congratulated Johnny for his heroic actions. He was a hero. The family lost their home and belongings, but they were all alive. Johnny spent two days in the hospital coughing up yuck. He recovered. Insurance gave the family a new start. Johnny, the baby of the family, had gone to bed that night a boy and woke up a hero.

THE GLEN CANYON UTILITY TUNNEL

Glen Canyon Dam holds back the Colorado River and forms Lake Powell, a giant reservoir. It was created in the late 1950's as part of the Central Arizona Project by Arizona Senator Carl Hayden. On the other side water is released and the river reforms and heads quickly toward the Grand Canyon. At the river side of the dam, at the base, there are buildings and a wide dirt parking area. The river runners use this staging area to launch river trips. The Bureau of Reclamation uses it to maintain the dam.

Access to the bottom of the dam is through a tunnel about a thousand feet long. It was dug through the east canyon wall with the entrance just west of the old Page Golf Course, near the sewer ponds. It was paved with a narrow but steep ditch on either side. The ditches had been put in a few years ago when a worker and his pickup was washed down the tunnel by a desert down pour. He and his truck ended up in the river. He drown. They dug the ditches on each side of the road deeper to divert the water from the roadway.

Raymond Garcia was part of the construction crew hired to replace some of wiring in the tunnel. The crew was assembling in the big parking lot at the bottom of the dam. He was in a company stake bed truck and entered at the top of the tunnel. The tunnel was lighted but it still took a second for his eyes to adjust. The road was narrow and paved with only enough room for one vehicle at a time. He hoped he didn't meet anyone; he didn't want to back up all the way back to the entrance.

Raymond tried to keep the truck to the fifteen mile per hour limit, but it gained speed quickly on the steep downhill grade. He moved his foot to the break and pushed down. The break peddle went instantly to the floor. He pumped it, but it didn't work. The breaks were out. The truck speeded up faster and faster. He struggled to keep the truck on the narrow road. He knew he was in trouble if a wheel fell into the ditch on either side of the tunnel. Faster and faster the truck gained speed on its downward high speed rampage. Raymond remembered the bulldozer parked near the exit to the tunnel. He then realized he was heading for the bull dozer at a

111

high rate of speed. He tried the emergency break, but it slowed the truck down only a tiny bit, not near enough. He panicked. All he could think about was the bull dozer waiting for him at the end of the tunnel.

Halfway down the tunnel, he decided to jump. He realized he was going to have to propel himself outward so he wouldn't fall under the wheels of the truck. He opened the door, hesitated and then pushed with his feet and jumped clear. Raymond was a powerful man and underestimated his strength. He had launched himself with such force that he overshot his landing zone. He drove the top of his head into the sandstone wall with great force. He then fell limply to the ditch and paved roadway. He didn't move.

Below his co-workers were milling around most with cups of coffee trying to wake up. Raymond's white company truck exploded from the tunnel at a high rate of speed and slammed into the bulldozer. The men ran to the truck and found no driver. The supervisor and another man took a truck up the tunnel and found Raymond lying in the road with his head hanging in the dry ditch. The supervisor, who was an EMT, stayed with him and the worker drove the pickup back down and called for an ambulance.

The Fire Chief and I were loading the fire hoses on Engine-Two. I stood on top of the hose bed and he fed me the hose. We had had a fire the night before and the hose was finally dry. The pager sounded and I climbed down off the fire engine. "I'm on the crew," I told him. He said that was ok, a Park Service EMT was on the scene and so we don't have to send a first responder. I pulled Rescue-One out of the building. The other two members arrived and we took off.

At the scene we found Raymond lying unconscious. I noticed blood coming from his left ear. There was blood in his nose and mouth. His pupils were unequal and his left pupil was unresponsive to light. He had abrasions to his right shoulder and upper arm. He opened his eyes. He did not follow commands and didn't appear to know where he was and who we were. These signs and symptoms indicated he had a serious head injury. He went unconscious again. We applied a c-collar and we placed him on a back board. We took a baseline set of vital signs, and put him on oxygen. He was a big, muscular man and lapped over on both sides of the backboard. In the ambulance we were preparing to continue treatment when he suddenly woke up. He yelled and tried to sit up. His large muscular arms swung about. He ripped the cervical collar off and threw it across the ambulance. I tried to calm him but he wasn't really alert. He was like a confused wild animal. Charlotte reapplied the c-collar and used a triangular to reinforce it. I tried to put the oxygen mask on him again, but he shoved it away. His eyes were glazed and he didn't understand where he was or what was happening. All he knew was that he wanted to run.

Charlotte and I struggled to restrain him, but he was so strong, it was hopeless. Just about then his left arm went out and hit me, Charlotte screamed as I flew through the air and hit the side door. It wasn't a sliding door. It was a regular door that opened outward. I was sure I was going out onto the road at highway speeds. I hit the door handle with my left side and my ribs exploded in pain. The door held and I bounced back and fell onto the patient who immediately shoved me off him. I landed on the bench seat in a heap. Just as I sat up the driver slammed on the brakes and I almost flew forward into the front wall but managed to hang on. "You guys ok?" the driver yelled back.

I regained my composure and noticed the patient was now laying still. "Yeah, get us to the hospital." I motioned for Charlotte to not touch him and I didn't either. The monitor showed he was breathing and I decided we were only two or three minutes from the hospital and didn't want him to go violent again.

We got to the hospital and unloaded him. He moaned but continued to lay still. I gave a report and made sure they knew about his violent outburst. We and the hospital staff gently slipped on restraints. He wasn't going anywhere now. I backed away and went to the locker room. I looked into the mirror and discovered I had a red mark on my left cheekbone that would be a beautiful blue in the morning. My left elbow hurt but didn't appear seriously injured. I lifted my t-shirt and found a bright red mark on my right ribs where I had hit the door handle. It hurt when I took a deep breath. I punched around and found it hurt a lot.

An RN walked in. "Are you ok Sharon?" Apparently she had been told of my bumpy ride.

"I think so."

"Let me see," she asked. She poked around and announced, "We should let the doctor look at this."

She took me to a private room and the doctor came in and checked my ribs. "I think you may have cracked a few ribs, Sharon."

I was beginning to believe he was right. "Nothing we can do about that," I commented.

"No, not really," he answered. "I'll get the nurse to tape the ribs. It will help. Do you need any pain meds?"

"No," I said. "I have some OTC (over the counter) that should work." I avoided narcotics and over the counter pain meds were all I ever took.

"If you change your mind, let me know." I thanked him and he left. The nurse came in and taped my ribs. It did feel better.

I walked out and a police officer approached me. "Do you want to press charges?" I sighed, how many people knew about this?

"No, of course not. He's got head injuries and I put myself in that position. I knew better. It was my fault, not his." Raymond had slipped into a deep coma and was flown out to Phoenix.

For the next week or so every breath I took I remembered Raymond. I couldn't take a deep breath, cough, sneeze or laugh without a sharp explosion of raw pain. It was horrible. I was reasonable sure it involved three cracked ribs. I had a huge blue burse on my cheek and my body was covered in other bruises. They healed quickly, but the fractured ribs healed much slower. Every time I thought I was almost back to normal, I would bump my ribs or cough and it would start all over again. Every day I would tape my ribs and spend the day trying to avoid a deep breath, cough or any contact to the injured area. Every time I had to lift my half of a two-hundred, fifty pound stretcher, I would take a deep breath, hold it and do the lift. I danced around trying to avoid contact to the tender area. Sometimes it worked, sometimes it didn't. Every time I answered a call without my ribs taped I was sorry I had not taken the time to tape them.

Eventually the ribs healed. Three months passed. Life went on. I occasionally wondered what had happened to Raymond, but for the most part he took a back seat in my busy life. One day I received a phone call at home. It was a friend of mine that was working on the tunnel project.

"Sharon, do you remember Raymond? You know . . . . . the guy that dove into the wall?"

"Sure I do."

"Well, he has spent three months in a coma. Yesterday his wife was sitting beside his bed and he sat up and said he was hungry."

"That's wonderful!"

"Sure is. He's got three small children. His wife never gave up hope. He remembers almost everything." He told me the complete story about the bad breaks and jumping from the truck. "Of course he doesn't remember the actual accident or the past three months, but he remembers everything else." I thanked him for calling. I was happy to find out what had happened to Raymond. I called the other people who were on the call. They were glad to hear he was going to be ok. God does work miracles and this was an example of one.

EXCUSE ME, MA'AM, YOUR AMBULANCE IS ON FIRE

In rural EMS resources are extremely limited. Backup may be over an hour away and sometimes not available at all. This is a story of one such time. Wahweap Resort and Marina is located about nine miles north of town. It is on the shores of beautiful Lake Powell. In the early years, the Park Service didn't have an emergency response team and the rangers, usually were first aide (Boy Scout level) and had no way to transport a patient to the hospital. They would do what they could with their training and meager equipment until Page Fire could arrive, usually around fifteen minutes after being called. Then they developed an EMS program, trained a few rangers to EMT level and purchased an ambulance. The plan was to use Page Fire as back up.

On this day the NPS ambulance wasn't available and PFD was called to building "Desert Rose" for a possible heart attack. I was driving the ambulance this time. Upon arrival the bellman led us up the stairs and down the outdoor walkway to room 234. Even before we opened the door I knew the man was at least a hundred pounds overweight. You see, I don't know why but the young, healthy, and athletic are usually given a first floor room. The guests who are older, in poor health, or overweight usually are given the top floor in a building without an elevator. This was just another one of many cases that supported my beliefs.

Mr. Otis was around seventy years of age, three-hundred and twenty pounds. His skin was the color of a piece of paper. His lips were a soft blue. He was sitting on the edge of the bed, leaning forward rubbing his left shoulder and arm. He was sweating and complaining of chest pain. These are classical signs of a heart attack. The EMTs quickly put him on oxygen and began assessing the patient.

"Excuse me, Ma'am." I turned around and the bellman stood behind me. "Your ambulance is on fire."

"What?" I said in surprise.

He kept his voice down, not wanting to interrupt the care of the patient. "It's on fire . . . . there's smoke and everything."

My stomach dropped. That was the last thing I expected to hear. I quickly left the room and ran behind him as he led the way. We hurried down the stairs into the parking lot. Sure enough, white smoke flowed abundantly from under the hood of the ambulance. "Wonderful" I sarcastically mumbled. The Park Service ambulance was in town being serviced. Page Fire's other ambulance was in Bitter Springs on a one car rollover. There wasn't anyone else to call. We were the only game in town. Unless the man with the heart attack wanted to hitchhike, it was looking doubtful he was going to get into town.

115

I ran over to the ambulance. I got the fire extinguisher and then I noticed it didn't smell like smoke. I slowly opened the hood. After the "smoke" cleared, I could see I had broken the upper radiator hose and the white smoke was actually steam. The vehicle should not be driven. It was about nine miles to town and the vehicle was hot and the day was even hotter. Without coolant, the engine would quickly overheat and freeze up. The engine could never be repaired. And if it froze up before we got to town, the delay could cost the man his life.

I looked up on the balcony in time to see them wheeling the man out the door on the gurney. I briefly considered having law enforcement transport him in a police cruiser, but DPS and the Sheriff was at the accident in Bitter Springs. Two NPS officers were in town with their out of service ambulance. The other ranger on duty was at a disturbance at Lone Rock. Page Police were ten minutes away but we could be in town in that amount of time. I had a decision to make. Did I gamble with this man's life? It was a gamble either way. I took a deep breath and made my decision. I quickly loosened the radiator cap and slammed the hood. "It's a radiator hose. Thanks for letting me know," I told the bellman.

"You want me to call a tow truck?" the bellman asked.

"No, we are going to transport the man to Page then get it fixed." He seemed surprised, but said nothing. He ran up the stairs and assisted the crew with the difficult task of bringing the large man down the steep, narrow stairs. The old movie "Mother, Jugs and Speed," came to mind. I always loved the scene where they are trying to get a large woman down a staircase. I didn't tell the EMTs about the ambulance. I was convinced this man was having a real heart attack, and if I had to sacrifice the ambulance, so be it.

I turned on the flashing lights and siren and took off. I drove fast, but not as fast as usual. I watched as the temperature gage steadily and slowly went up. I got on the radio and asked Al, from the city garage to meet us at the back door to the ER.

"Something wrong?" an EMT asked as he stuck his head through the small window from the passenger compartment to the driver compartment.

"No. How's he doing?"

In a soft voice he answered, "Not that good. Get us there as quick as you can."

". . . workin' on it," I answered. The ambulance continued to move forward and the temperature needle continued to go up. I am at heart a gambler. That day I won. We reached the hospital and Al was standing there, tool box in hand. We unloaded the man and I let the other two

EMTs take him inside. I told Al what had happened. He wasn't happy, but he didn't yell.

The City of Page didn't know it, but at that moment it didn't have ambulance coverage. Al called the mechanic working on the Park Service ambulance and told them what was going on. They quickly put it back together and got it running. The rangers staged at the bridge, ready to head either way, out to Wahweap or into Page. Al went to work on Page Fire's ambulance. It took about an hour to find the parts and get a new hose installed. We were back in service by the time Page's other ambulance pulled in with the woman from the one car rollover.

Our patient was indeed having a heart attack. He was stabilized and flown out to a Phoenix Hospital later that afternoon. I don't know the outcome but I would like to think he fully recovered. The citizens of Page never knew how close they came to calling for an ambulance and not getting one.

THE COP SET ME UP

It was a bit after six o'clock on a cold, dry winter morning. I was staggering about the kitchen preparing my husband's lunch. He had eaten his breakfast and was in the bathroom shaving. The scanner was active. A Page City policeman (name withheld for reasons that will become obvious) had discovered a semi broke down in the westbound lane of Highway 98. It was just inside the Page City limits. The semi was heading into town when the engine quit running. It was now blocking the westbound lane and traffic had backed up behind the stalled truck. It was still dark. At this time of day, about one-hundred and fifty people are heading east, toward the Navajo Generating Station, going to work and many other people were heading to work in town. It is as close to a traffic jam as Page gets.

I listened to the officer on the scene who went about making a bad situation worse. I couldn't believe the decisions he was making. It didn't have to be a big deal. If he had just let the west bound people sit for about five to ten minutes, until a second officer got there, it would have worked out just fine. But, no, he decided he would, by himself, make the highway a one lane road. He decided he would let a few west bound cars go, and then a few east bound cars go, etc. This would have worked, except he failed to take into consideration a number of factors. It was dark. He wasn't wearing a reflective vest and didn't carry a flashlight. He had not set out flares and he was standing beside the semi at the bottom of a hill. West

117

bound traffic could not see oncoming traffic due to the semi and the hill. The long line of traffic heading to work, east bound were all traveling around fifty-five mph and couldn't see the problem ahead due to the hill. Flares would have warned them, but there were no flares.

Maurice walked into the kitchen and picked up his lunch. "Be careful, Honey," I said. "A police officer has set up an accident waiting to happen." I explained the problem. Maurice shook his head and said he would keep an eye out as he approached the area and left. I had a bad feeling. I hurried into the bedroom to get dressed, preparing for the coming ambulance call.

Maurice was driving toward the scene. He was in a long line of traffic heading eastbound. He slowed as he crested the hill. It was very dark. He could see the semi at the bottom of the hill, but he couldn't see the police car parked snugly up against the back bumper of the semi, making his flashing lights visible mainly to west bound cars only. He could see headlights in the westbound lane, but couldn't tell if they were moving or sitting still. He could not see a police officer, anywhere. He was forewarned so he knew the situation, but visually, he knew the other people had no idea what was going on. Maurice slowed down even more, irritating those behind him.

The officer decided it was time to block the east bound lane and let the west bound lane cross the center line and go around the stalled semi. As Maurice began to drive past the semi-truck, the officer, dressed in a dark blue uniform and no reflective vest or flashlight, suddenly appeared in front of his car. Maurice said the officer just suddenly "jumped out of the darkness with his hands extended outward," trying to get Maurice to stop. Maurice braked quickly. Those behind him followed suit. Then Maurice, unable to completely stop, swerved to the right and missed the officer standing in his lane by inches. He swore as the car fishtailed and kept his foot on the accelerator. Behind him was a long line of vehicles on the far side of the hill that had no idea a problem had developed in the darkness of early morning. If he had stopped he would have been car number one in a multi-car pileup. He continued on, peddle to the metal.

A west bound pickup (vehicle #1), following directions of the officer, pulled around the stalled semi, crossing the yellow line, into the eastbound lane. A car (#2) heading east bound, going around fifty-five miles per hour, topped the hill completely unaware of the situation and slammed head on into the pickup. The east bound pickup (#3) following the car, hit the rear of the car (#2) which then slid off the road into the desert. The sound of screeching breaks filled the early morning scene. Break lights flashed bright red giving a slight warning to those following. Cars and pickups slid in various directions, each desperately trying to avoid the pile up. The east bound pickup (#3) then backed back onto the roadway and continued on east bound, leaving the scene of the accident.

Suddenly the pager went off announcing a three vehicle accident. I looked at the clock. Maurice had been gone less than five minutes. He should be at the scene, at this moment. Was he in the reported three car accident? I hoped not. I hurried out the door. My heart was pounding, not from excitement, but from fear the cop may have killed my husband.

I pulled up on the scene in Rescue-Two and quickly scanned the area. Was Maurice involved? I was relieved to see none of the crushed vehicles were a yellow Cadillac. The officer was running around like a chicken with his head cut off. He was at a complete loss as to what to do and had no idea he was responsible for the accident. I ignored him. The car (#2) was crushed in the front and damaged in the back. As I waded through debris that littered the roadway, I saw the woman sitting behind the wheel. It was Molly Dennison's daughter. Molly was a PFD EMT. I couldn't remember her daughter's first name but her married name was McDougal. She was heading to work at the plant that morning. She was unconscious and badly injured. Her knees had gone into the dash as it folded inward and the steering wheel had pushed into her chest. Blood matted her long blond hair. She was wearing a seat belt and still had a cigarette in her hand as it hung out the window. I took the cigarette out of her hand and put it out. Gasoline and antifreeze covered the roadway.

The attack truck had set up, and was ready to drown the area with water if something flared up. It was very cold and I wasn't that fearful of fire. It would have taken a blow torch to get a flame going that cold winter morning. I looked up and saw the second ambulance arrive and they went to care for the man in the pickup (#1), who was also badly injured, but not as bad as Molly's daughter (in vehicle #2). I was told about the pickup (#3) that left the scene of the accident. The pickup would have to be someone else's problem, I had my hands full. I slipped a c-collar on Molly's daughter's (driver of #2) neck and she moaned. She wasn't alert and didn't recognize me. We put her on a backboard and took her out of the car, and then put her in the ambulance.

En route the EMT took vital signs as I cut her clothing off and completed the examination of her injuries. I followed treatment protocols. I also called Page Hospital to let them know what we were bringing in. At that time, a doctor was not at the hospital 24/7 and the doc on call would have to respond from his home. I wanted a doctor standing at the ER door when we arrived. The second ambulance was close behind us and we both hit the ER within minutes of each other. Both patients were badly injured and Air Evac was called. Molly arrived. It was hard, but I didn't do the

119

regular song and dance I usually did with relatives of the injured. I told her everything. She took it bravely and went to be with her daughter.

Both people recovered after a long recovery. I don't know much about the male patient other than he recovered. The woman lived with pain for over two years and was off work for many months of rehab. The officer was never blamed for the accident by anyone of any authority (at least not publicly). The scary thing was, I don't think he believed he did anything wrong. Both drivers got tickets of some form or another. The pickup that left the scene was never identified. The stupid officer left the Page Police about eight months later to go to work for another small community in the Payson area. May God have mercy on them.

I still blame the officer, who will remain nameless for the purpose of this story. I know the officer didn't intend to hurt anyone but two innocent people paid dearly for his stupidity. I still thank God Maurice wasn't involved. It would have been difficult if Maurice had been the bloody driver sitting behind the steering wheel of the car when I arrived. I didn't know it at the time, but in a few years I would arrive at a two car collision and find my husband was one of the patients. But that's another story.

THE INDIAN PRINCESS

The man and woman lay on the living room floor on a soft sleeping bag. The thick comforter that covered their half clothed bodies was warm and comfortable. One lone candle flickered and lit the room in a soft faint, romantic light. They lay in each other's embrace, kissing passionately. Suddenly, the front wall at their feet exploded inward as a car ran through the wall, shoving the book case into the room, launching the television, books, DVD's and VCR into the air. The couple tried to get out of the way, but there wasn't enough time.

It all began three hours before. Lars was one of the four million visitors that come to Page to enjoy the many tourist related activities. He was in search of adventure. He was from Norway, twenty-two years of age, tall, blond haired, and blue eyed. He spoke English fairly well. He had walked into the Windy Mesa, a local biker/cowboy bar. He didn't exactly fit in, but he was non-threatening and personable enough so no one paid him much attention. He sat at the bar, ordered a drink and watched a group of men play pool. A white cowboy was playing pool with two Navajo

Indians, one dressed as a biker and the other in western attire. The cowboy's girlfriend appeared to be a mixture of both races dressed in tight leather pants and a tiny leather halter top.

This was America. He craved to taste, feel, experience America from a more personal level. Tourist traps didn't appeal to him. He looked around the crowded bar. He noticed a number of pretty Indian women. Their hair was coal black, their skin was a beautiful brown, and when they smiled their black eyes glowed and white teeth glistened. He had never slept with an Indian woman. Were they different? Probably not, but it would be something to write home about. "Hi Guys, guess what? I slept with an Indian Princess."

After a few unsuccessful attempts, he managed to attract the attention of a Native American woman. She was a dozen or so years older than he, a pretty woman and she seemed quite willing. "My name's Tawny," she said in a sexy voice as she snuggled close to the young man. They drank and laughed for hours. Finally, the time came, he made his move and she accepted. She and Lars walked a bit unsteadily to her car. She lived in the small Native American community of Le Chee (Leche-e), just outside Page. Lars was excited. He was on his way to an Indian village and had visions of a tepee or maybe one of the hogans he had seen in Kayenta. He was a bit disappointed when she drove up to a two story frame house on a paved road and parked on the street under a street light. Oh well, no teepee but she was still an Indian.

Tawny told him to be quite as she opened the door. It was a regular looking home with a southwestern decor. "The kids are asleep upstairs, but we have the living room to ourselves." She opened the closet and took out a thick sleeping bag and a big comforter. She made a bed in the middle of the living room floor. Lars looked around. On the west wall, the front of the house had a big shelving unit used as an entertainment center. It was loaded with a stereo, television, VCR, DVD players and lots of CD's and DVD's. Books lined the smaller bookshelves to the left and right of the entertainment center.

"Lars?" she said. Lars turned around. She sat on the makeshift bed, smiled and reached her hand up in invitation. Just then a loud snore vibrated through the room.

Lars was startled. "Who else sleeps here?" He looked around and his gaze fell on a man that lay sleeping on the couch across the room.

"Oh, that's my brother, Leo. Don't pay him any attention. He's drunk and won't wake up till in the morning." Lars hesitated, but gave in to temptation and joined her on the floor. Little did either of them know that only a couple miles away a full size car loaded with drunken teenagers was heading their way. The car swerved back and forth across the center line, barely missing a pickup. The teens were laughing and extremely drunk. They turned into Le Chee (Leche-e) and speeded down the narrow residential street. They came to the end of the cult sac and the driver whipped the wheel to the left, the car spun and skid. The driver floored the gas pedal and the car leaped forward, over the curb, across the lawn and into Tawny's house, through the wall and into the living room. The teenagers jumped out and ran away, leaving Lars and his Indian Princess under the car, tangled in the comforter and sleeping bag.

The Navajo PD had arrived before the PFD ambulance. Many homes in the community do not have addresses but the house was easy to locate. We just followed the rotating red, blue and white lights that lit the area. Neighbors stood in their lawns watching the excitement. We pulled up and got out. The officer approached us and gave us a short report. I listened to his report as my eyes scanned the scene. "The kids fled the scene. We are looking for them. There are two people injured . . . . They don't look too bad."

We thanked him for the report and approached the house. The car was almost completely inside the house. I decided to use the door. Inside was a confusing environment. It looked as if a bomb had gone off. A middle age woman, an elderly woman and about eight children were on the upstairs landing leaning over, looking at the accident scene. They were all talking at once and one of the older children was taking pictures. I bet show and tell next week was going to be interesting.

CD's, DVD's books, papers, the shattered bookcase and various pieces of electronic equipment littered the room. I picked a path across the living room to the woman lying under the car. She lay on a beautiful Indian rug, with her legs under the front end of the car, still tangled in blankets. The wheels had not run over her. There were no obvious injuries but she was hysterical and crying. She was dressed in black lacy undergarments. She companied of mild rib pain. Lars had slipped on his pants and his shirt hung unbuttoned. He was barefooted and stood awkwardly about ten feet away. He had a bump on his forehead. He later said he sat up in time to be hit in the forehead by the front bumper. He complained of a headache and neck pain.

Everyone's attention was directed towards Lars and Tawny. No one had noticed her brother. I heard a moan and looked over. The area wasn't well lit. I left Tawny in the care of my partner. I walked over to the couch that lay tipped over backwards into the dining room. The thirty-two inch television had flown through the air and landed on Leo. He had a large laceration to the side of his head, probably caused by the flying VCR or DVD player that lay near him. He now lay on the floor tangled in the power cord of the now shattered television. He was still very drunk, but awake. He moaned, completely confused. Who were all these people? Why did his abdomen and chest hurt so badly? Why couldn't he take a deep breath? Who was the half-clothed white guy standing in the corner?

Lars at first refused treatment, but as his headache grew to unbelievable proportions. He changed his mind. He was back boarded, put on oxygen and vital signs were taken. Lars vital signs were elevated but within normal limits. He passed the neuro exam but his neck pain was of concern. I applied a cervical collar, placed him on a backboard and applied an ice pack to the bump on his forehead in an attempt to slow the swelling. He and Leo were transported in the second ambulance. Leo was injured the worst. He had been asleep and caught a thirty-two inch television in his abdomen and chest. Even that wasn't enough to sober him up and he wiggled about on the backboard and clawed at his oxygen tubing. He kept asking questions in an attempt to make sense of this confused mess. It was hard to tell if the confusion was due to alcohol or the blow to the head. The female EMT tried to answer his questions as she cared for him, but it wasn't easy. Lars talked a mile a minute to the male EMT. He was hyper and his story was stocked full of details.

It took a little time to get Tawny untangled and out from under the car. She complained of rib pain but appeared to have escaped serious injury. She was back boarded and loaded into Rescue-Two. Her vital signs were within normal limits. She was crying and very emotionally upset. Tawny told me how she had begun to believe she was going home alone from the bar that night . She was delighted when this perfect specimen of a young man had taken an interest in her. Her boyfriend had left her a couple of months ago and she was lonely for the company of a man. "Do you think he will still be interested after this is all over? We could maybe go back to his hotel room, couldn't we?"

I didn't think he would still be in the mood with the headache and all, but I couldn't rob her of all hope. "Maybe?" I answered. She closed her eyes and sobbed. She continued to cry all the way to the hospital. She never asked once how her brother was doing or mentioned the destroyed house. All she had on her mind was the interrupted romantic interlude and the possibility of reigniting the flame.

Leo spent two days in the hospital due to four broken ribs and major abdomen, chest and shoulder bruising. He couldn't take a deep breath, had multiple lacerations, lots of stitches, and a headache that took days to subside. He was expected to fully recover. Lars and his date were roughed up a bit but not seriously injured. After discharge, Tawny tried to interest Lars in a second try at romance, but he had a huge headache and a bump on his head the size of a large plum. The mood had passed and he declined the offer. Tawny gave him her cell number but I doubt he called. Lars had craved adventure and he got it, just not what he expected.

CAN THIS RELATIONSHIP BE SAVED?

Marcy and Gary were in their early thirties. Gary was in construction and Marcy waited tables off and on. They had been playing house for almost ten months. Their relationship was volatile at times. On a Tuesday, around four in the afternoon they were in Gary's pickup heading south on Seventh Avenue (now known as Lake Powell Blvd.), the main street of town. Witnesses said the pickup pulled up at the Elm Street light and stopped. The witnesses said the woman in the vehicle was yelling and screaming to top of her lungs. Profanity filled the air as she swung her arms about, this way and that. The man just sat still, tightly gripping the wheel with his teeth clinched. As the light changed the pickup moved forward slowly. The man reached over, opened the passenger door and shoved the woman out. Marcy landed on her bottom in the middle of the main street. She had a shocked look on her face that was quickly replaced with pure anger. The witnesses called for an ambulance. I was a brand new EMT and almost fell over my own feet getting out of the house and down to the station. I had no idea what to expect. I had only been on a handful of calls and none of them had been exciting. Maybe this one would be.

The officer on duty was Officer McMillin. He had been around from the very beginning and no one messed with him. He was genuinely concerned when he pulled up and saw the woman sitting in the middle of the road. She was about one-hundred-ten pounds with sandy brown hair that hung to her shoulders. He approached her and kneeled down beside her and asked her if she was hurt.

Marcy had had about all the men she could take that day and unloaded on the officer. "The &@!*&%^ pushed me out of the &(&%$#%^ truck! That #$@!(*&^+!" She started to get up and he touched her elbow to assist and she jerked away. "Keep your #@!^%$* hands to yourself you #@!*&^$# stinkin' pig!" Then she made a serious mistake. She kicked him in the shin.

Officer McMillin grabbed her arm, swung her around and slammed her face down on the hood of his patrol car. She screamed and burst loose with more profanity. The ambulance drove up in time for us to see her swing her foot back and kick him again. She lifted her head and he slammed it back down on his hood. As we walked up I saw him trying to

124

cuff her and she somehow twisted around and clawed him on his wrist with her fingernails. Now he was also swearing just as loud as she was. I stood back and let the more experienced EMT handle this.

"If she's well enough to fight, she doesn't need to see a &%$#^7&* Doctor!" announced the officer in a loud angry tone. I looked around and saw a crowd gathering. None appeared to be on the woman's side. There we stood in the middle of the street watching the officer and the woman engaged in mortal combat. The officer grabbed Marcy and threw her roughly into the back seat of his patrol car. She fell on her back and kicked out at him but missed his chin by inches. He told us in no uncertain terms our services were not needed. We took the hint and left.

Normally this should be the end of the story, but it isn't. The woman was booked in jail for assaulting an officer and disorderly conduct. She remained defiant, screamed and yelled through the entire booking process, testing everyone to the limit. She was put in a cell and night fell. The old Page jail at that time was located in a large warehouse type building built of fabricated metal. The majority of the building housed the city garage, the front part housed the Page Fire Department and the rear part was the Police Department and jail. The jail cells were more or less cages and sound carried through the metal structure, echoing back and forth. Marcy wouldn't let it go. She continued to yell and scream insults aimed at her boyfriend, the officer who arrested her, all police officers and all men. Her shrill voice echoed through the entire building. The other prisoners, all men, quickly got angry. They couldn't see her but they sure could hear her. "Shut the bitch up!" one inmate yelled. Others took up the chant. Most of them had been drinking and/or had their own problems and just wanted to go to sleep but that was impossible with her screaming. They began to boo her and yell insults. Twice the officers had to go back and make everyone be quite. As soon as they left she would start up again and then everyone would jump in with their insults.

Marcy was losing her voice from all the yelling and screaming. And she didn't want to sleep on the lumpy mattress in the jail cell. She realized she wasn't going to get released, at least that night, so maybe a nice soft hospital bed would do. She started to yell and wine about her injured elbow. She even complained about her two broken nails. No one cared. She then lay down on the floor and laid there for a while pretending to be unconscious. The dispatcher had seen her on the monitor carefully sit down and then position herself on the cleanest part of the bare concrete floor. She ignored her. The other inmates were thrilled, it was quite at last.

When that didn't work, Marcy took off her panty hose, reached up as high as she could and tied one toe to the bars. She tied the other end around her neck and slouched down, pretending to hang herself. Her feet touched the floor with her knees bent and she was careful to keep her airway open. She let her arms dangle limp at her side and hung her head to one side. She wasn't sure, but she thought that is the way it would look if it was real.

The dispatcher couldn't ignore this new antic and she called in the officers and paged an ambulance. The officers ran into the jail portion flipping on lights and the other inmates moaned and complained. They opened her cell and "cut her down." She fell limp into the officer's arms. I was still on call and quickly arrived at the jail. I had never seen such a thing and thought it was real. The other EMT acted as if it was and I became more certain it was real. What I didn't notice was the EMT take the woman's hand and held it over her face and dropped it. It mysteriously slid to the side, not striking her flat in the face. I later learned that was one test to check if the patient was really unconscious. We took her to the hospital and afterwards the EMT explained the woman's attempt to get out of jail. I felt stupid for being fooled. Over the years I learned to view similar situations with skepticism.

My part in this story is over, but there is more. The next day McMillin and the Police Chief decided to let the charges drop. The woman was more trouble than she was worth. They released her. She called her boyfriend Gary, but he didn't answer. She called her female friend to drive her home. Marcy lived with Gary in a trailer park down off the mesa called Vermillion Trailer Park (known today as Lake Powell Mobil Home Village). When she and her best friend pulled up at space 129 they both got a surprise. Gary had taken all her belongings and tossed them out on the cement patio, hooked up the thirty-four foot trailer to his pickup and had driven away to parts unknown.

Marcy went ballistic. She screamed and began spewing profanity. Her friend couldn't quiet her and a neighbor called the police. When the call came into the police department the dispatcher looked up at McMillin and smiled. "Your lady friend's boyfriend has left taking the trailer with him. She's having a tissy fit. The neighbors want her removed." The Police Chief laughed at McMillin's obvious distress. "Now don't get too close to that kitten, she has claws and whatever you do, don't bring her back here!"

McMillin reluctantly drove down and met with Marcy. He explained the trailer was Gary's and he could drive off with it if he wanted too. She admitted her things were all there so the officer said the matter was closed. She and her friend spent the next half-hour loading the stuff into the friend's pickup and Marcy went to stay with her friend. Gary was never seen again.

A FAMILY DISASTER

I had been on foot near the bottom of the bike path down by Vermillion Trailer Park (Lake Powell Mobile Home Village) taking some pictures for an upcoming court case. I walked back to my car parked down a dusty road about a football field away and got inside. It was just after one in the afternoon and I was hungry. I put the camera away and pulled back on the road. As I was nearing the Highway 98 turn I heard on my scanner Page Police Officer Brody Smyth call the dispatcher. Brody was about five foot eight inches tall. He was young and a new police officer. His wife and they had just had a baby. He became an EMT at eighteen years old and rode a bicycle to the station when his pager went off. His first year out of high school he had seen a PPD officer in a struggle with a very angry man. Brody had jumped off his bicycle and leaped into the brawl and helped the officer subdue the man. The officer was very grateful. A few years later Brody looked the officer up and asked about how could become a police officer. The officer and the police chief helped Brody get into the Police Academy.

Brody was a good officer. I knew him well because he had been one of my EMT students. Today it surprised me to hear him scream into his radio. His voice betrayed the seriousness of the situation. "Get me an ambulance to Highway 98 MP 298 for a 963. (a motor vehicle accident with at least one dead)." The dispatcher asked for more information. His voice was strained and loud, "Get me a $#@&% damn ambulance, we have a woman and baby laying in the road @!*&$@ ....there's %$@!# others, some kids.....@%$*(&#. "

I turned onto Highway 98 and responded. The first out crew had just gone on an airport to hospital transfer and had not called back in service yet. The dispatcher paged for a second crew. The first crew realizing they were actually available for call, radioed and asked "Should we respond? We are 10-8." The crew was made up of two EMT's, Connie Miller and Gordon Taylor. As I rounded the slight hill and curve I could see Brody standing in the road. He was talking on the radio.

"Hell yes! Get your fuckin' butts down here! Send everything you got damn it! We got people all over the damn road.....shit......" Brody had lost it.

I keyed my radio as I parked on the down side of the hill (to be out of the way of responding emergency vehicles) and said into my radio, "Rescue-Two, roll." I thought they might need a translation on Brody's radio transmission. I then told the dispatcher, "continue to roll the second ambulance."

I could not see the victims or the car, but I knew by Brody's tone it must be horrible. Brody is a calm man, seldom excited. He was a good EMT and police officer. His use of profanity over the radio and the higher octave to his voice told me this was a bad one.

"Rescue-two copies, roll. 76 to mile post 298, Highway 98." I hurried and got my equipment and rushed forward. I topped the small hill and looked upon the scene. What I saw was total carnage. A small tan pickup had rolled two times in the middle of the road, coming to rest on its wheels. The camper shell was peeled open like a banana. The officer had just driven up on the accident, seconds after it happened while on routine patrol.

A seventeen year old girl had been driving. Her mother was sitting in the middle of the front seat holding the driver's two week old daughter bundled on a cradle board. The grandfather sat by the passenger side door. In the bed of the small pickup were grandmother and her grandchildren, seven month old boy lying in an infant seat, but not strapped in, a five year old girl, a four year old boy and a three year old girl. The children had been sick and had come into town to see the doctor. No one had had a lot of sleep with the sick children. They were heading home when the driver fell asleep and rolled the pickup. The people inside were thrown to the four winds.

The grandfather lay in the oncoming traffic lane, very dead. He had hit the rear view mirror and then the door post on his way out the passenger window and then hit the pavement with killing force. He lay very still with the rear view mirror embedded deeply in his forehead. There was almost no blood; his heart had stopped almost immediately. The mother lay on the center line. She was bloody and the blood formed a river and flowed down hill. Her eyes were open, fixed in death, as her brains lying on the pavement beside her.

The officer had picked up the two babies and made the hysterical seventeen year old girl to sit down beside the road and hold them. She sat crying, staring off into the desert, seemingly unaware of the babies she held in her arms. The grandmother was with the small children. The three year old girl was screaming and lay in the road beside her grandmother who gently stroked her hair. The four year old boy also cried loudly clinging to his grandmother. The five year old girl sat holding her broken arm. She sat near the driver, her older sister.

There is no more helpless feeling than to have far more people to care for than you are humanely able to handle. I forced myself to ignore the children, they were crying and that meant they had an open airway and were conscious. I ignored the two obviously dead people in the road. The officer had already told me he had checked them and said they were dead. I believed him.   I walked over to the seventeen year old driver and sat down. Most of the cars had stopped and a line was forming, but a car crept past us, weaving around the wrecked pickup and the bodies lying in the middle of the road. "Brody, go stop traffic. I'll get this." He hurried off. I think he was glad to be freed from what he saw. He ran to direct traffic and left me alone with seven patients.

I looked around. I decided to focus my attention on the babies. I had one oxygen mask and two unconscious babies. The boy's eyes were half shut and he lay limply in his sister's arms. I asked a bystander to get the car seat now resting in the desert. He brought it to me and I put the limp boy in it. He didn't move. I strapped him in the seat and then used a baby's blanket lying nearby and some tape to secure his head to the car seat.

The girl was so tiny. She had been strapped to a cradle board that had shattered on impact with the pavement. I took her from her mother. Her thick black hair was clean. I still remember the dress, white with little blue birds and pink flowers. I noticed a horrible depression above her ear and swelling on the left side of her head, just behind the ear. She lay still. Her breathing would stop for a few seconds and then resume. I put oxygen on her. Her tiny left arm was drawn up to her chest and her hand was bent at the wrist pointing toward her feet. This is abnormal flexion called decorticate posturing indicated bleeding in the cerebral hemispheres of the brain or internal capsule. The other arm was stiff at her side with the wrist bent and the hand point outward. This posturing indicated a bleed midbrain, brainstem and/or pons. Both indicate extremely serious brain damage. The baby was dead. She was still breathing, but she was dead.

I checked the boy. He didn't have a mark on him, but his breathing pattern was the same as the girls. They both stopped at once and I panicked. What do I do if they don't start up again? I can't do CPR on two babies at the same time. Which one would I choose to live and which one would I have to let die? He took a ragged breath and she immediately followed. They continued to have apnea events, but luckily never at the same time. They continued to breathe irregularly, but they were at least breathing on their own.

I traded the oxygen mask back and forth between them. It didn't seem to do any good. They were both dying and I knew it. I wish I hadn't known. I felt emptiness in the pit of my stomach when I realized nothing I did or anything the hospital would do would really make a difference. They were going to die. They looked so innocent, so sweet and smelled of baby powder.

The five year old girl came over and sat down beside me. I turned and looked at her. She was thin and her huge dark eyes looked up at me like a wounded fawn. She held her injured arm up for me to see. It was defiantly broken. Tears ran down her cheek. I couldn't do a damn thing for her. I had two dying babies. "Honey, just hold it still. We will take care of it in a few minutes." Anger flashed in her eyes. She looked at me like I was the Wicked Witch of the West. I felt like it. I turned my attention back to the babies and ignored her pitiful pleas. She got up and returned to her grandmother's side.

The first ambulance arrived with a two person crew. EMT Connie Miller was driving and Gordon Taylor was in back. I gave Gordon the boy baby and told him, "Get him in R-2 and on oxygen. He has serious head injuries." Gordon quickly did as told.

Brody came up. I told him I needed another person to go to the hospital in the ambulance to care for the girl baby. "I can't do it. I have been assigned other duties." He turned and walked away. I knew he was having a problem emotionally with this call. His son was just a tiny baby and he could identify too closely with the tiny victims of this accident. But I needed one more EMT. We would have to deal with his emotional issues later. Brody's supervisor walked up.

"I need Brody in the first ambulance to the hospital. Can that be arranged?"

"I'll release him. He's not going to be happy."

"I know, I don't have any other options." Brody walked over to Rescue-Two and reluctantly climbed in. I walked over with his tiny patient. I handed the tiny baby girl up to him. He took her in his arms. "She's got serious head injuries. Get her on oxygen. You may have to do CPR."

"SHIT!" He gave me a dirty look and turned around with the baby and sat down on the bench seat. He stared down at the tiny baby, fear was in his eyes. I knew he could do it, he just didn't know it.

A man came up and introduced himself. "I'm a doctor, can I be of help?" The three year old girl was almost back boarded and she would go in this ambulance.

"Get in that ambulance and tell me the babies aren't as bad as I think." He instantly obeyed. I wanted to be wrong this time. While the doctor was checking the babies, I had done a head count and decided a plan of evacuation. No text book can ever prepare you for this type of decision. I just took a plan and went with it, babies first, children second, adults last. Like it or lump it that was the order. We were delaying Rescue-Twos departure for a couple of minutes so a third patient could be loaded. She didn't appear injured and her grandmother said she was nauseated from her illness not the accident. Just be sure her grandmother was right she needed to be checked at the hospital.

Miller, a police officer and I boarded the three year old girl on her side, because her only injury appeared to be she was sick to her stomach but she required some spinal precautions to be taken. She was secured to the backboard. There were only two ambulances available and so each ambulance would have to speed to the hospital, off load their patients and turn around and hurry back to the scene. If I sent three in the first ambulance I could get it done in four trips.

The doctor found me. He motioned me away from the others. I went a few steps away as Miller finished taping the girl on the board. "You better get those babies out of here. They are bad." He shook his head. The look in his eyes told me everything I feared. Why couldn't he have told me I was all wrong? I thanked him for his help. Big city medics always complain about bystanders, I love them. They are willing to help. All they need is direction. In the middle of nowhere, they are part of the system and can help fill the manpower gap. The girl was carried to the ambulance and loaded on the bench seat. "She's stable. She just needs to be checked for possible head injuries. She was sick of her stomach but her grandmother thinks it's because of her illness. If she throws up at least she's on her side."

A bystander carried the four year old boy to R-2 and tried to put him inside. I ran over and took the boy and told him "No. The boy will have to go on the next ambulance." I held the boy in my arms and he clung to me, laid his head on my shoulder and sobbed. I looked up and saw the newspaper reporter snap my picture. I don't know why but that angered me and I turned around and avoided him and his camera, protecting the small boy by blocking him from view of the camera. I stood at the back door of the ambulance. "Remember, one tiny puff from your cheeks, and five compressions with your two fingers just one finger below the nipple line . . . . one puff, five compressions, got it Brody?" (Today CPR is done differently, but at the time that was protocol.)

With a voice dripping in anger he replied through clinched teeth, "I'll get you for this."

I slammed the door and the ambulance left, code three with red lights and sirens. Inside the ambulance, Brody was terrified of the baby girl and asked Gordon, "Can we trade?" Gordon agreed telling him the boy "wasn't a lot better." When R-2 arrived at the back door to the hospital, Gordon leaped from the vehicle before it stopped and ran inside with the baby girl in his arms. She was sinking fast.

I was using a husband and wife bystanders as assistants. The man took the four year old boy back reluctantly and the wife talked in Navajo to the grandmother. I assigned the doctor to keep me informed about any change in patient conditions. He wandered around and would come back with reports. He fit well into the system and the couple did also. In rural settings you have to use what you have and I learned fast to integrate the bystander into the rescue process.

Rescue-1 (the second ambulance) arrived and I assigned EMT Charlotte Garrison to the five year old girl and told her about the possible fractured arm. I suggested she use the male bystander and police officer to backboard the girl. I took the four year old boy from the male bystander's arms and laid him on the stretcher. He was scared and complained of stomach pain. EMT Laura Wells got in and examined him. The girl was put on the bench seat and the ambulance left. If there was anything I would have done differently in this entire call it would have been to backboard the four year old boy. I still don't know why I didn't. Thank God he had nothing broken and my momentary lapse in good sense and protocol didn't cost him.

I sat down with the grandmother and with the female bystander's help, questioned her. She quietly asked me to check her husband and daughter that lay in the road. I knew they were dead, I think she did too, but the old woman still hoped for a miracle. I left her and went to the man. He was very dead, but I went through the motions and checked for a pulse and even used the stethoscope in a bazaar way looking for a heartbeat. I then checked the woman the same way. An officer and I covered them up.

I walked back to the old woman, now strapped to a backboard, and as gently as possible, I shook my head, looked sad and told her they "had passed" (the Navajo way of saying they were dead) and there was nothing I could do. She understood and closed her eyes and didn't speak after that. I then went to the seventeen year old girl. I told her she could help by telling me where each person was sitting before the accident, what happened and the names, ages, addresses, and relationship of all the victims. She was in shock and kept wandering off mentally, but I was able to get the information. Officer Kemper kneeled nearby also writing down the information.

Rescue-2 came back and the elderly woman and the teen driver were loaded inside and taken to the hospital. Neither of them appeared injured. The old woman appeared to lose any will to live and the girl was hysterical and in emotional shock. She just stared off into space.

I picked up equipment and hurried to the hospital. I found every patient and left a copy of who they were and any information I had on them. They were all family and it was complicated. The elderly couple were the parents of the deceased woman lying in the road. They were the grandparents to the children, including the seventeen year old girl. They were the great-grandparents of the baby girl.

The deceased woman lying in the road was the mother of all the children and the grandmother of the baby girl. Her husband was a

132

highway worker and was being notified by a relative. It would be at least an hour or so for him to get here. The seventeen year old girl was the mother of the baby girl. The other children were her brothers and sisters. Her husband was a student at Tuba City High School and a Navajo Officer went to find him. I couldn't imagine facing this problem at seventeen years of age. At seventeen the most important decision I had to make was what to wear that day.

I remember at the hospital walking into the room and finding the girl baby on a bed. Her lovely white dress with pink and blue flowers was stripped off and she was naked. Two nurses were taking turns bagging her. She had stopped breathing on her own soon after arriving at the hospital. She had been intubated and with the bag valve mask they were forcing air down into her lungs in a rhythmical pattern that resembled a normal breathing. The nurses talked to each other about normal routine things and even laughed once. I knew they weren't being cold. They were protecting themselves from the horror that lay on the bed, the dying two week old child. They didn't want to think about it and so they shut her out. They just squeezed the bag mask every three seconds to inflate her lungs.

Later, the ward clerk told me she was passing by as the infant girl was being readied for Air Evac to a Phoenix area hospital. She said everyone knew the child was dying, but the mother didn't seem able to accept it. The Air Evac nurse gently laid the limp infant in her mother's arms. The girl began to cry as she touched the baby's face and ran her finger down her arm to her hand. She sobbed uncontrollable when her daughter's tiny fingers didn't wrap around her finger. Everyone just stood there with tears in their eyes. They all knew this was the last time this young mother would hold her baby in her arms alive. The ward clerk turned and ran down the hall to the lounge and cried in secret. The baby died in-flight to Phoenix. The baby boy was put on a respirator and after a few days, was declared brain dead. The respirator was turned off but he continued to breathe for three more weeks and finally died.

I wish I could end this story on an up note, but there isn't one. The family had just built a large home with four bedrooms at Shonto. They moved away and left it abandoned and no one dared venture near it. A place with so much sadness wasn't a place a Navajo wanted to live. They feared it could be haunted because of the large number of dead that died at the same time and all related to each other and all living under one roof. The young girl was blamed by the family for the death of her grandfather, mother, brother and her own newborn daughter. She was an outcast. This is an unbelievably heavy burden for a seventeen year old girl to carry around for the rest of her life. The marriage ended. She moved to Phoenix and one of her family members told me she started drinking. I don't know

133

if that's true, but I don't find that hard to believe. She wasn't welcome at her family home anymore.

No one in a Navajo family will talk about the dead. The grandmother just sits quietly in dignified silence remembering that in one split second she lost her husband, daughter, one grandson and one great-granddaughter. The traditional Navajo's feel there is little one can do to change fate. She accepts it, but she doesn't have to like it. The ones that died were the lucky ones that day. The accident destroyed the entire family.

I tried to forget the smell of baby power and the soft and beautiful baby girl and the sweet baby boy I had held in my arms. I also tried to forget the five year old girls accusing look as I ignored her pain. I tried to forget the lost look in the grandmother's eyes when I had to tell her that her husband and daughter were dead.

I almost managed to forget but then my husband came home about a month after the accident and told me there were flowers, artificial flowers placed in a make shift monument sitting off in the sand at the scene of the accident. I drove out there and tears came to my eyes as I stood at the side of the road and looked out into the desert. I know the seventeen year old girl put them there. They were small blue, white and pink flowers. The colors of blue, white and pink were the colors of the tiny flowers that were in the dress in which she had dressed her tiny daughter for the last time that fateful morning in July.

A MORNING PERSON

Laura Wells was Miss Perfect. Her frosted short light brown hair was beauty shop perfect, her children were perfect, her huge house immaculate, her husband was boring but near perfect. Laura lived in a world that was only colored in two hues, black and white. She alone knew what was right and wrong and cut no one slack if they had a different set of morals, opinions or went to the wrong church. Her way was the only way.

But, regardless of how staunch and uncompromising Laura was, she was a very good EMT. She gave her all and that was quite a lot. Laura had gone to college to be a registered nurse, something she never failed to bring up with great regularity. She failed to mention she had the education, but she never took the test and therefore was never licensed to work as a nurse. She often offended other EMTs in the process of

134

handling a call. She wasn't a good team player unless she was in charge. Over the years I learned to ignore her complaints about the incompetent EMTs with which she was forced to work, and the complaints of the EMTs about her uncompromising and pompous attitude.

Laura took everything very seriously. Her perfection was something she nurtured and treasured. But sometimes even perfect people have a bad day, and when they do, it's amusing to the rest of us.

Laura was an early riser. One morning she was up, dressed in a perfectly matching outfit and her hair combed to perfection when her pager went off. Laura grabbed her neatly ironed and folded jumpsuit that lay by the front door and rushed outside. She jumped into her car and discovered she didn't have her car keys. She jumped out and rushed to the door and found it locked. She beat on the door. But her near perfect husband had already left for work and her perfect children were still soundly asleep in their clean and orderly little rooms.

Laura suddenly realized she had made a mistake. Horrors! She looked around and realized that at this hour there was no traffic on her street. "Maybe a neighbor could drive me," she thought. Laura ran across the street and pounded franticly on her neighbor's door. No answer. She spun around on her heels and ran to the next house and beat on its door. Still no answer. She couldn't think of a Plan B so she ran to the third house, but no one answered. Laura was desperate when she beat on the forth house. That neighbor happened to also be an early riser and answered the door rather quickly. Laura babbled out between gasps for breath that she had an emergency call and had to have a ride. The neighbor said, "Come on, let's go." He and Laura rushed to his car.

As they were pulling away, Laura noticed that the doors to the houses she had beaten upon earlier were now all standing open and sleepy people, dressed in robes and semi-conscious stood looking up and down the street for whoever had woke them up by pounding on their door. Laura slid down in the seat as they drove past. She never could bring herself to tell them what she had done. The fact that she had made a mistake lay buried until now. It was just too good a story to pass up.

I SAID, GET DOWN ON THE GROUND!

I was baking a cake when the scanner came to life and the faceless dispatcher alerted police to a stabbing in Vermillion Trailer Court (Lake Powell Mobile Home Park). A woman had stabbed another woman and an ambulance was needed. I hurried from the kitchen and on the way out the front door, I told my husband, "There's a cake in the oven, check it in about fifteen minutes. Just set it on the table to cool, I'll ice it when I get back, love you." He smiled and went back to his newspaper.

Is the scene safe? We always think about that when responding to this type of call. I listened to police traffic as I *slow rolled* to the scene as the PFD first responding EMT. I heard Officer Prim ask, "Has the woman with the knife left the scene?"

"Yes," the dispatcher replied. I sped up a bit, but kept listening.

"What's the victim's condition?" he asked.

The dispatcher explained she was calling the call back number, a pay phone by the trailer court office, for an update on the situation and would relay the info when she got it. The other responding female officer, Sherry Carter called in on the radio. "I have her." Sherry was not a very good officer, but she managed to stumble by.

"Code-4?" Prim asked.

"Code-4" Sherry replied. I breathed a sigh of relief and continued to the scene.

I saw Prim pull in, directly in front of the trailer. I parked one driveway down to allow room for the responding ambulance. I got out, walked to the trunk of my car and opened it to get my jump kit. Then I heard Officer Prim's voice boom loudly. "Get down on the ground!" I slowly raised my hands skyward and slowly turned around. I saw he was standing by his car, pointing his gun directly at me. I stood still. I knew this man well. He was one of the better PPD officers. Why had he drawn his gun on me? Lots of things go through your mind when looking down the barrel of a gun. This was the second time in my life I was standing on the wrong end of a loaded gun. I was amazed at how large the black hole of the gun looks. I knew it was hardly larger than my thumb, but none the less, it looked big enough to pass a football through. I didn't move. This had to be a misunderstanding. It was a mistake, but until Prim also knew that, I was in danger. I trusted him not to pull the trigger unless I moved quickly, so I stayed frozen. I had no intentions of lying on the ground, even though he continued to shout.

"I said, DOWN ON THE GROUND!!!!!!" I continued to stand frozen to the spot. Then my eyes focused on a woman standing between Officer Prim and me. She was a Native American, about eighteen years old, dressed in jeans, t-shirt and tennis shoes. I hadn't seen her before. My attention had gone to the gun, not the space lying between he and I. "DOWN ON THE GROUND. DO IT, NOW!" Now I understood. He was pointing the gun at her, not me. I just happened to be directly in the line of

136

fire. His eyes had focused on the young woman as she ran across the street and not on me.

I continued to stand still as she slowly lay down on the pavement. He rushed forward and handcuffed her. If she was the one who had stabbed the woman in the trailer, then who did Sherry have? Sherry drove up. She got out and walked to Officer Prim. He turned on her with an anger I seldom saw in him. "WHO THE HELL DO YOU HAVE IN YOUR PATROL CAR?"

". . . . The woman who made the call from the pay phone."

"I thought you had the woman who did the stabbing," he said in a slightly calmer voice. She shook her head "no" and averted her eyes. "Damn it, next time, make yourself clear." He was still mad. Sherry apologized for her poor choice of words. It could have been a fatal misunderstanding, but luckily it wasn't.

They helped the woman who was still lying on the ground to her feet and into Officer Prim's patrol car. I moved and waved, "Can I go inside to the patient now?" Officer Prim saw me for the first time and immediately realized what had happened.

"I didn't see you," he sheepishly said.

"I know, but for a minute, I almost got down on the ground." He and Sherry laughed. I hurried inside. The two women were sisters. The older sister had told the younger sister she had to move out. The two women had augured and began to shove each other about the kitchen. The younger woman grabbed a steak knife and stabbed it into the older sister's left thigh and ran out the door. She ran to a friend across the street, and then when the police arrived, she decided to return and face the music and was caught while crossing the road. I kneeled beside the patient. She was about twenty years of age, 165 pounds, long black hair. She lay on the kitchen floor. The knife lay beside her. A small stream of blood slowly flowed from the wound in her thigh. I cut her jeans and bandaged the stab wound and stopped the flow of blood. The ambulance arrived and took over care. I collected my things and walked back to my car.

Prim came over. "Sharon, I'm sorry, I didn't see you were in the line of fire. Did I scare you?"

"You bet you did! I thought you had lost your mind for a minute until I saw the girl."

"Yeah, she just burst from the trailer over there and rushed into the street, I didn't know what to think. I focused on her. . . . . . . I just didn't see you. I should have, but I didn't."

"I'm ok. It's alright." I drove back home and found the un-iced cake half eaten, sitting on the table. I cut myself a piece, poured a glass of milk and took a break.

MY HUSBAND ISN'T FEELING WELL

The small car had left the road at around forty miles per hour. The passenger wheel had dug into the soft sand and the vehicle flipped onto its side. It was on the north access road, the northern end of Lake Powell Boulevard. Page sits on the top of a mesa, a flat topped mountain. The two access roads are steep and located on the north and south end of the business section of town. Homes and a few businesses had built up at the bottom of the mesa, but most businesses, hotels and homes were on top of the mesa. In a few years that would change, but for now it was just desert. The north access road came down the mesa and took a tight curve near the bottom. The small car didn't make the turn and now lay in the soft sand. The driver had crawled out and when I arrived as first responding EMT for the fire department, he was walking around. When the ambulance arrived he was quickly back boarded while standing. He was being loaded in the ambulance when my pager went off for a second ambulance. I knew there was no one signed up and if no one "volunteered" and just came down, transport of the second patient would have to wait till they were clear of this patient.

"Get him to the hospital quickly. No one's signed up for the second ambulance." They understood they might have to do a quick turnaround at the hospital. I loaded my jump kit into my vehicle and got in. I turned on the lights and sirens and rushed to the location. "Ill man," told me nothing. It could be almost anything, but it sounded routine. I beat the officer to the scene. I went inside a nicely maintained doublewide trailer in Lake Powell Mobile Home Village. I was greeted by a well-dressed woman around fifty years in age. She did not appear upset.

"My husband isn't feeling well," she said in a clear and calm voice. "He's in the bedroom, last door at the end of the hall." I didn't notice any stress in her voice. Nothing to indicate it was anything but a general illness. Officer Prim arrived and stood nearby listening. There was a lot of flu going around and as I hurried down the hall I expected to find a man lying on the bed coughing and running a fever. Nothing could be further from the truth.

I reached the door and opened it. Sitting on the edge of the bed was a man in his early fifties. He turned to look at me as I took one step into the room. He had a rifle on his lap. I came to a screeching stop. The officer behind me ran into me. He too saw the gun. We stood so near each other I could feel each breath he took. He whispered "Sharon, if I say move, go to your left and flat on the floor." I could feel him remove his gun from the holster. The gun was hidden from the man's view by my body.

138

My mind raced. This wasn't good. I'm between a disturbed man with a rifle and cop with a gun. "Your wife says you aren't feeling well."

"I'm not. Life sucks." He looked down at his gun and back up to me.

"Maybe I can help."

"I don't know how. I lost my job, the bank repossessed my truck and my wife won't stop nagging."

"This is a temporary problem."

"Maybe, but I'm tired. I just want out." He fingered the gun but so far it wasn't pointing at anyone.

"It doesn't have to be this way. Set the gun down and give me a chance. You do have other options."

"I don't think so," he said in a quite sad voice. The officer's muscles tightened as the man picked up the rifle but still didn't point it in any direction. I glanced quickly to my left and saw the area was free of furniture and although I would at first be out of the line of fire, there wasn't anything to hide behind.

I tried again. "I can help you, but the gun makes me nervous. Just lay the gun down and we can discuss some options." He sat silently for a full minute. The officer and I stood still and allowed him time to think. He moved and I almost dove for the floor, but then it became apparent he was laying the rifle on the floor. "Now kick it away." He did. I walked over and quickly picked up the gun and left the room. The officer rushed forward and shoved him face down on the bed and handcuffed the man. I sat the gun in the living room just as the ambulance drove up. I radioed them to stage where they were parked. I returned to the bedroom.

"Are you alright?" I asked the man. He looked up at me as the officer pulled him to a setting position. He looked defeated.

"I guess so."

"The cuffs are uncomfortable I know, but its procedure." He shook his head in understanding.

"We are going to take you to the hospital. There we can arrange for you to meet with a counselor. They can give you hope and offer an alternative to suicide. Give it a chance."

He weakly smiled at me and was escorted by the officer outside and into the ambulance. I found his wife and began to get some information for my paperwork. She appeared unconcerned. She had just watched her husband come close to killing himself and watched him walk out the door handcuffed and still didn't seem as interested as the neighbors who stood outside watching. I wondered what this man's chances were without this cold woman's support.

I got his name, date of birth, mailing address and an uneventful medical history. She continued to show no emotion whatsoever. She answered the questions in a casual, unconcerned manner. I began to see this man may be married but he's really alone in his emotional struggles.

He signed himself into Aspen Hills in Flagstaff. I don't know the details of his treatment but I saw him in the grocery store a few months later. He saw me and looked down at the floor, obviously embarrassed. I just walked by him and didn't say anything. In a small town I learned to not just blurt out things in public that should be kept confidential. If the past patient doesn't initiate the conversation, I just walk on by or if I know them we discuss general, safe topics. Unless they broach the subject, it's not discussed. I don't remember him being a patient again. Apparently he had decided to give it another try. Perhaps he found a reason to continue living. I hope so.

SOME PEOPLE SHOULDN'T DRINK

Keith was a thirty-two years old Anglo male. He had lived in Page for three years and liked it. His wife had left to care of her mother in Texas for a few weeks and Keith was suddenly alone. He hadn't been alone for over five years. He was enjoying his new found freedom. Keith was paid every Friday. He celebrated his new freedom by going to the Cove, a local watering hole. He knew almost everyone there and drank till 1 am, closing time. He paid his tab, said goodbye to his buddies and staggered around in the parking lot until he stumbled upon his car. It took three tries to get the door unlocked and getting in was awkward. Keith was drunk, very drunk.

Within five minutes of Keith walking out of the Cove, my pager went off. The report was a two car collision. I was all snug in my bed and got out reluctantly. Soon I was on the ambulance approaching the scene. The scene of the accident was only about a half block from the Cove. The road passes by the Cove, the police station, a clinic and a small church. There isn't a lot of traffic at this time of the morning. The road takes a slight uphill path that gently turns to the left. Obviously the blue car (driven by Keith) didn't turn to the left. Instead, he kept going straight and rear ended the gray car parked at the curb.

The driver of the blue car was sitting on the curb, leaning forward with his head in his hands. As I walked up, he looked up at me. His chin, nose and both palms had road rash. He had obviously gotten out after the accident and fell flat on his face. He had a wound in his hairline and blood

140

dribbled down his face and onto his blue shirt. "My name is Sharon; I'm with the Fire Department. I'm here to help. Is that alright with you?" Before I touched him, I had to get his permission according to the law.

He was a couple beats off, but he answered, "Yeah. It's ok. I'm Keith."

"What happened, Keith?"

Again, he was slow to respond. "I don't know. He just crossed the line and hit me." I had heard that one before. According to Kevin, the parked car had leaped out in front of him with no warning. A firefighter placed his hands on each side of Kevin's head and held it still. This provided some cervical spinal stabilization.

"What hurts the most?" I asked as the other EMT began taking his blood pressure.

"My head hurts."

I examined the wound in his hair. It wasn't that big, but head wounds bleed a lot. I put a dressing over the wound to stop the bleeding. "You're going to need some stitches," I said. He mumbled something I didn't understand.

"Vital Signs within normal limit," announced the EMT. We placed a cervical collar around his neck and got him on the backboard with spinal stabilization. He remained cooperative through the process. We were on the backside of the hospital so transport time was only a minute or so. At the hospital he received five staples in his head and a ticket for DUI.

This call was routine. It didn't stand out from other such calls. I quickly forgot about Keith until his next payday. They say "When the cats away, the mice will play" and Keith decided to play. Friday rolled around and Keith once again showed up at the Cove. At closing he walked rather unsteadily outside. "Hay, Keith, you need a ride?" his friend asked.

"No, my car's totaled, but I dug out my old bicycle. It works pretty good." Keith staggered over and climbed on the bike. He took off down the street. Now it's a proven fact, intoxicated individuals should not drive a car or attempt to ride a bicycle. But of course this obvious fact didn't enter Keith's mind.

"Beeeeeeeeeeeeeeeep! We have a report of a man lying in the street . . . . . . " The sound of my pager was loud and piercing. I sat up in bed. I got out and glanced at the clock, ten minutes after one in the morning that almost guaranteed alcohol was involved.

As we drove up on the scene, I couldn't help but notice the accident had happened in almost exactly the same spot of the accident one week earlier. Red, blue, and white lights lit up the scene in an odd disco fashion. I got out of the ambulance, grabbed the jump kit and oxygen bottle. I then hurried to the man sitting on the curb. A bicycle lay near him. When I kneeled down beside him I noticed it was the same man from last week. "Keith?"

He looked up and smiled a weak smile. "Hay, it's you again."

"I was about the say the same thing. What happened?"

"My bicycle hit a little rock and bumped the curb."

"What hurts?" I asked.

"I think I broke my wrist." He was cradling his left wrist and arm. I took a look and didn't see any deformity. He had good movement and feeling in his fingers. His pulse was strong. I splinted it and we put him on a backboard in spinal immobilization just in case.

At the hospital his neck and back was ok, but he had cracked his wrist and the doctor applied a plaster cast and took the staples from his previous accident out of his head. I was beginning to think if his wife didn't come home soon, she just might find herself a widow.

Another week passed. Keith wasn't the type of person that learned from his mistakes. His wife was due home Sunday. He decided to hit the Cove one last time before she returned. The night went well, he had a good time. His left wrist still hurt, but he was right handed so he managed. Closing came at one in the morning, my pager sounded about ten minutes after the hour.

As we drove up, it was the same location and same patient. This time he was walking home and his foot missed the sidewalk and he stepped off the curb and fell into the street. A car almost ran over him, but managed to stop and the driver called the ambulance. As I approached him he looked up and smiled. "We have to quit meeting this way." I laughed. This time he had a bump over his left eye that was growing larger by the minute. His eye would be swelled shut before the sun came up. His left elbow as painful and his left hip hurt. For the third time this month we transported Keith to the Page Hospital Emergency Department.

His elbow and shoulder wasn't fractured but his left arm was put in a sling. His left hip also wasn't fractured but he would limp for a few days. His left eye was swelling shut and the bump above his eye was huge. His fractured wrist and head wound had not been reinjured.

I wonder what his wife said when she returned to find the car totaled and her husband looking as if he had been sacking wildcats. I have the feeling she grounded him and made sure he had the supervision he so desperately needed. To my knowledge, Keith was never a patient in our ambulance again.

SHE'S DEAD, VERY DEAD

It was an ordinary day at the station. We had had no calls that warm summer day. Suddenly the door to the office flew open and two men burst into the room. They were big men, dressed in work clothes and both could use a bath and shave. The tallest man did the talking. His eyes were enlarged with excitement and his words tumbled out in a jumbled mess.

"It's bad, it's really bad . . . ." He was wringing his hands.

"What's bad?" I asked.

"The accident. . . . . it's bad. . . ." the shorter man pointed south east. Stress showed on his face as he nervously bit his bottom lip. He was restless and shifted his weight from one leg to the other.

"Where's the accident?"

"Out on 98, she's hurt really bad," his words trailed off, he gestured by drawing a line across his belly, his eyes glassed over and he was again seeing the horror he had left behind on the roadway. The look on his face told me this was worse than bad.

"Where on Highway 98? Before Kaibito? After?"

The man said nothing, he was lost temporary. The other man answered. "Before, I don't know exactly, about twenty miles east of Page, something like that."

"Call dispatch and have her page the ambulance," I said to the secretary. I then turned back to the two men. "How many people are hurt?"

"Three . . . . well the woman, she's . . . . torn in . . . . half . . . ." The second man had gotten the words out, but he refused to say anything else. He too just couldn't put into words the horror he had witnessed.

I got up and left them. I was driving that day and hurried to the ambulance, Rescue-Two. I started it up and pulled it out outside. I then loaded the suction machine. The other crew members arrived. Connie Miller was in the back. She was an old pro. Mitchell Hammerman was a rooky. I told them what we had. Connie climbed in the back, Mitch looked uneasy.

I pulled out, turning on the red lights and we headed to the scene. We all realized that if indeed the woman had been torn in half there was absolutely nothing we could do. But there were two more people hurt. We all silently prepared ourselves for what awaited us twenty miles out.

We topped a hill and suddenly there it was. To my right lay a car on its wheels. It was sitting about twenty feet off into the sand. Two people were about fifteen feet behind the car, one laying and one sitting. Several bystanders stood around. The same spaced look was in their eyes. They all turned and watched us get out of the ambulance. Each expecting a miracle we didn't have. I sent Mitch and Connie over to the two on the ground. A bystander I knew as a local from Page walked over to me and offered to help. "Do you know how to use flares?" I asked him. He said he did. The hill I topped just before the accident was now a hazard. On coming vehicles wouldn't see the ambulance. It was parked as far to the right as I could get it, but because of the soft sand, it still hung over into the roadway. I gave him the flares and instructions on where to place them.

As driver, I had to check the dead. I walked over to the car. It had obviously rolled and landed on its wheels. In my years on the ambulance, I had seen a lot but this was indeed horrible. The lower half of the woman lay on the driver's side by the front finder. On the feet were white tennis shoes and the woman was wearing blue pants. It looked like our CPR doll, Annie. I had trouble believing this was a human being. A piece of cardboard had been placed over the lower part of that half. Human tissue clung to the driver's crushed finder.

I walked to the other side of the car. Another piece of cardboard had been placed over the upper half of the body. Medium length sandy blond hair fanned out from under the cardboard and a small white hand lay delicately in the sand. The rest was hidden from view. In all honesty, my curiosity got the best of me. I didn't have too, but I had to look. I lifted the cardboard. The woman looked perfectly normal as she lay face down, except the lower half was gone. She had been severed in half at the waist. Her intestines hung out on the sand. There was no noticeable blood. Death had come instantly. I lowered the cardboard.

The bystander returned to report mission completed. He looked down with pain in his eyes. "I covered her up. It was awful." I went back to the ambulance and found two sheets. I came back. The bystander looked at me with horror in his eyes. "You aren't going to uncover her again are you? I don't think I can look at her again."

"You won't have too." I held one end of the sheet and opened it up to cover her. "Now just pull the cardboard out gently. He did it and I covered her. No one had to look at her again. We did the same for the lower half on the other side of the car.

I went to the other EMTs. The female victim lay staring up at the sky. She answered questions in a robot manner. She showed no emotion, and never asked about the other woman. It was apparent she had already seen her friend. The male patient sat up and he also answered questions is short, quick sentences. He said very little also. He sat staring at the two white sheets about thirty feet away that covered his friend.

We found out the dead woman was driving. They left the roadway and the car rolled several times. He gave us her name. It was hard for him. He didn't appear injured and refused any medical help regardless of how much we tried to encourage him. The woman was put on a spine board. She was like a zombie.

Somewhere in the process, Connie and Mitch both whispered to me they too wanted to look at the woman. EMTs are a curious lot. I understood their morbid curiosity because I also had the same affliction. Connie discreetly went over and peeked then came back. The live victims didn't see her. Then Mitch went over. I was worried about him. He was only eighteen and this was about as bad as it gets. He stood looking down at the sheet. He took a deep breath and lifted the sheet just enough to see her head and lowered the sheet again. He hurried back to the live patients.

I went back and completed the investigation. As driver, we try and get a quick guess of how it happened. The best I could come up with was the car rolled end over end in a slightly cocked position, driver's finder, and passenger tail light. On the first roll, the woman was ejected out the passenger door and thrown onto the sand. The car continued on and the driver's finder pinched her as it landed on her, tearing her in half. The lower half of her body became stuck to the finder and was carried with the car on one last half roll, and as the car landed on its wheels, the lower half fell from the finder, thus leaving the upper half on one side of the car and the lower half on the other and blood and tissue on the finder.

The ride back was a hard one. Everyone was quiet taking their cue from the two traumatized patients in the back. Neither appeared injured physically but emotionally they were seriously injured. At the hospital the patients were taken into ER-1 and 2. I explained to the head nurse what we had left behind. I expressed my concern and suggested a counselor be called later. She completely agreed.

For the record the officer's didn't agree with me and said the woman's seat belt tore her in half. I just don't agree. There was no blood or tissue on the belt and where did the blood and human flesh come from on the finder? Oh well I guess it doesn't really matter what the reports say in this case. The woman was very dead.

The male patient seemed to come to grips with what happened. He had problems but they appeared to be of a normal nature as he started working through the tragedy. The woman lay in bed staring at the ceiling. A psychologist was called the next morning. Over the next three days extensive counseling with her helped bring the tears and the verbal expression that was needed. The normal grieving process began.

The two witnesses that reported the wreck, worked for Peabody Coal (Kayenta Coal Mine) one of our EMTs Gordon Taylor was a good friend of the taller man. He went over to the man's house. The man had kept silent at home about the accident. He couldn't tell his wife of the horror he had seen. He felt it unfair to submit her to that and besides, he didn't want to show the fear and weakness he felt concerning the matter. When Gordon came in and offered to listen, the man was so relieved. He blurted out the story and Gordon listened. The man then went over and over it, again, trying to get it straight and in perspective. Gordon knew and understood and just sat and listened. After the man was through Gordon explained how EMTs deal with this. He explained what was considered a normal reaction. The man began to see what he was feeling wasn't bad, it was normal. He felt better.

Gordon made several visits to the man's house. The man recovered. The second witness was approached by Gordon and he too eagerly told the story. He had already begun to work through it and needed only a little assistance. The EMTs on the call didn't have serious problems. We all remember the call, but it didn't cause any lost sleep. Mitch told everyone he had lifted the sheet and saw everything. I let it go at that.

The two officers that investigated the accident were friends of mine. It's hard to talk to ordinary people about something like this. A husband or wife is usually of little help, even if you choose to bring them into it. You have to be in the business to understand what is required of us at times. After church a few weeks later the officer took me aside. He told me he wanted to thank me for the sheets. They rolled the victim onto the sheet and used the four corners to move the body so the wrecker could tow the vehicle. He told of the horror he felt at carrying half the woman away and discovering her intestines had fallen out of the sheet and he was stepping on them as they tangled around his shoe. He said he and the other office had to stop and throw up. They then scooped the intestines up and tossed them in the sheet and carried her away to await the morgue. Without the sheet, the job would have been far harder. He said the hardest part was going back for the second half.

I understood what he was going through. I shared my personal conflicted feelings with him. He understood and realized he wasn't alone. We both felt better having talked about it. We never discussed it again.

HE LIKED FIRE TRUCKS THE BEST

Sheppard was our family dog. He was a mix of Border Collie and Austrian Sheppard. He looked like a Border Collie with long thick fur, black with white and brown markings but he was a big dog like the Austrian Sheppard. He weighed around eighty pounds. I know most dog

146

owners brag about how smart their dogs are, but it's been proven a Border Collie is one of the smartest. He hiked with the boys, even allowed himself to be pulled up steep cliffs on ropes. He seldom barked and was loyal and protective of our family. He was a good dog.

Late one night my pager sounded. I jumped up and ran into the hallway. Sheppard always slept in the hallway stationed in the middle between all three bedrooms where his human family slept. He had heard the pager sound and now stood on his feet to the end of the hallway waiting for me to exit the bedroom. I hurried down the hallway with him on my heels. I quickly slipped on the jumpsuit and my shoes. I grabbed my keys and noticed he stood by the door, his tail wagging, hopping from one foot the other and the look of anticipation on his face.

I had to smile, "Ok, let's go," I said as I opened the front door. Sheppard hopped happily to the car. It was a convertible and he loved to ride in it. He would never jump out, growl or bark at anyone walking close by. He climbed over to the passenger seat and jumped to the floor board and held on. He had learned I drove fast going to an emergency and the only way he could maintain his balance was to lay in the floor.

We arrived at the fire just after the police. I parked a half block down on the same side of the street as the fire. "We're here, Shep," I said. He jumped up in the passenger seat and looked around. He loved the flashing code lights. Police or ambulance was ok, but when he saw the fire, if a dog could smile, he smiled. He loved the fire trucks the best and he knew one was on the way. "Stay," I said to him and got out and walked toward the burning trailer. I could see a person lying on the grass and an officer kneeling beside him.

"Page (dispatch) F-3 is 10-97 (on scene). It's a fully involved single wide trailer with at least one injured."

"F-3, Dispatch copies." I also knew all responding fire personnel also heard my report. As I approached the injured man I could see he was dressed in jeans only. He had obviously dressed quickly to escape the fire.

"My name's Sharon. I work for Page Fire. Is there anyone else in the trailer?"

"No, my wife's visiting . . . . " He coughed violently. He continued "her mother in Salt Lake (City, Utah)."

"Are you injured?" I asked as I visually looked him over for obvious injuries.

"I just got too much smoke . . . ." he coughed. "And I twisted my ankle on the front steps."

The smoke was drifting our way and the flames were hot as they fed on the trailer. "Let's move him across the street," I said to the officer. He and I each took an arm and helped him up. We limped him across the

147

street to his neighbor's lawn. The officer took off to get the crowd that was forming to back up. The fire chief drove up. The first in fire truck was only a couple of blocks away.

I put the man on oxygen. He continued to cough but he began to breathe better. I noticed a small laceration to his forearm and a second degree burn to his right hand. I was bandaging them when the officer walked over. "The chief says you should move your car."

"Here," I said as I tossed him my keys. "Can you move it? I'm kind of busy here."

"Sure." He caught the keys and hurried to move the car. I thought I had parked in an out of the way spot, but apparently the chief had a plan to park an engine there or pull off the hydrant nearby. I continued to treat the patient. The ambulance would be there shortly.

Sheppard was having a wonderful time. He saw the flames grow bigger and two more cars with red, white and blue lights flashing arrived. He loved the lights, the people running about and the excitement of the fire scene! Just then a man approached the car. Sheppard turned his head in time to see the man do the unpardonable sin, he touched Sheppard's car handle. Shep spun around and with hind feet on the passenger seat and front feet on the driver's seat he snapped out at the intruder. The man dressed in navy blue pulled his hand away from the door handle. He was obviously angry. Sheppard couldn't imagine why the man would be angry. He was the one who touched the car. Sheppard stood growling a serious warning. The man left. Sheppard turned his attention back to the fire. He could hear the fire engine in the distance. He got excited. He loved the fire engines the best.

The officer walked up and tossed me the keys, "Here, you move your own car. Your damn dog almost bit me."

"I'm sorry. I forgot I had brought him along. Stay with him for a minute." I got up and ran for the car as the fire engine's siren got louder. I jumped in the car and drove it down the block and pulled it onto a side street. Sheppard still had a ringside seat, but here he and the car would be out of the way. I petted him on the head. "Good boy Sheppard. Are you having fun?" He wiggled and wagged his tail. He moved to the back seat and stood looking over the trunk of the convertible as the fire engine arrived. He was so excited.

I returned to my patient and allowed the now angry officer to leave. It was my fault, not the officer's or the dog's. The ambulance arrived and took over care of the man. I assumed Medical Control for the remainder of the fire.

The trailer was a complete loss. It burned fast and the department could only save his neighbors trailers on each side, a storage shed and the man's car. When I returned to my car, Sheppard was still watching but with far less enthusiasm. The excitement had died down and cleanup was boring. He was glad to see me and sat up in the passenger seat on the way home.

The story doesn't end here. The fire department office was small and contained four desks all in one room. People dropped by often and the phone rang off the hook. It was hard sometimes to get something done. Around six weeks after the fire, I lay awake. I had been on a call a couple of hours earlier and couldn't get back to sleep. I got up. I decided to go down to the office and work a bit on the fire pre-plans project. It was a useful system. The Chief and I would each take a building, let's say the Page Boy Motel as an example. What fire hydrant should the first arriving engine pull off of? Where do they park? Where does the second arriving engine park? What is their assignment? Where should the ambulance park? How many rooms did it have? Two to four people per room equals how many possible people to evacuate if there was a fire? What if it's snowing, where would you evacuate them too? It was complicated to plan and compile, but once done, no responding vehicle need to clutter the airways with questions. All they had to say was they were en route and report when they arrived at the scene. They already had their orders. Command could cancel the pre-plan with a simple order over the radio if an unanticipated event caused the pre-plan to not be the best way to go. Three fire chiefs used the plans even after I left. The current Fire Chief is a micro-manager and prefers to command without pre-plans. It makes him feel important and powerful to have responding units ask him for orders.

It's time to get back to the story. I awakened Sheppard when I opened the bedroom door. He had not heard the pager go off, but he knew I was going somewhere and maybe he could go for a ride. I let him come with me. It was two in the morning, dark and the station wasn't in the best side of town. I could use the company and protection. He knew he wasn't going to an emergency so he sat up in the passenger seat looking around during the trip. He was very interested in the two coyotes wandering down the middle of the street, but didn't bark and stayed in the car. Page had been invaded by coyotes ever since the short sighted Department of Health decided to poison the prairie dog settlement. They were worried about the Bubonic Plague. The plague is alive and well in northern Arizona and the fleas loved prairie dog holes. Prairie dogs are the favorite food for coyotes. No one knows how it happened but the coyotes discovered cats taste like prairie dogs. Everyone's pet cats were in danger of becoming lunch for hungry coyotes. And when the sun went down the coyotes moved into town. In Page the household cat was an endangered species.

I opened up the door and entered the dark office. I switched on the lights and locked the door. Once inside the PFD office, Sheppard lay beside me, facing the door leading to the city garage. As I have noted previously, the fire department shared a building with the city garage. That door remained unlocked. My back was to the door.

Remember the Page Police Officer Sheppard almost bit at the fire? Well, he parked at the back of the city garage and went inside to use the men's room. He noticed a light under the door to the fire department office. He wasn't aware of my habit of sometimes working in the wee hours of the morning. He wandered over and listened. He couldn't hear anything. He reached out for the door knob and opened the door. I didn't hear the officer on the other side of the door but Sheppard did. When the door suddenly opened he launched himself into a flying leap, aimed at the intruder's neck. He had full intentions of protecting me from harm. The officer was met with a frightening sight. All he saw was an animal in mid-air heading toward his neck with large snapping teeth. He screamed and slammed the door. Sheppard crashed into the door, quickly stood up and barked twice.

I jumped up. "Sit, Sheppard." I opened the door and the officer was sitting on the floor with a shocked look on his face. I burst out laughing. He was screaming profanity to the top of his lungs. The profanity was strung together in a very creative way with no recognizable English in-between. It made no sense but defiantly conveyed his anger. "Are you alright?" I asked between burst of laughter.

"@$#%%^*&!@$#, I think so," he said as he rose to his feet. He brushed off his behind and calmed down a bit. "What the hell are you doing here this #$@!&%^$# time of night?

I explained how this wasn't that uncommon. Sheppard had positioned himself between me and the officer. The dog's ears and tail were lowered and he continued to growl a deep threatening growl.

"He doesn't like me much, does he?"

"No." The officer was right. Sheppard liked the other officers, but for some reason known only to him, he didn't like this man.

"Well, I don't like him much either."

"Seriously, he was just trying to protect me. I'm sorry you were Startled, but he was just doing his job.

"Yeah, I guess so," the officer said. I promised to call dispatch the next time I decided to work in the middle of the night. After he left, I petted Sheppard. He lay down beside me and placed his head on my foot and drifted off to sleep. He died many years later in his sleep with his head placed on the top of my husband's foot. He was quite old. He was a good dog. I miss him.

DODGING LIGHTNING BOLTS

"He probably took it," said Vicki, PF's Administrative Assistant.

"Who?"

"You know, Roger."

I was digging through my desk in search of chocolate. "I was sure I had a Snicker's bar in here, somewhere," I said as I peered into one of my desk drawers. Yes, I did know. Whenever the Fire Chief got hungry he had no problem going through everyone's desks in search for food. Chocolate was high on his list. "Damn it. That makes me mad. It wasn't his to take. I paid for that candy. In all the years that tightwad hasn't even bought me a cup of coffee."

Vicki walked to the window and looked out. "Looks like we might need an ark." The storm had hit with a vengeance. Black clouds filled the sky and lightning bolts struck earth over and over again. It was the middle of August and my two sons were at a friend's house. A loud clap of thunder sounded and we lost electricity. Then another flash quickly followed by the loud roar of thunder. I don't like thunder. It comes from my childhood, something I should have outgrown many years ago but didn't. The adult in me faced the event with outward calm and control, but the little girl in me still huddled in fear.

All around town the lightning wrecked physical and emotional damage. Light poles were struck, one actually caught fire. A transformer was smoking and the green metal transformer box was now black around the edges. Children and adults ran for cover. The lightning hit the flagpole of the McDonalds. The pole was in the center of a pretty round brick wall and it had been filled with dirt and flowers. The wall blew outwards sending chucks of brick and dirt flying. A clump of flowers landed on the hood of a red car. The drive through microphone stopped working and the electric went off. Page was without electric power. The hospital, PPD, FD and Safeway grocery store were on emergency power. Then the rain hit. It was a desert downpour, heavy and the streets ran like rivers. My pager went off. "We have a report of a child hit by lightning at Page Rock and Sand in the industrial park." I didn't want to go out in the storm, but I didn't have a choice.

The other two crew members quickly drove up. We got in Rescue-One and headed out. Page sits on a flat topped mesa and the industrial park is located just south of the town, off the mesa. As we reached the edge we could see down into the industrial park. Bolts of lightning were flashing downward, striking the Industrial Park many time minute. I didn't like this. "Do we get hazard pay?" asked the male EMT in humor, but I failed to see the humor at the time. I tried to think about something

151

other than the lightning storm. Page Rock was owned by a polygamist family. Page is about a hundred miles from the polygamist stronghold of Colorado City. Some of the polygamists live in Page. One man my husband worked with at Navajo Generating Station lived in Page with his first wife and two daughters. He worked four days a week (ten hour days). On Friday he and his family would pack up and drive to Colorado City. There his first wife would take the girls and go visit her mother. He would go visit his second wife (his first wife's sister). Later he added a third and fourth wife and was forced to quit his job and move back to Colorado City.

My mind wandered to the last time I went to Page Rock. It was a fourteen year old boy who had fallen in the rock crusher. There were two double wide trailers parked at the site and a large rock crusher standing on an elevated platform. When we got there, we were taken to a cave carved in the side of the red sandstone cliff bordering the business. The cave was large, about twenty foot wide and fifteen foot deep. In the walls of the cave, shelves had been carved. Oil lamps sat on the shelves. The outside edges of the cave were lined with sleeping bags. In the far corner was a bucket that smelled of urine. Apparently around a dozen boys lived in this cave. A number of them were hanging around. They were thin, about ten to fourteen years of age. They all wore faded jeans, cowboy boots and long sleeve cowboy shirts with the neck buttoned up to the top button. This was typical polygamist attire.

The boy was lying on a sleeping bag. He was alright except for a scraped shin where his leg had slipped into the intake portion of a rock crusher. His foot was bruised, but worked well. The man who insisted he was the boy's father refused transport. He had called for an ambulance before he had realized the boy was not seriously injured. I bandaged his left leg and we left.

I called child protective services when I got back to the office. I seldom called child protective services but it was illegal for children to operate a rock crusher. It was far too dangerous for someone so young. I also wondered if working boys that young all summer and making them live in a cave was within the law. The agency worker and a police officer arrived the next day and the boys were gone, every one. The cave was vacant. It seems they had been sent to work at the business for the summer. They received no pay except Colorado City money that was accepted only within the polygamist community. This is legal. This also made sure the boys couldn't save their money and run away with a secret girlfriend. When the situation became common knowledge, the boys were sent back home to Colorado City a polygamist community on the Arizona Strip.

My thoughts returned to the present as we pulled into Page Rock and Sand. We were motioned to a white double wide trailer on site. We pulled up and got out. The hairs on the back of my arm stood up because there was so much static in the air. Lightning continued to flash, almost one after another. It was a bit unnerving. We were soaking wet when we entered the living room and saw our patient. She was a small, pretty girl dressed in a pink dress. Her father said she and her older brother were playing outside when the storm hit. While running for the trailer, a wide, bright lightning bolt struck just in front of them. They were soaking wet and running through mud puddles. The strike knocked them both to the ground. The boy got up and managed to drag his sister to the trailer.

Her father, his two wives and around nine children stood and watched as I knelt beside her. I don't know which woman was her biological mother, but both women look very concerned. They were dressed in long cotton dresses, one in pink the other in blue. The dresses had white collars at the neck and puffy sleeves. There were ruffles around the long sleeves and the hem that stopped inches above the ankle. A sash at the waist tied with a bow in back. They were wearing tennis shoes and their hair was long and tightly curled up off their shoulders held in place with many hair pins. It's an odd hair style that is hard to explain. Kind of an exaggerated blend of a late 1940's to early 50's hair style.

The patient was named Emily, she was nine years old. She was dressed in similar style to her mothers except she had a pair of long pants under her dress. Her eyes were open but she didn't see me. I spoke to her, but she didn't hear me. She tossed her head from one side to the other with a panicked, confused look on her face. Lightning had damaged her central nervous system. She was alive, but unaware of what happened. She was confused and very deaf. I began to check her over. Lightning isn't like electricity. This was not a direct strike. The girl had been in front of her brother when the lightning struck the wet soil near her. She received a large jolt but not as much as a direct hit. That was why she was still alive. Her brother was a couple of steps behind her and that's why he had escaped injury. The lightning in this case followed the damp outside skin. Her dress was cotton, but the metal zipper up the back had burned her back. The elastic waist and legs of her panties were melted into her skin. The metal hair barrettes she had holding her braided hair had touched her neck and left burns.

The little girl was very restless and began to grunt and groan. Since we were basic-EMTs the best thing we could do for her was provide immediate transport. Her father carried her outside to the ambulance. Rain continued to fall and lightning was everywhere. I felt very uncomfortable. I jumped in back and continued to monitor her. Her heart rate was fast, but regular. There were no changes during transport.

The hospital was on emergency power when we pulled up. Again her father insisted on carrying her into the hospital. She lay limp in his arms, her head moving back and forth as she tried to make some since of what was going on. Her burns were treated. She was held in the ER till the storm passed and then she was flown to Phoenix Children's Hospital.

One full year later I heard she wasn't completely recovered, but functioning reasonably well. She didn't remember that day. Her sight become normal and her hearing returned. Some of her fine motor skills took longer to return. She had to learn to read again. Even a year later, she would often be at a loss for the right word to say. The last I heard, her short term memory was affected, but the doctors expected it to improve eventually. The polygamists that owned Page Rock and Sand tried to stay out of the limelight due to their unusual lifestyle, but it just didn't work. They moved back to Colorado City a little over one year after the accident. Multiple wives and more children than you could possibility imagine was normal for them. Women were not allowed to progress further than the sixth grade and were considered little more than "baby making machines." She only had two more years of school anyway and hopefully finished the sixth grade as originally planned. According to their custom, at around fourteen years of age or so she would be married off into a polygamist household. She was pretty and if her problems became permanent disabilities, at least they were not generic so her babies should be normal. Whatever her possible weak areas might be, she would have the help of the other "sister wives". I am certain she did alright within the limits of her religions boundaries.

After the call, I went back to the office. I did my research and discovered the guilty culprit who (probably) took my chocolate candy bar hated chocolate covered raisins. He thought they felt like eating chocolate covered bugs. Guess what chocolate delight I kept in my desk drawer from then on? It wasn't a Snicker's bar. Problem solved.

WOMEN HAVE TO BE SHOWN WHO'S BOSS

We had just delivered a patient to the Page Hospital that had been mauled by a Rez dog. The tourist had pulled over and stood beside the road to take a picture of a beautiful sandstone cliff. A flea infested Rez dog

154

with ribs showing walked up to her looking for a handout. She took pity on the malnourished animal and made the mistake of tossing him a few crackers and then attempting to pet him. His life was a hard one and I believe he thought she was going to take back his crackers. His lips curled up and his teeth were bared. He snapped out and caught her right hand in his mouth. She screamed and struggled to free her hand. The dog let go. She spun around and the dog got her on the calf of the leg. She screamed again and ran for the car. She jumped in and began to cry. Her husband had used his cell phone and called us. We took her into town and delivered her to the hospital.

We were trying to get the rig back in service. Rescue-Two was heading west on Highway 89 for a reported dirt bike accident in Big Water, Utah. They would be gone at lease another forty-five minutes. Park Service was suffering a man power problem and their ambulance was currently unmanned. We were the only ambulance for around seventy-five to one hundred miles in any direction. Our pager sounded.

"Beeeeeeeeeep! We have a report of a woman with a possible fractured arm." It was a local address. We threw the ambulance back in order and rushed out of the hospital parking lot.

We arrived quickly. The husband was standing in the open doorway and let us in. His wife was sitting at the kitchen table cradling her right arm. She had her head down and didn't look up. She was obviously in pain. I was on the ambulance on this call and went to the woman's side. I kneeled down, "What happened?" I asked.

"She fell," the man answered.

"Where did you fall?" I was trying to find out how far she fell.

"Down the back stairs," answered her husband. "She a klutz and falls all the time." RED FLAG! He was doing all the talking and described her as falling down all time. I had seen this before in domestic violence cases. I wasn't sure, not yet, but I begin to listen to the way he worded his responses, his tone, and mostly her expression. She kept her head down and let him do the talking.

"Could I see the stairs?" I asked. He led me to the back door just off the kitchen. He opened the door. The home was a single wide trailer sitting about four feet above the ground. I looked down at six wooded steps leading to an unfenced, sandy back yard. The steps were covered in sand that had not been disturbed. There were no foot prints at the base of the stairs either. I could see a large indention in the sand about five feet from the base of the stairs and small footprints leading away from the indention to the road in front of the trailer. It didn't take CSI training to see what happened. The husband was a big, muscular man and his wife was a small woman, weighing less than ninety pounds. He had picked her up and threw her out the door. She missed the steps and landed in the sandy yard. He then locked the door. She got up and walked to the road and circled around and re-entered the trailer. Why? I don't know. She should have kept going at top speed as far as she could away from this man, but abused women often go against logic and choose to stay with an abusive spouse for a number of reasons. It's a complex issue and I will leave the explanations to the experts.

I had a problem. This man was violent. I didn't want to set him off. My crew had one man and one woman plus me. Men such as he tend to view the EMT male as an intruder. The female EMT and I were just stupid women and he knew how to handle stupid women. I was suddenly afraid. Calls such as this can end in someone being attacked, stabbed or shot. I couldn't call for police backup with the husband standing there and besides, it could take too long for them to respond. If I confronted him with my suspicions, he would become uncooperative and possibly violent. He was one big dude. I decided to get out of there as quickly as I could without raising his suspicions. I stood with my back to the man looking out at the yard. I closed my eyes, composed myself and turned around. I smiled and faced the husband. If he thought I was dumb, why not use that to my advantage. "Looks like a four foot fall. She's lucky her arm was all she hurt." He accepted my comments and had no clue what I was really thinking. I walked over to the crew. "Let's get her in the ambulance." She was quickly loaded and he followed in his truck.

On the way to the hospital I took vital signs and looked for other injuries. She had no other complaints of pain except her arm. She had some bruises on her arms and legs in different stages of healing. I tried to get a story out of her, but she lay there, eyes closed and didn't say much. At the hospital I took the doctor aside and explained what I had found and what I suspected. He said she had been seen in the ER before for another fall a few weeks before. He talked with her and then called the police to report a case of possible domestic violence.

It was a messy scene. Eventually it ended in the police dragging off a screaming husband, with his sobbing wife and an ER staff standing clear of the altercation. This one ends like so many other similar cases. Everyone wanted to help but the wife didn't want help. She refused to testify against her husband and his charges were dropped. She went back to him. They moved a couple of weeks later to parts unknown. I wonder if he's still beating the hell out of her?

FIRE IN THE HOLE !

It was around the year 2000, in Page, Arizona. Helen, a woman who worked at a local grocery store, lived in the Lake Powell Mobile Home Village. One morning, she went outside because she smelled smoke. She lived on the outside border of the Park. A drainage ditch bordered the west side of her back yard, running north/south. Some children had set on fire the twigs and dry grass in the drainage ditch. A black plastic pipe about two and a half feet wide ran east/west and dumped excess rainwater into the drainage ditch. The plastic pipe was buried under her yard and was now on fire.

Helen called the fire department and then walked out to the center of her back yard, watching the fire in the drainage ditch. She had no idea the plastic pipe ran under her yard. She was dressed in slippers and a house coat. Just as the police officer drove up, the ground beneath her feet gave way. What she didn't know was the fire had moved up the west/east pipe and melted where she stood and the heat had weakened the plastic pipe. Her foot dropped though the thin layer of dirt and grass and went into a burning fire. She screamed as the young policeman ran for her. He ran like a quarter back with the football. He was focused on the woman. He could see the flames as they licked out the hole, trying to set on fire the hem of her housecoat. She screamed as her foot burned. She tried to pull the foot out, but it was stuck. Black smoke engulfed her as she struggled to breathe and pull her foot free. She was seconds away from death by fire. The officer made it to her and entered the black toxic smoke. He ignored the flames licking out of the hole at his pant leg and grabbed her and pulled. Her foot was stuck. He later told me, "I wasn't leaving without her, even if I pulled her in half." Well, he almost did that, but her foot pulled free and they both fell to the ground. I drove up in time to see them scurry to their feet and burst into a run. Each step they took they feared the ground would give way and plunge them into the burning hell that roared beneath the grassy backyard.

I listened as the two hyper people told me the story. The officer was a true hero. He risked his health and safety to pull her free from an almost certain fiery death. I bandaged her burned foot and gave him oxygen to help his cough. The officer was fresh out of the academy and this was his first day as a police officer. Helen was grateful and thanked him over and over again for saving her life. His supervisor came to the scene and with a smile on his face he said, "Well, you're quite a show off. Only two hours into your first shift and you save a woman's life. I suppose you want the rest of the day off."

The young officer laughed then said, "No way, I love this stuff."

Fire trucks arrived and extinguished the fire in the drainage ditch. They had to trace the pipe and see how far the fire had extended. They discovered the fire had made its way across two yards before being stopped. Both the woman and the police officer quickly recovered. I must say, I have never seen anything like this before or since.

RATTLESNAKE BITE

Navajo's have a rich culture. Many Navajo's have accepted mainstream religions and still respect and believe the traditional Navajo beliefs. Most of the beliefs don't conflict. There is a time and place for everything and the back of an ambulance isn't the place to debate religion. I want my patients to feel comfortable. I have learned to show respect for other's beliefs. Not all people are religious but many are and when religion plays an important part of their life, the topic comes up at times during an emergency or a long range transport. Patient care sometimes goes beyond medical treatment. People are complicated. They are not a broken machine, they think and feel and their perspective, emotions and beliefs can affect how they respond to treatment, especially on long range transports. A million things are zinging around in their head as they try to cope with their situation. I have found if I can help lessen the patient's stress level, my patient is more cooperative and responsive to medical care. Often there is little I can do, but sometimes I can help. This time my care involved more than medical intervention.

Isolated small communities do not have the luxury of huge Trauma Centers. Patients transported from an accident scene often end up in a clinic with no beds for overnight stays. This day I asked to transport a man about thirty years old from Inscription House Clinic to Flagstaff Hospital (about one-hundred and seventy-five miles one way). He was bit on the hand by a rattlesnake. He was stable. His hand wasn't badly swollen. He was lucky; he had received only a little venom and would recover with his hand intact.

The patient began to tell me about his Navajo beliefs. He said that he was bitten by a snake and now he was dirty. His wife couldn't get near him, couldn't hold his hand, and couldn't touch him in any way. He couldn't hug his children either. He was dirty. He had driven himself to the clinic trying to save his family from becoming contaminated. He explained that the only way he could become clean again was to have a ceremony performed by a medicine man. It would be a complicated

158

ceremony and cost him a lot of money, but it had to be done and soon if he was to rejoin his family. At his request, I called his brother on the cell phone and explained the problem and let them talk. The brother lived near the Flagstaff Hospital and he said he would go get the medicine man and meet us at the hospital. I called the hospital emergency department and explained. They said they would have a room available so the ceremony could be performed in private. The hospital staff understood and allowed cultural differences to be accommodated as much as possible.

When we arrived, his family was waiting at the back door, standing fifty feet away and waved at him as we wheeled him into the hospital. The room was ready. About ten candles were burning, the brother and the medicine man went into the room and pulled the curtains. Sounds of a rattle and soft chanting drifted out into the ER and the smell of candles. I gave my report to the doc and went outside. His family came up and asked about him. They were waiting for the brother to come out and tell them they could now come in and be with the ill man. I told them he was stable and as soon as the ceremony was over and the doctor had treated his snake bite, they would be allowed in. His wife smiled and thanked us. I was glad I could help reunite this family.

IT'S A SMALL WORLD

It had been a busy morning. Gus Garnett, a PFD EMT, had lost his pager. We had collected a number of people to help find it. We decided to set it off and the beeping would alert us to its location. The trick was to find it before the batteries ran out. We stationed people at his place of work, inside and out, by his car, in his house, in his back yard, his garage, the fire station, etc.

I was standing in the fire bay when the pager was set off. I didn't hear anything. No one else heard anything either. We all began walking around listening for the beeping sound. I hurried all around the station but I didn't hear anything. At his place of work they come up empty too. At his home his wife, son, one firefighter and the Rescue Chief wandered inside and outside his house.

Suddenly, the firefighter heard something in the back yard as he neared the garden. He bent down and listened to the faint, muffled sound. "Guy's I think I hear something." They ran over and watched as the firefighter fell to his knees and began to dig up the newly planted garden.

159

"Hay, I worked half a day yesterday getting the garden planted," complained Gus.

The firefighter felt something and held it high into the air, "I found it." Two weeks before the Rescue Chief had lost his pager as well and we found it had been knocked off a table at his home and landed behind the sewing machine and the wall. This was getting old and the Fire Chief made a point of telling everyone to start paying more attention to their pager.

I had just received word the missing pager had been found when my own pager sounded.

It was a fairly routine call to Wahweap. The tour boat threw up a huge wake. Often it would cause a smaller boat to lunge upward off the wake and then come down hard on the other side. People inside would fly up off the seat and then come down hard. It was (and still is) common for this to result in damage to the lower spine (compression fracture). NPS usually handled medicals within the recreation area, but they were on another call, so we were called. We arrived at Wahweap and hurried out on the dock. We found our patient by the marina store.

She was about thirty, average size, dressed in a bathing suit. She had managed to walk off her boat and sit down at a picnic table. But, the pain became very intense and she laid down on the bench part of the picnic table unit. She lay on her back, her feet out on the bench and her arms hanging down to the deck on either side. She didn't know it but she had instinctively self-splinted her back. She looked up at me with eyes filled with tears, fear and pain. I introduced myself and began to question her. We connected well.

Then National Park Service arrived, two men in ugly gray shirts and army green pants, badges, guns, and an attitude. They approached me and said in a condescending voice, "Thanks, we can take it from here."

The patient looked at me confused and shifted her gaze to the ranger that had unceremoniously moved me aside. He began to speak with her as if he was interviewing a criminal. She obviously didn't like him. She interrupted him, looked back at me and asked "Do I have the right to choose who takes care of me?"

I was between the rock and the hard spot. Both rangers looked at me. I hesitated. It was the ranger's area. PFD had been invited but later dismissed and we were quickly becoming an intruder. We were called by NPS and we came, but rangers had become available and NPS had the right to dismiss us at any time. I decided to tell the truth. "Yes."

"Then I choose you (me), and you (rangers) go away." The rangers gave me a shocked look and backed off. My crew and I moved in and put the woman in full spinal precautions. It wasn't easy since she was lying on the narrow bench that was connected to the picnic table. We transported her to the hospital. I knew the top park ranger would be calling the Fire Chief. I did nothing wrong and I knew the Fire Chief would simply tell him the patient has a right to chose and perhaps Park Service should look into why she chose Page Fire over the rangers.

At the Page Hospital, the patient was diagnosed with spinal compression injuries to her lower back. We parted ways and I thought I would never see her again.

Three years later – Anaheim, California. My husband, two sons and I were on vacation, staying at the RV Park across from Disneyland. I was walking down to the office and I heard my name called out. "Sharon?" I turned around and there stood a woman with a big smile on her face. "Imagine, meeting you here. How are you?" the vaguely familiar women asked. I began to talk to her, but I didn't recognize her. "You don't remember me do you? she asked, still smiling.

I shook my head "No, I'm sorry."

She just smiled. "I injured my back at the lake......."

"I'm sorry, but I go on a lot of calls ...."

"I'm the one laying on the picnic table and wouldn't let the rude rangers treat me."

I broke out in a big smile, "Yes, I do remember you! You got me in trouble."

She laughed, "The rangers were sure mad....." She laughed again.

"How are you doing?" I asked. I was happy to find out she had completely recovered. She thanked me for taking care of her. We had a good visit. It was a happy ending. It is indeed a small world.

DID ANYONE EVER DIE IN HERE?

It was the Third of July, nearing sunset. Tuba City had a great firework show set off at the high school after dark on the fourth. Locals were not allowed to set off their own fireworks but many did anyways. I was about half way through my paramedic duty shift. I heard a pop nearby and peeked out the window of quarters. Gunfire in the neighborhood wasn't uncommon so I was interested in what had made the sound. Across the street three little boys were celebrating the coming holiday. The smallest boy around four years of age had climbed a ladder and sat on the roof of the front porch. The older boys, around nine and ten years of age,

161

stood in the sandy front yard lighting firecrackers. The fireworks would shoot into the air and explode in a shower of bright colored sparks. The littlest boy would giggle and clap. Their parents were inside the house and chose to let the boys have their fun. The fireworks were small. I played with fireworks as a child and I still have ten fingers so I decided to stay out of it.

I stood watching the show for a few minutes. One missile almost hit my car, but since it missed, I still decided to stay uninvolved. Then suddenly the small boy on the roof began to yell. The largest boy climbed the ladder and helped him to the ground and the three boys ran into the house. A few minutes later a Navajo Police cruiser drove slowly past the house. I heard the police traffic on the scanner. He was looking back and forth, searching for a reported illegal fireworks show. He left the area and the boys came out. They helped the little one back on the roof. Now I understood. He was the lookout. From his perch on the roof, he could see any approaching officer. They started to set off fireworks again. Then they stopped and ran inside the trailer. An officer drove by twice then left. They came back out and started again. This went on for a couple of hours.

My pager went off around the boy's bedtime. The hospital had a long range transport from Tuba to Chinle Hospital, around a two hundred and forty mile round trip. My EMT partner came out his room. He had been awakened by the pager. He stumbled over to the fridge and found a half-eaten submarine sandwich and a can of Pepsi. He tossed his snack into an insulated lunch bag and hurried outside with me right behind him.

At the hospital we found our patient in the ER. He was around forty years of age. He had wrecked his car. His injuries were not life threatening, but his arm was badly broken. Tuba Hospital was full and didn't have any beds so he was being transferred. The trip would take a little over an hour. I got all the paperwork, a report from the nurse and called medical control at Flagstaff Medical Center with a report of what I would be transporting. It was a simple transport and the call to Medical Control took only a few minutes.

We were in the ambulance and on our way in a short time. Some patients want to sleep. But most want to talk and he wanted to talk. He was a Navajo and lived in Red Lake. He was friendly and we had something is common, he had been an EMT. "Has anyone ever died in this ambulance?" he asked.

"Not on my watch," I told him.

"Good," he said. "When I was an EMT, I lost a patient in the back of my ambulance. I tried CPR, but everything went wrong. I know she was dead long before we reached the hospital."

"That's rough," I replied.

162

"Yeah . . . . She followed me home." He waited for my reaction.

I wasn't surprised. I have worked for years on the reservation. I am aware of their beliefs. Traditional Navajos believe they can be oppressed by those who have died. "What happened?" I asked.

"Everything. The truck quit running, my mother fell and broke her hip, my teenage son wrecked my Dad's car, my wife had a miscarriage and our sheep started dying for no reason. It was bad, really bad."

"What did you do?"

"We scrapped the money together and got a ceremony done. She left. I quit the business. I'm not an EMT anymore. I can't risk that happening again." I couldn't blame him. After working on the reservation for almost ten years, I may not completely understand it but I too am convinced there are things that go bump in the night. The patient I transported had told me a story I had heard before. The Navajo's have some serious concerns about the dead. The way it was explained to me, the Navajo's believe we all have good and bad inside us. They believe the good goes to what an Anglo would call "heaven." They believe the bad part is cursed to wander the earth. They don't speak of the dead in fear the dead will hear their name said out loud and then the bad part of a loved one, friend or neighbor might follow you home. If the person wasn't really that bad, it may be only a mischievous present, if they were evil in life, they could cause many terrible things to happen.

One of the Navajo EMS offices has an elderly Navajo woman "ghost" that moves furniture around their office and rearranges things on their desk. They didn't think it was serious enough to pay for a medicine man to come over and run her off. The door to the back bedroom would not stay shut. They decided to just leave it open. They ignored the faint figure that appeared in the doorway occasionally. They decided to leave the furniture the way she liked it and ignore the stapler that appears just right of the phone every morning, regardless of where they left it the evening before.

In general Navajo's tend to be superstitious. My mother was superstitious so I understand the concept. I once transported a six year old child with pneumonia. Her mother believed it was her fault that her daughter was so ill. "I knew better, but I cut her fingernails after dark." I had heard the same thing before. Navajo's can't cut a person's fingernails or hair after dark either without bad luck following. Bad moons also bring bad luck if someone is out after dark. Often people I pick up after dark, either in their home or from an outside location, have a smudge of ash on their forehead between their eyes, similar to the mark found on a Catholic's forehead on Ash Wednesday. They believe it wards off the curse

163

of a Bad Moon. Apparently it didn't work if I was called but to many it is very important.

The trip was uneventful. At Chinle we delivered him to the emergency department. He was scheduled for an orthopedic consult. We said our goodbyes and left him in the competent hands of the ER staff. By the time we got back to quarters, the boys had gone to bed and the fireworks show had ended for the night.

THE FIRE BREATHING DRAGON CALLED"FLASHOVER"

"Come on Honey," said the child's mother as she dug in her purse for the keys. "We have to get groceries before daddy gets off work." The girl was around three year old. She walked into the living room dragging her doll's blanket. She carried her doll in her arms. The chill of early spring still made it necessary to start a fire in the mornings. The morning fire was embers now. The little girl walked toward the fireplace and peaked in. She liked it when the flames danced around and she was disappointed the fire wasn't blazing. She had watched her mother and father start the fire many times. She knew how to get the fire to burn, but she wasn't supposed to do it. She turned and looked at her mother. The mother had moved to the kitchen and was searching for her keys. The little girl looked back at the fireplace. She tossed her dolls blanket into the fire place. The flames sprung to life.
"Come on Honey," said the child's mother, not noticing what the girl had done.

The tiny girl turned and hurried out the door with her mother. The fire grew larger as it consumed the blanket. The blanket was only half in the fireplace and the tail hung outside and to the side. As the fire ate its way down the tail, leaping flames caught the newspaper and then the drapes on fire. The fire on Thunderbird Street had begun. Neighbors were the first to notice smoke seeping from the cracks around the windows. The alarm was sounded and the fire engines rolled. The fire chief, in order to gain access, broke a small window and opened the back door. He foolishly, in the heat of the moment, used the radio he held in his hand and managed to slice his hand open. He knew better. He shoved a garden hose into the house.

I arrived and immediately saw the fire wasn't that big. It involved the corner of the living room and part of the breakfast bar. The burning drapes had set fire to a spot on the ceiling, but that was all. It wouldn't

164

take a lot of water to put this one out. I saw blood running down the Chief's arm. I approached him with my kit. As he yelled orders in his radio, I chased his waving hand around and bandaged the wound. The entry crew went in through the back door. It opened onto a long hallway that ran from the back master bedroom to the living area with bath, washroom, and child's bedroom opening onto it. All the doors were closed. Three firemen entered and drug a hose with them. There was a shortage of firefighters and their backup, Mark Teak stayed just outside the back door with a charged line.

I usually don't get that close to a working fire when assuming the Medical Control Sector, but this one was small and Mark wasn't wearing his gloves and got a large splinter in his hand. I walked over and pull it out and covered it with a band aid. I gave him my turnouts, gloves and helmet. I held the hose while he put them on. Mike took the hose back. "Now keep the visor down too," I said as I reached up and lowered his visor.

"Yes, mother," he said.

Then it happened. A Page Police Officer, in misguided heroism, kicked down the front door. A gust of fresh oxygen fed the small hungry fire. I heard the door kicked in and peaked in the door and looked down the hallway. "What was that?" I said to Mark as he peeked around me. I could see the three firefighters were on their hands and knees and they were almost to the living room. They certainly hadn't made the noise.

Then everything happened at once. It appeared to happen in slow-motion. The living room exploded in orange and yellow flame. The fire rose to the ceiling. Black smoke with balls of orange and yellow fire rolled along the ceiling toward the back of the trailer. It resembled an angry churning flash flood of roaring water. The sound was loud like a freight train. The flames followed the ceiling, setting on fire the upper molding strips and the top half of the paneling that ran down the hallway. It was beautiful in a strange way. It appeared to move in slow motion, graceful billows of black, yellow and orange, dancing down the hall toward me.

Flashover! I had never seen it before, but I knew what it was. I was in the wrong place and I was about to be engulfed in a ball of flame. This was bad since I had just given my turnouts away. I watched in fascination for a split second and then my well-developed sense of survival sprang into action. I withdrew from the door way, spinning around and flattened my back up against the side of the trailer. I yelled, "Get back . . . !" to Mark who was knocked backwards by my hasty retreat.

The rolling ball of flame hit the master bedroom door at the end of the hall and exploded. It instantly set the entire door on fire. The left over flame from the flashover shot out the open back door like a dragon's breath. It flashed by me as I pressed my back up against the wall. Mark disappeared from sight as the flames totally engulfed him. Mark had managed to stay on his feet and rushed forward with the backup hose fully open. The firemen inside had flattened themselves on the floor as the flame flashed over their heads. Now the hallway was a blazing tunnel. The molding strip was made of plastic and melted and dripped on the three men crouching in the hallway. Captain Alto had been bringing up the rear and was a little slow in issuing the command to abandoned ship and the two fire fighters in front of him climbed over him and hurried for the exit.

I stepped back from the now burning trailer. The back door frame was now ablaze. Mark pumped water into the hallway to provide an escape for the firefighters that were now beating a hasty retreat. They exited in reverse, feet first. They seemed to all tumble out at once onto the ground and then get to their feet and hurry away from the flames. All hell broke loose. The fire was no longer small. The limited manpower was suddenly an issue. And if at that moment any member of the fire department could have gotten their hands on the "helpful" policeman, he would have died a horrible death. The fire was now fought differently. A firefighter joined Mark and they attacked the fire driving it back down the hallway to the living room. Another hose went in the front door, now hanging by one hinge, thanks to the hyper police officer. The fire was driven back to its original area. That area had already burned and there was no more fuel, so the fire monster died of starvation.

The front of the trailer was destroyed, as well as the items in the living room and kitchen. But the rest of the belongings were saved. I was in the wrong place at the wrong time. I let my guard down, thinking it was a small fire, forgetting how quickly things can change. I knew better and should have never taken that chance with a working fire. I had given my protective gear away and if Mark hadn't been dressed in the turnouts he would have been swallowed up by the Dragon's fiery breath and would have suffered serious burns. Luck was with me that day. I got to witness a firefighting event that is by far the most spectacular to see, a flashover, and I lived to tell the story.

THE KEY DID NOT FIT

John Hail was as big as a bear and as strong as one. He was a great EMT/Firefighter and was well liked. One evening we were partnered together. We received a call to Wahweap Resort and Marina on Lake Powell. It's about ten miles north of town. The report was woman with a

166

server asthma attack. Asthma causes inflammation and narrowing of the airway as a result of an allergic reaction to environmental pollutants, stress, pollen, some chemicals, and food allergies to name a few of the causes. Usually the Park Service handled EMS calls at the resort, but apparently they were one short a crew this time.

I pulled up at the new fire station and rushed inside. The EMT who was driving was already behind the wheel. I was riding "shotgun" as John climbed in the back. With red lights flashing and siren blaring we pulled up to the edge of Coppermine Road. To our right the road started down a steep hill. It was impossible to see oncoming traffic. They couldn't see us either. It was a blind spot of enormous size. The old Fire Station was very old, cramped and inadequate, but I never liked the new station. It didn't feel right and I found it strange that it was built on the far west side, nowhere near the center of the town and at the top of a hill that didn't allow a clear view of traffic. Having to stop and slowly pull into traffic slows emergency response and creates a potentially dangerous situation. I once suggested a flashing light to warn oncoming traffic, but the city council has never been known for its common sense and found other projects on which to spend the money. Today, years later there is still no light.

"Cross your fingers," said the EMT driving as he inched slowly onto the road. No one was coming. We were en route. I stuck my head through the small window connecting the cab with the passenger compartment. "John," I said, "When we get there I will need the drug box. Can you take these keys and get it out of the compartment?"

"Sure," he said. He took the keys and went to a locked compartment in the wall on the driver's side. It was located at the foot of the stretcher on the driver's side of the ambulance.

"The key doesn't fit," John announced.

"Maybe I gave you the wrong one. Try another one." I was a reserve paramedic at the Page Fire at the time, a contract paramedic at a local coal mine and ran as a paramedic for an independent ambulance company so my key chain had a lot of keys. I watched as John struggled with the keys. He tried them all and none worked. I had to have the Albuterol for a breathing treatment (SVN). It opens the bronchial tubes and allows an asthmatic patient to breath. Without the drug it would be about as good to transport her in the back of a car. "John, I have got to have that box."

"I know, but the key doesn't work." He handed me the rig of keys. I looked them over and found the key and handed it to him. "I'm sure this is the key."

John took the key and tried again. We left town behind us. There was very little traffic. John giggled the key in the lock. It didn't work. He did it again and again. The compartment door remained tightly closed. "It won't work."

I had to have the drug by the time we arrived. "John, no matter what you have to do, I have to have to have that drug box when we arrive."

"Ok," he said. I glanced out the front windshield and saw we were approaching the turn off to the lake. This was before they built the guard house and demanded money to enter the Glenn Canyon Recreation Area. At the time National Park Service could not charge anyone to enter a recreation area. They could only charge for National Parks. But a few years later the law as "interpreted" in another way and they started charging a high fee to enter. Many locals who had limited income can still view the lake from afar, but not up close due to the charge. NPS about five years ago decided they needed more money in addition to the entrance fees. They put "donation" envelopes in every hotel room. They only got eight dollars. So the next season NPS decided the donation program should be made more "convenient" for the visitors. They decided to automatically charge two dollars a day on all room, boat rental, and some other activities. Locals call it the "Feed a Hungry Ranger" Program. Of course, technically it was "a donation" so if the tourist requested for it be removed, it would be removed. But the name they gave it was vague and non-descriptive and of course no one was told the charge was an optional donation. So only a few tourists who questioned the charge and locals who knew about it requested it be removed. NPS was thrilled when donations went up.

Suddenly a loud ripping sound came from the back. I looked back and saw John holding the door to the compartment in his huge hands. Splintered wood lay scattered about. The compartment opening now had ragged edges were the door had been ripped out, hinges and all. "I got it open," he said.

"I can see that," I answered. I had not expected him to rip the door off with his bare hands, but I now had access to my drug box. "Thanks John." John was a brute and after all is said and done, I told him "No matter what you have to do . . ."

Just then the dispatcher called. I picked up the radio mike and answered. "Medic-Two."

"Medic-Two, you are cancelled. The Park Service got a crew together and they are going to handle the call."

"Medic-Two copies, we are cancelled, returning to station, available for call." When we got back to the station I climbed in back to survey the damage. It was a sight to behold. I swept out the splintered wood. John commented about the broken compartment door. I had been giving some thought to the situation. "John, you did exactly as you should have. You found a way to access the drug box. If the Fire Chief gives you any grief, you tell him you were just following my orders. I will talk to him in the morning and let him know what happened. Thanks for getting me my drug box. Even though we were cancelled, my key didn't work and we might need that drug box on the next call."

The next morning I went to the fire station and found the Fire Chief, Leo Cain. He was the kind of man who seldom smiled, growled often and led by intimidation. If someone disagreed with him or did something he didn't like he would start to yell. He had discovered that if he yelled loudly, most people would back down. If they didn't he just yelled louder and louder. His favorite position for a discussion was him leaning over his desk looking his advisory in the eye and yelling to the top of his lungs. He firmly believed "who yelled the loudest won the argument." If you somehow won the disagreement or refused to back down, you were put on his list. You did not want to be on his list. He never forgot or forgave. To my knowledge everyone on that list eventually was fired or forced out of the Fire Department one way or the other.

I had known Leo for years before he became chief. He had worked for NPS and in the course of doing our jobs we came in contact with each other. Probably because of our previous working relationship, we got along well and he never personally gave me any problems, but his policies and his "whip and chair" type of leadership made working for him difficult. He was not the popular choice for the position of Fire Chief and some theorized he somehow kissed the right butt or had some compromising photos of someone to be appointed Fire Chief by City Council over the protests of many. He was very good at fighting fires and even though he was a bit prone to micromanage, he handled Incident Command well. On paper he did his job well but there were a few skeletons in the closet. Many people believe him to be a seriously dangerous and disliked man so they tiptoed around him, being careful to "not to poke the tiger with a stick".

That morning I found him in his office. "Can you come with me? I have something to show you." He got up and followed me into the ambulance bay. I told him about the call and about my inability to access my drug box. I opened the ambulance and told him, "I told John that no matter what he had to do, I needed that drug box."

"So he ripped the door off . . . . ."

"Yes."

The chief sighed. Firemen were traditionally rough. They often don't have a gentle bone in their body. He wasn't surprised. "Well, the reason your key didn't work is because we changed the locks yesterday. I assume you didn't get the new key."

"No. No one called me and when I came on duty Jones didn't mention it. I don't want you to blame John for this . . . . this . . . . destruction. He was only following orders and we all had the patient's best interest at heart."

"I know. I'll get someone to repair the door." He took me into his office and gave me a new key.

$8.26

During my career I have met many battered women. One stands out in my mind. Her name was Rosie. She lived in a small three bedroom house (Indian Public Housing) in Tuba. She was forty-two, five foot tall and overweight. She didn't drink alcohol. Her "common law husband" drank enough for both of them. He had slapped her teenage son around a number of times and finally she sent her oldest child to live with his grandmother a few blocks away. She was absolutely terrified of her live-in boyfriend. Each call, her injuries were worse.

One week I went on a call and he had hit her, knocking her to the ground. He then kicked and kicked her. Then he stomped repeatedly on her knee. He was mad because they had $8.26 cents, just enough to buy a bottle of liquor at Antelope Hills, a trading post just off the reservation. She made the mistake of telling him she couldn't go get his alcohol today, something about her grade school children. He began to yell and threaten her. He didn't care if they didn't have a car and it required her to walk to Highway 160 (a few blocks), hitch a ride west to the junction (thirteen miles). Then she would catch a ride going south on Highway 89 (twenty-two miles) to Antelope Hills. Then buy the liquor and hitch back home with the alcohol tucked under her blouse. She was risking jail if caught with the liquor on the Reservation, but she feared him more. That day she had limped to her neighbor's house and called the ambulance. The ER x-rayed the knee and put a serious brace on it and told her to keep off it as much as possible and come back next week.

Next week arrived and I got a call. Rosie's boyfriend had $8.26 cents again and wanted her to go get him a bottle. Her knee hurt and she could barely limp around the house. There was no way she could hike to the highway and hitch a ride. He exploded in anger and knocked her to the ground. He then repeatedly stomped on her injured knee. I guess he was mad at it because it was the reason she couldn't get him alcohol. He had inflicted the injury to it to begin with, remember? I found her hiding at a neighbor's house, screaming in pain. He really hurt her knee this time.

I usually don't offer advice but this time I had too. I told Rosie, "He's going to kill you one of these days." She shook her head in agreement. "You don't have to put up with this." She began to cry. Before the short ride was over, she agreed to meet with a worker of Family Harmony (Navajo's family service organization). I explained to the nurse in the ER. She made the necessary calls and they came to the ER. The police were called to arrest her boyfriend. She promised to get a restraining order against him. He was black, not Navajo, so she also filed papers to have him thrown off the reservation and he would face arrest if he sat foot on it again. It took a long time of abuse for her to find the strength, but Rosie finally stood up for herself. I honestly believe that day I helped save her life.

NO SCENE IS EVER SAFE,
BUT SOME ARE SAFER THAN OTHERS

EMTs and Paramedics deal with volatile personalities and step into situations full of conflict with confusing and incomplete stories. Danger is a part of the job and to tell the truth, it is exciting. Many jobs are stressful, but most don't involve the worker facing a life and death situation. In EMS if they do it wrong they won't get fired, they die.

This story takes place in Vermillion Trailer Court (now called Lake Powell Mobil Home Park). Two men, Vince and Wally, had been watching the football game. A few beers too many lead to an argument that turned to physical pushing and shoving. Wally ordered his guest to leave. As the two men continued to shout obscenities at each other Vince was escorted to the door. As Wally stood on the porch, Vince walked down the steps, mumbling. He was really mad. He reached into his pants and withdrew a knife and spun around. He jabbed upward in an attempt to stab Wally below the sternum, hoping to hit his heart. The knife hit the sternum, a flat bone, and slid off causing minor skin tearing. The second stab was caught by the Wally as he struggled to disarm the attacker. The knife cut into the flesh of his hand, but he knew if he let go, he was a dead man. He managed to pull the knife from the attacker's grasp. Vince turned and ran, screaming, "I'm going home to get my gun!"

171

I arrived as EMT first responder and found Wally sitting on the steps of his trailer. Blood ran from many cuts on his hands and forearms. He and his clothing were covered in blood. An officer drove up and hurried over. I kneeled down and began bandaging his wounds as I listened to the story. I quickly realize the scene wasn't safe. The attacker had promised to return with a gun and we didn't know where he was right now. As I quickly bandaged his arms and hands, an officer stood over me with a shotgun cocked.   He looked back and forth. He was very alert, providing me and the patient some protection, but we all knew this wasn't enough if the man decided to be a sniper and take a shot. If Vince really wanted Wally dead, he would not be happy that I was helping Wally. Talk about stress. I felt as if I was standing in the patient's front yard with a bull's eye on my back. The radio came to life. I told the responding ambulance to pull up, but don't get out. I would walk the patient to the ambulance. The ambulance pulled up, we quickly walked up and the patient got in, I told the driver to take off right now because the scene wasn't safe. Doug Alton sped off to the hospital. I got in my car and quickly left the scene. Only a minute or two later I heard on the radio the man was caught with a rifle about a block away. We got out of Dodge just in time.

THE EASY WAY OR THE RIGHT WAY

When the sales clerk at the local department store is feeling a little lazy, the worst thing that can happen is the department may not be as neat and well organized as usual when the store opens the next day. When the cook at the local pizza parlor is having a bad day, well, the world won't end if he forgets the extra cheese. But it's a different ball game when the person handling a medical emergency can't or won't get their act together. Emergency Medical workers are human. But the majority of the public think they can walk on water and raise the dead. They can't. They are good, very good at what they do, but it takes effort, constant training, quality review of calls, and once in a while, a boss that will kick them in the ass and tell them to shape up or get out. I was the ass kicker in the PFD Rescue Division. The EMT's were good and usually I had to use a fine toothed comb to find a problem, but this time was different. Sometimes they would forget to do something, but almost always it was something small that really didn't make much difference one way or the other. But occasionally they blew it.

172

I carefully reviewed their written reports. If the report was used in a court case, the report would be blown up to four feet by six feet and every small mistake would make the medic look stupid or incompetent. The report would be all you had to refer to if you were sued or asked to testify in a court of law. If an EMT treated a newborn baby, in Arizona the parents had eighteen years to sue, and the baby then had an additional three years to sue. Our memory can grow vague after twenty-one years, so written reports are important. On a copy of the reports I would mark with a yellow highlighter spelling and grammar mistakes and return it to them. My yellow highlighter was joked about but mostly feared. One time I asked a male EMT ". . . you did 'what' to a woman in a blanket?" He read his report. *"I then raped the woman in the blanket."* He turned red and stammered. He corrected the report to read *"I then wrapped the woman in the blanket."*

I also checked quality of treatment given. One time an EMT named Sara Simmons blew it. She was an average EMT and the oldest one we had working in our department at the time. She had seen her fiftieth birthday a few years before. She was short and a bit heavy. She dressed impeccably and her hair, makeup, and accessories were always perfect. She sold Avon on the side and did quite well. She was sociable and easy to talk too. Although Sara did well as a member of the crew, she had not yet mastered the art of *being in charge*. She tried, and usually managed to provide adequate care. But her desire to do things *the easy way* at times interfered with her reaching the higher level of competency she could have reached with a little more effort.

One such time involved two men, whose pickup had hit a guard rail down by the Glen Canyon Bridge. One man was of average size and the other was over three-hundred and fifty pounds. Both were in the same accident and both had the same complaints, but Sara, for the sake of convenience, dropped the ball. The average size man was found outside the vehicle. Sara put a c-collar on him and his head was held as he was log rolled upon a backboard, carefully maintaining spinal integrity. His head was secured to the board and he was transported using the backboard as a big splint for his neck and back.

The three-hundred and fifty pound man had felt the urge to lie down after the accident and had crawled into the back of the tiny camper. He filled the small compartment. Sara checked him over and knew getting him out of there would be very hard, and damn near impossible with the limited number of manpower they had on the scene, if they were to go for complete spinal precautions. Sara decided to let the patient move himself to a sitting position on the tail gate of the pickup and then stand up. He then turned around and sat on the backboard they had placed on the gurney. They delivered him all packaged just like the other guy. Some places allow EMT's to clear c-spine in the field, but Arizona wasn't one of those places. Some EMS responders bend the rule almost to the breaking point and don't board all patients or do it in a sloppy, easy manner by allowing them to move to the backboard on their own power. I found the practice common in Phoenix, but my department knew it wasn't acceptable.

When I reviewed the report I saw at once there had been a serious breach in SOP's. I called her in for a talk. "Sara, why did you take spinal precautions on the one man and not on the other?"

"Oh, I did it on both."

"No you didn't. It's true you delivered both men to the hospital strapped on a backboard, but you let one stand up and move himself."

"Well, he was really big and we couldn't lift him." Her eyes told me she knew she was in trouble and she also knew I wasn't going to buy it.

"If you needed additional help, why didn't you just use your radio and call me or another staff member?"

"It was really late, and. . . . .well . . . . . "

"That isn't a problem Sara, you know that. You could have paged the duty crew to help. Time wasn't a serious consideration in this call. You could have waited for them to help. You were only about a hundred feet outside the city limits."

"I didn't think of that." She tried to think of something to say that would get her off the hook." He was a very large man. I just thought we could let him move himself. It was the easiest way to get him out of the camper shell."

My eyes flashed. That was the wrong thing to say. I had to learn to walk again after a serious accident that involved spinal cord and nerve damage. I know firsthand what it is like to not be able to take care of yourself. I personally know the pain and humiliation involved in just sitting there and letting others do things for you. No, you could never convince me that spinal precautions were no big deal. "Both men were in the same accident and they both presented with the same symptoms and complaints. Just because one man is overweight isn't a valid reason to take that kind of chance with his quality of life."

She sighed then said, "OK, I won't do it again."

"That's not good enough Sara. You have to understand, we can put one-hundred people on a backboard and ninety-nine won't need it. But we do it for the one out of a hundred who does need it. (See the story "The One in a Hundred.) You see, we can't tell which one he is. No one deserves to be forced to live the rest of his life in a wheelchair or on a respirator just because of your convenience." I was getting wound up, bring out the soap box. Sara didn't like my tone of voice or what I was saying. She knew I was right but she was defensive and wanted to just get this over with and get home. I wouldn't let her go, not till she understood she was to take spinal precautions on all patients that "may" need it regardless of race, creed, religion and weight. I continued. "I am not doing this for this man. He was one of the ninety-nine. It didn't matter in his case. But you just might meet that one in a hundred next time and it will matter." At the time I didn't realize how prophetic my statement turned out to be.

Less than a week later, Sara was on another call. A car had rolled near Cedar Ridge. It was around forty miles south from Page. She was in charge again and my words still rang in her ears and some self-righteous anger still remained inside her. The car lay on its roof about thirty feet off the roadway. The man inside the vehicle was conscious. Sara crawled into the glass strewn car and checked him out. This man was average size, but the car's roof was caved in and there just wasn't a lot of space to move around. Getting him out wasn't going to be easy, not if she decided to do a full spinal immobilization on the man.

She later told me she remembered my words. "Convenience isn't a valid reason to not do something that should be done." She looked around in the dark mass of twisted metal. She crawled back out. She looked up at her partner, "Get me a back board, KED, cervical collar and head immobilizer." The driver sighed and turned around to go get the requested items. He wasn't that excited about what he knew lay ahead. "Oh yes, and bring something to get this windshield out. We will bring him out that way." Sighing again, the EMT hurried off.

The windshield came out fairly easy. The man didn't. They couldn't get the backboard inside the car because of the way the metal and seats had twisted. So Sara, doing the best she could and using a great deal of imagination, managed with help, to get him in a KED. His head and back was held still during the process which is no small matter. They then moved him outside the car and onto the backboard. "Probably all a waste of time," the other EMT thought. So did the police, so did everyone. But Sara wasn't about to face another ass kicking incident in my office. Even if the man didn't have any symptoms of spinal injuries, the car was destroyed and he defiantly rolled it several times. She stood stubbornly to her decision and defended it afterward when the others complained.

The next day I sat in my office working on next week's training drill when Sara came in. "I wanted to let you know something. You know I was really mad at you the other day."

I smiled. "I know."

"Well, last night your words came back to me as I lay in that overturned car. I really wanted very badly to let that man move himself out of the car, but after what you had said, I took the hard way and we did full spinal precautions on him."

"That was the right thing to do."

"Yes, it was. You see he was the one in the one hundred. He didn't have any symptoms at the scene. But en route he started to complain a little. At the hospital they found he had fractured C-2, 3, and 4." Cervical vertebras two, three and four are in the neck. That information even caught me off guard. C-2, 3, and 4? The bones were broken and sharp. The thin spinal cord, the size and texture of half cooked spaghetti was just sitting there still intact but surrounded by sharp bone fragments. One wrong move and the man would have been a paraplegic, living the rest of his life on a respirator, unable to move anything from the neck down.

I smiled. "Good work Sara."

She smiled. "I just wanted you to know, it did sink in. I couldn't have lived with myself if I had caused that man to become paralyzed. I'm glad you yelled at me."

"I just want you to be the best you can be. I'm glad you listened. It isn't easy being boss and doing what has to be done when you know you are going to hurt you friend's feelings in the process."

"Better my feelings hurt than that man being paralyzed." I felt good. If I did nothing else during all those years, I was directly responsible for a man that is walking around now, leading a full life when he came so close to being forced to live a life that many would consider not worth living. Sara kept improving with time and by the time she moved away, she was a good EMT and never let convenience color her judgment when it came to patient care.

BABYSITTING GRANDMA

I was working at the Page Hospital Emergency Department as an ER Tech. One day just before lunch, a pickup pulled up at the emergency entrance and a young teenage girl ran into the foyer and retrieved a wheelchair. I went out as an elderly woman was being helped from the vehicle. She appeared to be in her early to mid-seventies. She was Navajo and dressed in traditional style. Her shirt was dark purple and made of soft velvet material. It was a type of tunic with a v-neck and hem that hung below her waist. Her skirt was full and made of a lighter purple with many, many tiny pleats. The skirt was long and stopped halfway between her

176

knee and ankle. She wore a large turquoise broach at the v-neckline and a beautiful turquoise bracelet. Her thinning hair was still black with only some gray. It was long and was rolled up and tied with a wool string at the nape of her neck to form a type of an oblong bun. She didn't appear to be in a life and death emergency. A woman wheeled her into the ER. I asked ". . . What's the matter?"

The woman began to explain, "My mother hasn't been feeling well for the past few days." The nurse on duty came over and took them into a room. I started to gather vital signs as she questioned them. The woman continued. "She won't eat. She just lies around not doing anything. That's not like her. I think she's sick." Her vital signs were normal and she didn't have a fever. She took only one high blood pressure pill daily and had taken it that day. She sat on the gurney looking around and didn't appear in distress. The nurse continued to question the patient's daughter. The mother didn't speak English so the daughter translated. The patient's son-in-law stood nearby with his teenage daughter and son. The other son, around eleven years of age looked bored. As they waited, the patient drank a cup of water and talked to her daughter. She did not appear to be in pain or discomfort. The doctor was called and examined her. He then left the patient and walked over to the nursing station and sat down. I walked over. He didn't appear happy. I asked him what was the matter.

"There's nothing wrong with her." He took out an admit slip and began to fill it out.

"Are you admitting her?"

"I don't have a lot of choice. She is elderly, her caregiver says she's not eating and isn't feeling well. I tried to talk the woman into taking her mother home, but she insists she isn't good at caring for the ill and refuses to assume responsibility. She demands I admit her overnight for observation."

"But what good will that do?"

The nurse walked up and joined us. "Guess who's going to Flagstaff as soon as they get grandma settled in a room here at Page Hospital?"

I took a guess, "Them?" indicating the room full of family members and the elderly woman.

"Bingo. Grandma didn't want to go so they brought her here, to the Page Hospital Resort," the nurse said.

"So this is all a game to get grandma a babysitter while they go on a trip," I said.

"Yeah," answered the doctor. "They know Medicare will pay for 80% of the bill and Medicaid will pay the rest. It's a cheap way for them to make certain grandma has someone to watch over her until they return."

"And we pick up the tab," commented the nurse. Grandma was admitted. The family kissed her goodbye and left for Flagstaff.

This began on a Friday. Grandma had been admitted for a twenty-four hour observation. Saturday rolled around and Grandma was still doing great and the doctor wanted to release her. The family couldn't be found. The cell number they left was turned off. Grandma ate like a horse. She watched TV and took naps. She was waited upon hand and foot. She took a warm bath each day, walked in the garden and enjoyed her stay at the Page Hospital Spa & Resort. Sunday came and went with no contact with her family. The doctor wanted to discharge her but without a caregiver, he couldn't. He couldn't even call for Arizona Adult Services because it was the weekend and there was only one woman who covered the entire northern half of Arizona. If she was working overtime on a case it would be one of abuse or neglect not overstaying her welcome at the hospital. Grandma was an adult and her children actually had no legal obligation to care for her. When the family returned from their trip they would come get her.

Monday morning arrived. After school had begun, the patient's daughter showed up at her mother's room. The woman knew Medicare would pay for three days only so she returned to pick up grandma before 11 a.m. on Monday. The elderly woman was checked out and taken home.

Medicare paid most of the bill and Medicaid picks up the co-pay for Native Americans, so Grandma's weekend at the Page Hospital Resort and Spa cost them nothing. While I worked at the hospital I saw this story repeated over and over again. The care was "free" as far as the families saw it and they worked the system. The fact they failed to understand was that the babysitting wasn't free. You and I paid the bill. This is only one of the many ways I saw the system perverted. Free health care isn't free.

THE WOODEN LEG

The EMT or Paramedic has to stay constantly alert for the unexpected. One such situation happened on a cool fall day. The trees had lost most of their leaves. The sky was overcast; a slight cool breeze blew from the south west. I turned onto Cedar Street and began looking for the address. It was a quiet residential area, plain cinder block, rectangular homes with two trees out front in every yard. I was responding as Rescue Chief for PFD. The call was for "a man lying in his front yard." I then saw him. The man was laying supine (on his back) "spread eagle." I got out with my jump kit and walked over to him. I kneeled down beside him. He was around mid-40 years of age, lying on the grass of his front yard. He was dressed in jeans, long sleeve plaid flannel shirt, tennis shoes. He had a full beard that had begun to turn gray. He didn't open his eyes when I walked up, but when I started talking he looked up at me. He was dazed and in a shaky voice, told me he was trimming the tree and fell out.

I looked up, to gauge the height of the tree. Directly above me was a chain saw. It was dangling overhead, held by the cord he had plugged into an extension cord. If the plug pulled out, the heavy saw would fall and I would get a chainsaw in the head. I had blindly walked into a hazardous situation. I had focused on the man lying in the grass and had not taken a minute to look around for other dangers. I knew better. I cradled his head on my forearms and my hands under his shoulders; I gently pulled him away from the tree. Another thing happened that was funny on this call. As I was checking him over, I discovered he had a wooden leg and that was part of the problem with him climbing a tree. R.J. was an EMT and worked for Fed Ex at the time. He drove up in the Fed Ex truck and jumped out to help till the ambulance got there. He was a brand new EMT and in his hurry to assess the patient, he told me the patient had a good pulse in both feet. That was a great trick with a wooden leg. He later became a paramedic, but never lived it down the fact that he felt a pulse on a wooden foot. The man had no serious injuries but minor aches and pains. And after being checked out at the hospital was released.

CHILDREN SHOULDN'T DIE

Did you ever get that gut feeling that something awful was about to happen? I felt it that day when my pager went off one Sunday afternoon. It was a clear but cold winter day. Some spots of snow lay on the surrounding red cliffs. I could see my breath as I hurried for my car. I wasn't on the duty schedule, but I drove down to the station anyway. Why? I don't know why, I just did. Call it women's intuition, lucky guess, ESP, or just plain weird, but I had a feeling this call was something more than it appeared to be. It was a reported one car accident with one dead and one hurt at the Little Cut. Don Alton was driving; Susan Elders and Gordon Taylor were in the back. It was a good crew.

At the station, I found the report hadn't changed much. There was now two dead and one hurt. Where did the second body come from? Or did the first injured person die and another injured person suddenly

179

materialized at the scene? Did I go with them? As Rescue Chief it was my call. On out of town calls I usually didn't go to the scene unless I was on the schedule. The original call and even the second report was something the crew could handle alone. But still I had that nagging feeling that I should go. Over the years I have learned to listen to that quite voice that comes from somewhere deep inside me. I decided to jump in the back. I seldom did this, but I knew beyond a doubt I should go on this call.

Susan Eldon was getting in back of the ambulance. I climbed up front. Susan and I were often in competition. She joined the department soon after I joined. She was short and a little stout, dark hair cut short. She was a no-nonsense person and made decisions quickly. She and I had both been up for the Rescue Chief's job, and I got it. She could have done the job as well. She was a good EMT and easy to work with. I trusted her judgment and respected her. Later, she convinced her husband to do what few of us women in Page could, she got him to bid on a job in Phoenix and they moved back to the real world. She went back to school and became a nurse.

On with the story . . . . The Little Cut is a path carved through a mountain by dynamite and a determined road crew. The highway passed through the steep sided "cut" and out the other side on its way to Page. The cut has been the site of many accidents over the years. It's downhill, sharp curves, and in the wintertime, ice covered in the areas where the sun never shines.

"We now have a report that there are two injured and only one dead at the scene," reported the dispatcher.

"Wonderful. They sure didn't need us; one of the dead has come back to life," I said.

"Sounds that way," answered Gordon Taylor. Gordon was in his forties, strong and opinioned. He drove heavy equipment. He and I had problems when he came to work at the department. We went through some bad times. He didn't like taking orders from anyone and a woman made it twice as bad. It finally came down to me telling him "I'm your boss Gordon. You have to make up your mind. Either learn to live with it or quit." I secretly hoped he wouldn't quit. He was a very good EMT and an excellent ambulance driver. He went home and three days later he came into my office and said he had thought it over and he could live with it. It's funny, but I liked to work with Gordon and I grew to think of him as a friend. I believe he felt the same way. What he lacked in social grace, he made up in skill.

My thoughts returned to the present. We now have the report of one dead and one injured . . . ." announced the dispatcher. My mind raced. Obviously whoever was feeding the dispatcher reports couldn't tell

180

a dead person from a live one. This worried me. That meant that we had two patients that somehow were hurt so bad that no one could make up their mind if they were alive or dead. We set up for the worst case scenario.

As the road crawls up the hill toward the "Little Cut", the road takes a long wide swing to the right. Just were the curve straightens up and enters the first cut, there was the accident. As we pulled up at the scene, I could see a new, large black pickup sitting on its wheels at the side of the road. The pickup had been traveling to Page and had just driven through the cut. The truck sat pointing west (it had been traveling East) in the soft sand of a wide spot about the size of a small house lot. The view of the entire Lake Powell/Page/Glen Canyon Recreation Area was breath taking from the scene but no one noticed that day. We hurried to the truck.

I was met by a man in is fifties. He was tall and wide. A woman I later found out was his wife stood beside him. They were Navajo Indians. She was dressed in traditional style clothes, velvet blouse, and long pleated skirt. Her black hair was pulled straight back and an elongated bun was arranged at the back of her neck. The man was wearing cowboy clothing.

"Our daughter is hurt bad, but she's breathing, now. . . . Our son is hurt real bad too . . . ."

I could see the girl so...."Where's the boy?"

"Over there....." the man pointed.

"Susan (Eldon), you take the boy, Gordon, you check the girl."

To the father, "What happened?" I asked.

"We slid on the ice and the truck rolled on its top." The father looked pale and I began to wonder if he was alright. The family had attended church that morning. They decided to drive into Page (from Cedar Ridge) to have a Sunday dinner with their family. Eleven people could not fit in the cab. So, Mom and Dad, plus three of the smaller male children, about four, six and eight years of age sat in the front seat. Adult son, his wife and new born daughter sat in the cab's back seat with the ten year old son. No one was wearing a seat belt. Their fifteen year old daughter and twelve year old son were riding in the pickup bed.

The truck slid on the ice, spinning backwards, leaving the roadway, rolling one full time then coming to rest on its passenger side. The fifteen year old girl and her twelve year old brother had been thrown out of the pickup bed as the truck rolled. "The truck landed on our daughter and son," The mother said. She was breathing fast and although she tried, her voice betrayed her fears. "We rolled the truck over on its wheels. . . . ."

181

". . . . . . And dug our daughter out," said the father finishing his wife's sentence.

"The officer said our daughter and son was dead, but she started to breath," added the mother. Now I understood why the report kept changing. I walked over to the girl and looked down. She lay in a hole, a small round hole in the sand. When she was thrown out of the pickup she landed on the sand on her knees. The truck rolled on top of her, bending her forward, face down in a tight fetal position. The force of the truck shoved her body into the soft sand making a hole with her in the center face down, in a tight ball. Gordon was working on the girl. Her long black hair had sand in it. She was small and pretty. She was in bad shape. Her respirations were labored, irregular, and noisy. I didn't have to examine her to know she was going to die and soon, unless she got to the hospital and even then I wouldn't place heavy bets on her long range survival. Chest injuries are real killers. Then with her head bent forward as she sat wadded up in the hole, thoughts of possible spinal cord injury sprang to mind. And let us not forget head injuries, after all a truck had rolled on top of her. This girl was seriously injured.

"How many were in the pickup?" I asked. The man and woman stumbled around for a minute counting and recounting.

"Eleven." he finally said. I looked around. There were people sitting, laying, and walking around the entire area. ELEVEN? This was just getting better and better. I didn't say anything at that time. I walked over to the boy. He too was shoved into a hole and lay wadded up in a ball, face down. He was twelve. Susan Eldon looked up at me. □

We had run so long together I could read her mind. He was dead and she didn't want him to be. "I can't get a pulse," she said. I bent down and felt the boy's neck. He was warm. Bubbles still clung to his lips, pink bubbles. I couldn't feel a pulse either. I moved my fingers again and again. I wanted nothing more than to feel a pulse. But it wasn't to be. There was no heartbeat. I leaned down and listened for breath, there wasn't any.

I looked up at the boy's parents, hope burned in their eyes. They hoped with all their hearts that I could do something for their son. I never felt so helpless in my life. I then noticed the father was rubbing his left arm and wiggling his fingers. His face was even paler and his breathing seemed strange. It appeared he might be having a heart attack. I had a decision to make and it wasn't going to be easy.

I looked down at the young boy. My youngest son was twelve. Damn. If we didn't do something and do it now, this boy was dead. If he had been the only patient, I have no doubt that I would have pulled him from the hole and started CPR. He had not been in arrest long. But he wasn't the only patient. His sister lay only twenty feet away and I could actually hear her struggling for each ragged breath. His father appeared to be having a text book heart attack. I could also see a woman around twenty-one lying on the ground with a year old girl sitting beside her. A young man was hovering over them. Another young man sat with an obviously fractured ankle and several children were running around probably uninjured, but then maybe not.

Decision time; I have one ambulance, eleven patients. I stood up. I looked at the boy's parents. "I'm sorry, but we can't help your son. He has passed (the Navajo way of saying he was dead)." We have to concentrate now on your daughter." I turned away from them, not wanting to see the intense pain in their eyes.

I walked over to the EMTs working on the young girl. "Susan, get the girl on a backboard, load and go." The decision had been made. I chose to leave the boy and go for the girl. His heart had already stopped. Her heart was still beating. With the limited resources we had, I was going for the ones we stood a chance of saving.

I ran to the ambulance and picked up the mike. I was breathing hard and my mind was racing. I talked as my eyes scanned the scene making plans. "...Page another ambulance, Rescue one will be bringing in a girl with serious chest injuries and a man with a possible heart attack. We have one 901 (death), two or three other adults with moderate injuries and about five or six children that don't appear injured but need to be checked." The hospital had to know we were going to descend upon them with a large group and they needed to get ready.

I went back to the parents. They stood looking down at their dead son. I took the father and led him to Rescue-One and sat him in the front seat. "Your daughter is under age and one of you should go with her," I said as I took his pulse. It was strong, but every once in a while it would skip a beat or speed up and then slow down. I didn't think he would leave the rest of his family behind unless I made it seem as if his daughter needed him more. I looked up at him, "Do you have pain in your left arm?" He shook his head *yes*. "Does your chest hurt?" Again he shook his head *yes*. "We will need to have you checked too. Just sit here. Your daughter will be loaded in a minute." He shook his head and stared straight ahead. He appeared to be secretly grateful I had taken him away from the horrible nightmare he was forced to live. He was glad he was being driven away from his dead son. You see, the father had been driving the truck. At the time I was a Basic EMT and couldn't do all the things I later could do as a Paramedic, so I put him on oxygen and left to check on what was keeping the crew.

The crew managed somehow to stabilize the girl's neck and spine and get her on the backboard without incident. She still breathed on her own, but it was getting worse. They had her on high flow oxygen but her color was bad. I grabbed a corner of the backboard and we quickly loaded her in the back. "I took your second jump kit and demand valve (oxygen). The second ambulance will be here soon. I'll stay with the rest." I looked at the girl who lay so still on the stretcher and then shut the door.

I took Don Alton, the driver aside. "Don the man in the cab with you is the girl's father. He's having chest pains and other classic heart attack symptoms. I can't put him in back with the girl. The stress is what's getting to him. Up front he can disconnect for a few minutes and regroup mentally. At the hospital get the girl inside and come back for him with a wheelchair."

Don looked at me with wide eyes? "And what do I do if he codes half way to the hospital?"

"You're good Don, think of something," I patted him on the back.

"Thanks, I owe you one." He turned and got in mumbling something I think I am better off not hearing. It was a gamble but I didn't think the father would go down for a while. I felt he was doing ok and would hold for the short ten mile trip. The crew in the back was very busy trying to save the young girl. The father would have been in the way. The father's condition would have probably got worse if he had been forced to watch his daughter struggle to live. If I was wrong . . . . well right or wrong the decision was made and the ambulance drove off.

I turned around and viewed the scene. Where do I start? Then it occurred to me, where in the world are the two police officers that was supposed to be at the scene? I looked around. I saw one taking pictures the other one wasn't in sight. It made me mad. There were eleven patients and he was taking pictures. I was now by myself and expected to examine and care for the remaining eight while the police wondered around with their fingers up their noses. In rural EMS police usually jump in and help, but not these two.

I picked up my equipment and walked over to the woman lying on the ground. She was the only Anglo patient. She was married to the nice looking young man that hovered over her protectively. (He was the oldest son in this family) I kneeled down beside her. "My name's Sharon. I work for the Page Fire Department. What seems to be wrong?"

"My hips hurt." She ran her hand across her pelvis. I reached down and gently compressed them. She sucked in breath. I stopped.

"Can you please check the baby?" The young father asked. I looked down at a lovely child of about a year. She was fat and smiling. Not a scratch on her no dirt no blood. She had been riding in the tightly packed truck cab and had not been thrown out. I checked her quickly and found no obvious injuries.

"She looks uninjured but just to be sure we will have a doctor check her over." I turned my attention back to the child's mother and asked a series of questions. I took her vital signs, which were normal. She could have fractured her pelvis but I didn't think so. She was alert and very stable. But when a mother lies down and doesn't get back up there could be a problem especially with her back. The mother had been thrown out of the pickup bed. But thankfully, the truck had not landed on her.

I then recognized the young woman. I knew her mother. It wasn't long before my radio came to life and the dispatcher asked as casually as possible ". . . 3312 is near the area and is asking if she might be of assistance?" 3312 was Lena, the Anglo woman's mother. She worked with the police department and apparently had heard about the accident. The radio message was in code asking about her daughter and granddaughter.

I am not supposed to notify family of patients from the scene, but Lena was one of us. It was time to bend the rules a little. "Thank 3312 for me (translation; polite response). I expected her call (translation; it does involve her daughter and granddaughter). But everything is under control (translation; they are alive and stable). When Rescue-Two arrives at the hospital we will know more (translation; Lena should meet the second ambulance at the hospital).

I turned my attention to examining the young husband. He insisted he was uninjured but he admitted to pain in his leg and elbow. It turned out he wasn't seriously hurt just bruised. But none of us knew that day that he had only two short months left to live. Sadly his wife and daughter lost him two months later when he dove into a pond and struck his head on the bottom and didn't come back up.

"A second ambulance is on the way. I have to check out the others. She looks ok for now. Just don't let her move and call me if she starts having any problems." I got up. It was apparent he didn't want me to leave but I did it anyway. There were other patients to check. I had to have an overall view of the scene and patient's conditions by the time the next ambulance arrived. I had to decide who needed what and who went next.

In an incident that involves this many people, it takes a while to completely understand the entire incident. I discovered this was one big family consisting of the parents and their seven children, daughter-in-law and granddaughter. As I checked out the second oldest son's fractured ankle I heard breaks and looked up. Two of the young boys around six and seven years of age, stood in the middle of the highway throwing rocks at each other. "I'll be right back," I told the man and hurried to the highway.

Where are the officers? I thought. They had set up cones and as I neared the highway I saw one standing at the side of the road watching the traffic crawl through the cut. The other was still snapping pictures some

185

distance away. Now through the years I have gone to a lot of accidents. Not all officers are created equal when it comes to ability, skills, experience or temperament. But these two took the cake. I didn't know either one. I was beginning to wonder if they even knew I was there. They just continued to wander around looking like they had no idea what they should be doing. If they had reported eleven people involved in the accident initially there might have been enough manpower to do CPR on the boy. My anger grew at their incompetence.

"Get out of that road," I yelled at the boys in my best mother tone. The two boys dropped their rocks and walked over to two additional boys. I walked over and I kneeled down in the sand and started to ask them questions. Neither of them hurt anywhere. None had any obvious bruising bleeding or any sign of injury. They had all been in the cab of the truck.

The mother walked over to me when I finished examining the boys. She touched my forearm and with pleading eyes "Maybe if you put some oxygen on him? Please? She pointed to her dead son. I felt my stomach turn and I wished I could perform miracles. No child should die.

"Come on," I said as we walked over to the boy. We both sat down in the sand. "He isn't breathing. If I put the oxygen up against his mouth he wouldn't breathe it in. I wish I could help him, but I can't. I am so sorry."

Just then the four young boys came over and looked down. "He's dead isn't he?" the bravest asked.

"Yes," I said.

"Oh. Bummer," he said. They turned and hurried off to play a game of chase. They obviously had no idea what death really was. They were too young to understand.

The mother reached out and stroked his shiny black hair. "He was a good boy. He liked to play the guitar. He loved the color red." She hesitated, and then continued, "He always went to church with us....." Tears formed in her eyes and ran down her cheeks. Tears formed in my eyes too. "He was always my happy child. He laughed a lot. He made us all laugh .... He was a good boy .... " Her voice broke. The family members they were going to see that day went to my church and I knew them. And the Anglo girl was the daughter of a woman that worked for the city whom I knew. I didn't actually know this family but in a way I did. This woman was only a few year older than I was, and my youngest son, Stephen, was the age of her now dead son. My oldest son, David, was the age of her daughter who's life hung by a fragile string. We had so much in common. I could feel her pain and understand it. "He's in heaven now." Her voice crashed and a quite sob came out.

"Yes he's with God now." We obviously shared the same religious beliefs. I tried to give her some comfort and at the same time to help my own emotions that were being stretched farther than I usually allowed them to be stretched on a call. I just couldn't distance myself from this family. They were too much like mine; the mother was too much like me. The mother and I sat there, both with tears running down our face. She seemed to get some comfort in the shared sorrow of two mothers sitting in the sand beside a dead child.

"F-3? Rescue-Two." My radio pulled me back to the job at hand.

"This is F-3 go ahead." I stood up and wiped the tears from my eyes. I turned around and could see the ambulance coming up the hill still about a mile and a half away.

"Where do we park?"

"Look for me." I walked to the road and waited for them. They arrived and out of nowhere came one of the useless officers.

"Need any help?" he asked as he snapped one last picture.

I couldn't hide the anger in my voice. "No, not NOW!" I turned my back on him and walked over and opened the ambulance door. Three EMTs got out. "The woman over there has a possible fracture pelvis. She needs to go on a backboard. See if her husband will let you check him out it's his leg and elbow. The baby's fine."

I went and got a pillow and went over and splinted the young man with the fractured ankle. After he was put in the ambulance a man came up to me. He was wearing a bright orange vest that said "ADOT" (Arizona Department of Transportation) on it. He had apparently decided I was in charge and completely ignored the two useless police officers. "I just graveled the curve." pointing to the icy dark Little Cut. I guess he was looking for a compliment such as *good job*.

I couldn't help it but in my frustration I lashed out. "It's a little late now don't you think? The boy's dead." I turned and walked away.

The rest of the family was splinted, vital signs were taken, and they were all eventually transported to Page Hospital. When we finally arrived at the hospital, we found out the girl had gone directly into surgery and the father whet straight into the big ER and was connected up to a heart monitor as IV's flowed into his arm. He was having noticeable problems when he first arrived but they cleared up after he calmed down and a little medication was given.

The Anglo woman didn't have a single broken bone but her burses were beauties. The young man's ankle was cracked but not seriously broken. All the others were completely uninjured.

After the two ambulances were cleaned up, the crews sat down to write the report. I assigned a number to every victim. I then drew a diagram that gave each victim's name, age, location before and after the pickup rolled. I gave the crews my scribbled notes and any additional information I had.

"My family is across the street at the pizza place. I'm going over there and steal a piece of pizza. I'll be back in a little bit." I left them with the paperwork. I walked across the road and into the pizza parlor. My husband smiled and waved me over to their table. My son David and Stephen sat eating pizza. I sat down. My husband didn't ask about the call and I was glad. I just nibbled pizza and listened to the boys and my husband talk, tease and laugh.

Guilt descended upon me. I sat here with my family but that woman was going to have to bury her son and maybe her daughter. Her husband had just suffered a heart attack and carried the guilt because he was driving. Why did she have to suffer that way and I still had my family? I thought of all of my faults that I tried to hide from others, but I knew they were still there, deep down, so it couldn't have been because I deserved good luck. Stephen kicked David under the table and David kicked back a little too hard. A minor fight erupted.

Gads it felt good to hear them bicker and fight. I remembered the young boy that now lay alone in the hole in the cold sand awaiting the medical examiner. Why did he die? Then a cold feeling swept over me. Did he really not have a pulse? Was it possible I missed it? Was he breathing? Did I make the wrong decision? Maybe he didn't have to die. Doubt swept over me in waves. Had I killed the boy by writing him off too soon? Was I responsible for that woman's grief?

My family chatted on. No one seemed to notice my struggle. I rethought my actions. No there wasn't a pulse. I didn't miss it. . . It wasn't there. Breathing? No. Was he salvageable with CPR? Probably not. I knew it when I made the decision. His sister would have died had she not been treated and transported at once. His father could have died as well. We were not set up to do CPR and care for two other critical patients. It had to be one or the other.

My self-confidence started to return. I know I did the right thing. The boy had no pulse, verified by two trained EMT's. The girl lived. The father lived. The family drew together and will get through the tragedy. I have replayed this accident many times in my mind. I would make the same decision, if I had to do it again. In multiple patient incidents where the number of patients overwhelms the system, hard decisions have to be made. Triage occurs and a different set of rules apply. I followed those rules.

My coping mechanisms are well developed. I worked through my self-doubts rather quickly. Things fell into prospective and life went on. I hesitated to put down on paper my human weakness but it wouldn't be fair to leave them out as they played too big a part in this story. To feel, to cry, to sympathize with others isn't a weakness, it's strength. I have learned to accept my human side as a normal and natural part of living. Thank goodness I never quit feeling sorrow for other's misfortunes and that ability to care is what makes me a good EMT/Paramedic.

There was fallout from this accident. I turned in the two officers. Their behavior at the accident was not up to standards. They had arrived just after the accident and found the truck on its top and was told the two children were trapped under the vehicle. The two officer s wrote the two kids off and walked away. The family rolled the vehicle back on its top and dug the girl out and then the boy. The girl started breathing the boy didn't. I fear he may have suffocated to death. In my frustration I hinted that if they had not written off the boy so quickly and applied skills they had been taught in their first responder class the boy might have been breathing when I arrived.

There were eleven, not two patients, and I still don't know why they couldn't have counted heads and relayed the information. If I had known the number of people involved, a second ambulance could have been dispatched a lot sooner. Then when they didn't even offer to help, until the calvary had already arrived, I really got mad at them. I had never reported an officer before and my complaints were taken seriously. They got in a lot of trouble. One officer finally had to bid to another area and the second was stuck here for a lot longer than he had planned. He hated me and that caused some difficulties since we ran into each other at other accidents. He would stock me if he saw me on the highway in my personal car. He wanted to write me a ticket so bad he could taste it. But I never gave him the opportunity. It was years later before his anger faded and others replaced me on his list. I learned afterwards that both men were rookies and it was their first serious accident. Usually at least one officer was experienced but this time they both ended up at this MVA. With hindsight in good working order I probably should have cut them some slack. It was their first serious accident but I still believe they should have known better.

Months later a man I knew that worked for the highway department told me that my harsh words at the scene with the man putting gravel on the road after the accident had hurt the man a great deal. He said the man had nightmares and felt guilty. His work had been affected and he suffered from depression. My words had cut deep and had left scars. I had not intended for my one emotional outburst to emotionally damage the man.

I called the man to apologize for speaking to him so harshly. I told him I know now it wasn't his fault. He was following orders and certainly didn't mean to hurt anyone. He had nothing to do with the decisions involving when and where to gravel potentially icy roadways. In all fairness they can't gravel all curves and icy areas. I told him I was sorry my words had caused him grief. I was stressed and spoke without thinking. I truly regretted I caused him such personal distress. He seemed relieved. Somehow, hearing me say it wasn't his fault, helped him put the incident behind him and allowed him to go on with his life.

This story wasn't easy to write. I let my guard down and allowed myself to become too involved. I paid the price. I learn from my mistakes. This job has a downside. The responsibility can sometimes weigh heavy on an EMT-Paramedic's shoulders. I wanted to show the good and the not so good part of making decisions that will affect others for the rest of their life. I honestly don't know if we won or lost this call. But once a decision is made.......once the words have been said, they can't be changed or taken back.

For a long time every time I would drive past that spot I would remember and all the emotions would come flooding back. At first the holes were still visible. I hated those holes. If there had been a place to pull off I would have stopped and filled them up. But there wasn't and it took a long time for nature to fill them. Today there is no physical sign of the accident; the holes had filled in with sifting sand. A small cross of rebar marks the spot. The officer now talks to me and the ADOT worker can sleep at night. But I still remember every time I drive past. The vivid memories, the emotions and feelings are dulled by time. But the memories still come back when I drive around that bend. I remember his thick black hair and his bright red cowboy shirt and his mother telling me he was her "happy child who made them laugh." I try not to remember, but I still calculate how old he would be if he had lived. He would have been thirty-eight at the time this book was published.

"WHY DID YOU CALL US?" An Abuse of the System

I never minded getting out of a warm bed to go to an emergency. I was also willing to risk life and limb driving code-three to an emergency. But, I have problems being polite to those who abuse the system. It has happened too many times to count. Here is a good example of the abuse by thoughtless people. This is the only story in this book about my time on a big city ambulance. The reason I have included it is because this story isn't

190

about big city or rural, it's about selfish people who feel it's their right to demand the unreasonable and your duty to give it to them at any cost.

In Phoenix, while a paramedic student, I was riding along with the Peoria Fire Department. We received an "unknown medical" call to a local address. We had no idea what type of emergency we were going to find. Was a baby not breathing? Had a beloved grandfather had a heart attack and was lying on the floor turning blue? Was someone bleeding to death? We drove code-three through the streets of Peoria. Some people would pull to the side, others didn't. We ran through red lights and drove on the wrong side of the road. I hung on as the fire engine roared through traffic.

We arrived at a small frame house in a Latino neighbor of Peoria. We pulled up, and with everyone carrying a piece of equipment, we rushed to the door. It was opened by a man of about twenty-eight years of age. "It's my mother, she cut her hand." He pointed to the kitchen. With visions of a woman holding a blood soaked dish towel to a bloody stump, I hurried into the tiny kitchen. Sitting at the dining table was a short, stout Latino woman of about fifty-five years of age. She was drinking a cup of coffee. She was perfectly groomed. Not a drop of blood could be seen. Since I was the student, I was supposed to handle the call with the paramedic watching closely, guiding me when necessary. The paramedic and the fire crew stood to the side, waiting to see how I would handle this. "I understand you cut your hand."

"Yes I did," she said and took a sip of coffee.

"Can I see the wound?" I asked. She held up her left hand, extending her index finger. I took a close look. "I don't see anything."

"There," she said, indicating the tip of the index finger.

I looked closer. There was a tiny, very tiny paper cut. The firemen were snickering at the situation. I was perplexed. But I had been on calls before where it wasn't obvious why an ambulance was called. I knew this woman called because she wanted something. I was just having problems figuring out what she wanted. So I asked. "I see the wound. It's rather small. Why did you call 911?"

"I need a band aid."

Some of the firefighters snickered, others hurried from the room before they burst into laughter. I looked up at the paramedic, "Do we even carry band aids?"

"I think so," he said as he opened the gray box. He dug into it and found a band aid. He handed it to me. I took it and applied it to the finger.

"Thank you," the woman said as she smiled at the now bandaged finger. We left and returned to the station. At the station I was told that the City of Peoria was tired of such calls and had just passed a new law, due to go into effect next month. The fire department would not charge

191

"real" emergency first response calls. They would even overlook calls that were called in with the best intentions and end up being nothing. But the ones who abused the system would receive a bill for the service. If that woman ever called again for a band aid, it was going to cost her over $300. I hope she called.

THEY CAME FOR HIM

This call is perhaps one of the strangest calls I went on over the years. I have decided to just tell you the story and let you make up your own mind. It was just after sunset on a warm July evening in Page, Arizona. Police were called to do a welfare check at a local trailer court. Neighbors had not seen Mr. Williams all week and they were concerned. When police arrived, the door was opened by Mr. Williams. But after talking to him for a few minutes, they decided to request an ambulance.

We drove Rescue-One up to an old thirty foot trailer. It wasn't hard to find, it was the only one with a patrol car sitting in front. I walked up to the door and a police officer met me and told me about why they were there. "He's not quite right. I don't know what's wrong."

I entered the small trailer. It was neat, dishes were washed, the stove top was clean, and the place was pleasant inside. A small man smiled at me as I entered. He was in his mid-forties, about five foot, four inches tall and one-hundred and thirty-five pounds, almost bald and wearing thick rimmed glasses. I introduced myself, he half stood up and shook my hand and smiled a warm smile. I immediately liked him. "Your neighbors were concerned about you when they didn't see you out and about," I said.

"I am sorry you had to come out, but I am alright. They are nice people. I am sorry I had them worried." I looked down on the coffee table in front of me and there lay a thick picture album. He smiled and opened it. "This is my family." He began to tell me about each of the people pictured in the album. His voice showed great affection. It was obvious this was his beloved family and the album was a treasure he valued greatly. I wanted to evaluate him and gain his trust, so I listened patiently as he gently introduced me to his beloved family. He sounded rational, sane and totally aware of who I was, where he was, and the situation.

I looked around and noticed all the windows were covered in aluminum foil. In Page we have people that work nights and cover their windows so they can sleep, but this was the living area and it looked strange. I guess he could see I was confused. "It's so they can't read my mind," he calmly stated.

"Who?" I asked

"You know (he gestures by looking upward)."

"No, I don't think I do."

"Them . . . . I'm tired of them intruding into my thoughts."

I hesitated and tried to think of a possible "them", but only one thing seemed to fit, ". . . . do you mean . . . . aliens?" (from outer space).

"Yes," he calmly said in a gentle, rational voice.

"So, they read your mind?"

"Yes, they do. The last time they took me, they put in an implant and it's driving me crazy."

"Does it hurt?"

"Yes, it hurts, right here." He pointed to his right ear.

I questioned him about the pain. "Have you seen a doctor about getting it removed?"

"Yes, but they couldn't see it on the x-ray. I guess it's transparent."

"If you have pain, perhaps you should get a second opinion. Now, you can refuse, it's your right. But if you would like a different doctor to check out your ear, I would be glad to give you a ride to the hospital. Maybe the ER Doc can find something the other doctor missed."

He thought for a short time. "I would like that. I have insurance. And they can't see or hear inside the hospital. But they might see me leave. I'm afraid if they take me one more time, they won't return me to earth." As strange as his words were, his voice, his manner, his actions appeared calm, gentle, and rational. He was easy to believe. But as a medic, I knew he could be delusional. I learned a long time ago, it works better to play into their delusion. The brief time I am feeding the delusion won't make a difference in the long term treatment. And there was always the chance he did have something wrong with his ear. He was in pain.

"Well, we could hide you?"

"How?" he asked. The plan was simple. We took him out on the stretcher, covered in a sheet. I know his neighbors would think he was dead, but the aliens couldn't see him. He liked the idea. We loaded him in the ambulance, keeping him covered and the police quietly followed us. Our orders were to stop and abandoned ship if the man went nuts (or aliens showed up). I tried to not laugh when I noticed the ambulance driver look up into the night sky. We continued on so I guess he didn't see any ships. We arrived at the hospital and took him in, still covered with the sheet. I had called ahead to warn them about what we were bringing in and the doctor was prepared and acted as if this was a weekly occurrence.

The doctor began questioning him. He continued to sound completely rational, cooperative, but concerned about the possibility of being abducted again. He defiantly wanted the implant removed. The doctor looked inside his ear and saw nothing. The CT machine was down, but would be up and running on Monday (it was Friday evening now). "There could be a number of things causing the pain. The CT will give us some answers," the doctor told him, "But, the CT is down. We expect it to be up and running Monday."

A new nurse walked up. She was an average sized woman of plain, ordinary appearance. No one knew her well, since she was new in town and had worked at the hospital for only a few days. When Mr. Williams saw her, his face drained of all color, his mouth dropped open, his eyes widened and he took on the appearance of a man who was completely terrified. His voice became loud and filled with raw fear. "She's one of them. She's one of them! Oh my God, they know I'm here!" He panicked.

The doctor looked at the nurse, who seemed surprised. "I think you should leave." She shook her head and left.

"Who is she?" the doctor asked.

"Susan something. She's new," answered the nurse.

"She one of them," his voice was now filled with hopelessness. "Now they will come get me. I know they won't bring me back this time." He was sad, and gave up his struggle. He appeared to accept his fate. "Thank you for trying." He lay back down and closed his eyes.

We went and finished our paperwork and he was given a trip back to his home by the police. He was told to come in Monday for a CT. But he appeared to not be interested. He quietly took his paperwork and left, all hope was gone from the little man. He had given up and was just going through the motions. He was so sad and looked so helpless. He had lost all hope.

On Monday, I got a call from the police officer concerning Mr. Williams. "Sharon, you remember the space cadet we met last Friday?"

"Yes, Mr. Williams. I was going to call later today and see if they found anything in the CT."

"He's gone. A half-eaten meal was on the table, and all his stuff was untouched. Looks like he just . . . . . disappeared."

"What about the photo album?"

"It was still there on the coffee table."

"He would never leave that behind. He treasured that album." I was absolutely certain he would have taken that family photo album if it had been any way possible.

"Nothing was missing, just him. No one, not even the nosey neighbor saw him leave. And you want to hear something else strange?"

194

"What?" I asked

"The nurse.....you know, the one he said was a Martian? Well, she's also missing. She didn't report to work today and she didn't even pick up her paycheck. The phone numbers on her resume don't check out. I went to her apartment and found only a mattress on the floor, nothing else."

I considered the situation for a minute. "Do you think?"

". . . . . That he was abducted by aliens? I don't know, but this is really strange."

It's been a number of years now. No one ever saw Mr. Williams or the nurse again. On a quite summer night as I look up at the beautiful night sky, I wonder . . . .

EVERYONE IN THE DITCH!

A wise man once said, "Never get into the front of the ambulance with someone that is braver than you are."

Rescue-Two roared through the Big Cut, sirens blaring and echoing off the tall sandstone cliffs on each side of the narrow road. The overheads (exterior code lights) rotated red, white, blue, red, white, blue, red ......etc. The reflections caused almost had a hypnotic effect as we sailed through the cut that had been made in the steep sandstone mountain to allow Highway 89 to access Page, Arizona.

Down the six percent grade we traveled, cars, pickups and semi's moving to the right, hugging the guard rail and using the slow lane to allow us access around them. The road was three lanes, two up and one down. We were traveling the wrong way (down) in the passing lane. The vehicles coming up the steep hill could see us and would quickly pull into the slow lane and allow us to pass. This worked fairly well except on tight curves where visibility was restricted. Then luck came into play. I sat up front riding shotgun with Patrick Simpson. He was a good driver, a bit fast but a very good driver. He reminded me of the way my husband drove a car. I liked riding with him. He was calm and relaxed, at any speed. My mind drifted back to the week before. Lady luck was with us.

It was a completely different story one week ago. I had been riding with another EMT driving. He was hyper as usual. When he was on a call he would never allow anyone else to drive. He thought he was fantastic, but nothing could have been further from the truth. We were responding down the same steep hill as we were now, but it was very different. He took corners too tight and stomped on the gas then the breaks, then the gas, making it turbulent riding in the back. I was hanging on for dear life when I heard Ken Connors who was riding in the passenger seat scream loudly, "Sharon, DON'T LOOK! DON'T LOOK!" Now I don't know anyone who would not have looked. I did.

I peeked through the opening and saw Ken with his legs stretched out stiffly in front of him, gripping the seat arm rests and the look of terror in his eyes. Coming up the hill was a yellow Volkswagen van. It was chuggin' along, trying so hard to pass the huge, long semi with double trailers creeping up the hill in the slow lane. The little van wasn't gaining much ground as we were closing in on him. Roger slammed on the breaks, locking it up. The tail swung slightly and I was flung back and forth almost torn in half by the seatbelt. The driver of the van saw us and decided to break. He too did a panic stop and with only inches to spare, managed to slip behind the semi into the other lane and allowed us to pass. We were quite a sight, lights flashing, siren blaring, breaks locked up and the look of panic on everyone's face as we slid by almost sideways past the semi and van.

Thank goodness, today Patrick was driving. We smoothly negotiated the hill and at Bitter Springs found ourselves on fairly flat ground. Patrick opened it up and we were in hyper-drive. We came up behind vehicle after vehicle. They would see us and pull over as far as they could. The road was only two lanes with a foot of paved shoulder and then loose sand. They would pull over and the oncoming traffic would too, then we would squeeze between them, side mirrors almost touching, straddled the yellow center line. It was exciting. I loved it.

We reached a very narrow bridge and I was certain there wasn't room for three vehicles to pass, but Patrick reached out and coolly grabbed the big side mirror and jerked it inward and we passed between a big black pickup and a full size car. If he had not pulled the mirror in, we would have exchanged mirror parts with one or both of the vehicles. We roared onward to the reported one car rollover. Car after car took to the side of the road and allowed us to rush past. I know they were thinking "I wonder what they are going too?"

Mile after mile we traveled down the highway code-three. Then the call came in, "No one at the accident scene, only the flipped over car." We were cancelled.

Patrick reached over, turned off the flashing lights and the siren. "There's Cedar Ridge Trading Post, might as well get some lemonade." I agreed so we pulled into the wide dirt parking lot in front of the old wooden structure. We got out and went inside. It was a typical trading post made of logs about 1,200 square feet. The building was built just after the War for Southern Independence (aka the American Civil War), around 1870. Pots and pans hung from the ceiling. Rugs, blankets, and towels were stacked on old rough hand chiseled shelves. Some coats, a few shirts and Levis were displayed on racks. This wasn't a tourist trap. It was a store to supply the local Indians with supplies. I loved to look at the silver and turquoise jewelry that lay behind a dirty glass display. The Indians would pawn it and most of it was of good quality. The grocery part was mostly canned food, bread and one small refrigerator with milk and soda. The white man, Trader Bill, behind the counter owned the trading post, fourth generation owner. Beans, rice, crackers, flour, corn meal, sugar and such were stacked high. He had only one more year on the 100 year lease and the tribe had told him they were not going to renew it. They were going to take the trading post and give it to an Indian that lived in the area. For one hundred years the Miller family had called Cedar Ridge home. There had been no complaints against Bill. His only sin was having white skin. After four generations, Cedar Ridge Trading Post would be out of the Miller family hands.

Patrick and I got tall lemonades and exited the store. It never occurred to us that in two years it would be burnt to the ground because the new local owners would refuse to pay a group of Native American thug's protection money. The people driving by were staring at us with angry looks. At first we were confused. Then a car pulled off and flipped us off (middle finger salute). "What's his problem?" Patrick said.

Then I understood. They had no way of knowing we had been cancelled. "They think we ran them into the ditch to get here for lemonade." We climbed back into the ambulance as the line of angry travelers drove past, staring at us with angry expressions.

Years later history repeated its self, sort of. I was in another ambulance, this time with Rick Stone. I was working in Tuba City, Arizona for a private ambulance company. We were based on the Navajo Reservation about eighty-five miles south of Page. Navajo Nation EMS was east on Highway 160 for a two car accident. We provided backup for Navajo Nation's 911. We were paged for a one car rollover on Highway 89 just beyond Cameron, about thirty miles from Tuba City.

Traffic was heavy. It was summertime and tourists filled the highway with cars and trucks many pulling trailers and boats. Native Americans were out on the road, usually driving to and from the only big city in the area, Flagstaff (seventy-five miles south). The road wasn't much wider here and it was impossible for a vehicle to completely get off the road. We passed an ugly green van with about a dozen kids inside. They were all staring at us with wide-eyed interest. We then came upon a pickup pulling a boat, they slowed down and then pulled off as far as they dared, and keeping only the left tires on the road as the right sided tires sank slightly in sand. Then we passed a semi, then another semi hauling a wide load, then a white car with an older couple behind the wheel. Each vehicle pulled off as carefully and as far as they dared to allow us to squeeze past. We inched our way through the maze. Lights flashing, sirens blaring, it was exciting.

Then the radio blared we were cancelled. No reason, just cancelled. We pulled off at Gray Mountain and turned around. We started back. Within three minutes dispatch called us to report of a car pedestrian accident back in Tuba City. Rick turned on the lights and sirens and we headed back. Suddenly, there was the wide load and then the other semi, the white car with the older couple, the pickup pulling the boat and then the ugly green van. They pulled to the side one by one and allowed us to pass. Everyone in the vehicles was looking at us, wondering where we were going.

Then, Navajo EMS said they were clear of the first incident and would take the car pedestrian accident. We shut down the code-three response and started a normal roll back to Tuba. Then, "Med-41, can you respond to a reported one car rollover with man lying beside the road wearing an orange traffic vest." It was just two miles past Gray Mountain Trading Post, that was behind us now. " We looked for a spot to turn around, there wasn't one. Rick turned around anyway. As he turned off the pavement our back tires were spinning on the soft sand before they were able to gain traction.

Lights came on again, siren blared and off we went back south down the highway retracing our path. Again, the green van pulled off, then the pickup pulling the boat, then the semi then the wide load and then the white car with the two retirees inside. This time we couldn't help but laugh. This was the third time we had run the same people more or less off the road. Five miles from the reported accident, we were cancelled by Park Service. It wasn't an accident. It was an old tire and a casually discarded orange traffic vest at the side of the road. No people, no car, no accident. Reaching to turn off the code-lights he looked at me. "We are going to drive past the same people again."

"Maybe they will not recognize us and think it's just another ambulance, not the same one......" I interjected.

We started driving back, we were driving in a non-emergency "normal" manner this time, and there they were, the white car, the wide load semi, the pickup pulling the boat and the ugly green van. I know some of them had to have recognized us. I know they were thinking, what on earth we were doing, rushing by them three times with lights flashing and finally meekly passing them as if nothing is going on? I wish I could have explained, but they will never know why we did what we did.

DUMB HUMAN TRICKS

It was early in the morning and Carl was half asleep as he stumbled from his trailer. He was on his way to work. He put his key in the car door and opened it. Carl took a sip of coffee and looked across the street. His face exhibited surprise as he spun around and ran into his house to call 911.

PD Anthony Santiago and I pulled up at the same time. We got out and stood for a minute taking in the scene. There was a young man, about twenty years of age. He was a large man. He had taken an extension cord, bent a tree over and tied one end to the tree top and the other around his neck. He was so heavy that when he pulled up his legs to hang himself, the tree would bend over and he would find himself kneeling on the grass. So, he decided to jump up and hope the cord would strangle him. Anthony and I stood and watched this huge young man jump up and down like a yo-yo on a string. No way was he going to kill himself, at least not this way. I struggled to not laugh. David Letterman's "Stupid Human Tricks" came to mind. Anthony and I walked over and I grabbed the man around his legs and lifted him up a bit (with the help of the tree) and Anthony cut the cord with is pocket knife. The man fell to the ground, crying.

The ambulance drove up and quickly we had him back boarded and in the ambulance. There was a red mark around his neck, but other than that, he appeared uninjured. I had to ask, "Why did you do this?" He told me that he had just married a beautiful woman. He went out and got drunk for the first time since the marriage and she refused to allow him in the house. He stumbled to his father's house and asked to borrow the truck, of course his dad said "no." Then he decided no one loved him anymore and he saw no reason to live. He was walking through the trailer court when he saw the extension cord and the tree and devised a plan.

"That is the most piss poor reason to commit suicide I have ever heard." I try to avoid editorial comments when dealing with patients, but this young man was so stupid I couldn't help myself.

"I know," he said through tears.

"Your wife and father still love you, they didn't want you to drink and drive. It's the alcohol they hate, not you. If you went to them and promised to not drink again, they would show you the love you want." I usually didn't play "Dr. Phil" but he was so young and so stupid. The mother in me took over and I had to do what I could.

"I could do that," he said. I don't have to have it (alcohol)."

"Then give up alcohol as an act of love for your new wife and father."

"I could do that," he said again. He got quiet. I don't remember ever seeing him as a patient again. I would like to believe he went home and begged forgiveness and made the wise decision to not drink ever again.

This day ended up being "suicide attempt day". I heard the report of an attempted suicide in process behind the golf course. That was an unpopulated rocky area that led to the edge of the Glen Canyon Gorge. I drove out to the area and saw the Sheriff driving at a breakneck speed over the flat sandstone rocks. In front of him was a beautiful sixteen year old girl. She was running like the wind for the seven hundred foot drop off. His car reached a place where it couldn't go anymore. He leaped out and ran for the girl. I hurried, but could see whatever happened would be finished before I got there. I too reached a stopping place and leaped out of my car. Ahead of me ran the girl and directly behind her was the sheriff's deputy.

The girl was racing to the edge and just as she reached the edge she leaped. I held my breath. The officer also leaped in an attempt to grab her. He caught her and together they went over the edge out of my range of view. I stopped. Had I just seen two people go over the edge of a seven-hundred foot drop to the Colorado River?

I hurried over a slight rise and saw they were still more or less on top. The rise had hidden a narrow piece of crumbly sandstone rock that lay a foot or two off the edge of the canyon. The girl and the officer lay in a tumbled heap only inches from death. I reached down and assisted him and the girl up to safer ground.

She was crying, he was obviously shaken but happy he had caught her. He was a hero, a true hero. The ambulance was called to transport her to the hospital. As the ambulance drove off the officer sat down on a rock. His hands were shaking and he came down quickly from the sudden surge in adrenaline he had experienced. We talked for a while. He was just now realizing how close he had come to falling to his death.

After a few minutes he stood up and announced, "I need a cup of coffee." I laughed. We left, he for the coffee shop, me for the hospital. The girl had taken some unknown drug at a party and then had a fight with her boyfriend. She had decided to kill herself. Her friends called the police when they discovered her gone. She had threatened to jump off the cliff and they believed she was heading that way. Thank goodness the sheriff had intercepted her. She was examined by a doctor and a mental health specialist. They both agreed she wasn't suicidal, just high. I believe they were right because the only thing she had asked me was if someone would drive her to work. The sheriff deputy was an unsung hero that day.

THIS ISN'T A NORMAL LIFE

My husband, Maurice, is a morning person. I am not. He greets the day with anticipation. I just struggle to keep awake and not hurt someone till around ten o'clock. I got up at five thirty and prepared him breakfast that morning. "Don't forget your lunch," I said as he almost left without it. He smiled, gave me a quick kiss, grabbed his lunch and hurried off. I wandered back to the bedroom and dressed without enthusiasm. In my mind I ran through the things I had to do today. I had an hour and a half until I had to wake the boys. The pantry was bare and grocery shopping could not be postponed any longer. This was the day the garbage was picked up and I made a note to remember to put it out. When the pager went off, it startled me. I hate early morning calls. I am not at my best. I searched for my shoes and slipped on the first pair I found and ran down the hall.

At the station, I discovered it wasn't really all that pressing an emergency. A man had died last night and his body was discovered in the park this morning. LARC, the Local Alcohol Rehabilitation Center, had recently shut its doors due to lack of financial backing. It was still cold at night. Spring was coming but hadn't arrived yet. The local police had spent most of the night transporting inebriated individuals to the local jail. They were given blankets and allowed to sleep the night in the warm waiting room. I guess they missed this man. The man was a local "drunk" that lived on the streets. He had gotten drunk the night before and passed out. Local Alcohol Rehabilitation Center (LARC) was closed. He lay on the damp grass all night and slowly died from exposure.

I got out of the ambulance and walked up the slight hill to the area where the body lay. Two police officers stood around. One had been taking pictures, the other writing down information. "Nothing unusual just appears to have passed out and didn't wake up." I looked down at the body. The man was in his late thirties. He was a couple inches less than six

201

feet. He was in good shape, muscularly built, callused hands and very dead.

We rolled him over on his side. I recognized him. He was "Eddie something." We slid the backboard that had been covered with a sheet under him. We laid another sheet over him and pulled the bottom sheet up over the top sheet. It formed a crude shroud. We only used the body bags for messy deaths. We loaded him in the ambulance and I crawled in back with the body. I sat looking at the white sheet that covered what only a few hours ago was a man. He had let alcohol rule his life and it eventually killed him, but he was a man just the same. I resented him and people like him being called "drunks." I wondered if anyone would miss him. Would a woman somewhere, a mother, sister, wife, daughter, shed tears at the news of his death? What was his last name? Why did he have to die in such a stupid way? Would it have made a difference if LARC had been open? I knew people dying of cancer or living in a body that was paralyzed or ravaged with disease who would have given almost anything for this man's physically healthy body and yet this man threw it all away by committing slow suicide by drinking himself to death. What made him make the choices he made? Would it have made a difference if he had passed out just a few feet earlier and not just over the top of the hill, out of the view of patrolling officers?

We unloaded him at the morgue and we quickly cleaned up the ambulance and finished the paperwork. The final chapter in a man's life, done, completed, over. I had seen many dead bodies by this time. This one wasn't really that different. I had these thoughts about him, but in a couple of hours, my curiosity would fade and I would get on with my life. I knew I wouldn't lose sleep over this, none of us would. But all the same it was an unnecessary death and we all felt it.

I hurried home and woke the boys up for school. I rushed into the kitchen and started breakfast. The boys came out. Stephen was grumpy. He was cursed with my hatred of mornings. David was more like his father, but he treaded quietly in the morning surrounded by two night owls struggling to survive in a morning person's world.   After they left the house became quite. I sat down and had a cup of coffee. I went to work and spent the morning up on the fire truck with tools in hand installing a new monitor gun. I then drove it out to the airport and connected it up to a hydrant and tested it. It worked much to my surprise. I then went home and fixed lunch for my boys. They were returning to school when my pager went off. I drove the ambulance code-three forty miles to a house on the Rez where a man was having a crystal meth moment. He threatened to kill me and when he lunged at me, the officer and other EMTs took him down.

202

We returned to town with him screaming threats and violently struggling to get out of his restraints.

That evening we sat eating an early dinner. I had barely taken a bite when I was called out to the local electric company warehouse. I arrived and found the Fire Chief and a police officer there. "Sharon, they found a bomb."

"Bomb? Then why aren't we staged back there?" indicating an intersection a block away.

"Oh, it's a little one, sort of. Come on, I'll show you." The Fire Chief led me into the warehouse. It was filled with shelving units with cardboard boxes and bins with fittings. We walked over to a huge roll of wire. It was on a round wooden spindle, with wire wound around it. Through the hole in the middle was a metal bar. The chief pointed at the metal bar. "That's the bomb."

I looked closer. It didn't look like a bomb. "Who put it here?" I asked. It was a long story, but apparently this type of explosive device was used during the construction of the Dam, many years ago. A hole would be drilled in the sandstone and this thin metal pipe filled with explosives was dropped into it. The metal pipe bomb would then be set off. The resulting explosion would create shock waves and instruments were used to determine density of the rock and other geographical findings.

"Why is it being used to move and spin a roll of wire?"

"They didn't realize it was explosive until now."

"It needs a dynamite cap and detonation cord, doesn't it?"

"Technically, yes, but it's old and therefore could be unstable. Explosives deteriorate with age. Here's the problem. We are near a residential area. I didn't think they were in danger because the explosion would be kind of small. But if this exploded the resulting fire would spread toxic smoke (burning wire) and might spread to other structures. The nearest bomb squad is in Flagstaff and can't be here till tomorrow morning.

"If we could get this bomb to the fire training grounds in the industrial park, we could rest a bit easier until the bomb squad gets here."

"How do we get it there?" asked a Fire Captain.

"It's been tossed around and misused for years. I doubt that it is that easy to set off. What if we put it in a trailer, lots of packing and just moved it," I suggested.

Lots of discussion followed. Pro's and con's were discussed. Finally, we all decided it probably wasn't that big a danger, but should be moved to a safer area. The Chief called the bomb squad and discussed our idea. They gave us their thoughts on the matter but stopped short of saying it would be ok. We decided to move it. The small open trailer was

203

brought to the scene. We took pillows and blankets used on the ambulance to pad the small trailer. It would make bumps less scary. We connected the trailer to the attack truck and only one man would drive it out of town, therefore minimizing the chance of multiple causalities.

Now, who would carry it out of the warehouse? A fire fighter? No way. They are rough and don't have a gentle bone in their body. I volunteered. No one had a problem with that.

I went back inside the warehouse. I walked up to the bomb and stood looking at it for a minute. What if I was wrong? What if this old explosive devise had taken all the abuse it could take and was ready to go off? The explosion wouldn't be huge but it would be enough to cause me serious injuries or maybe death. I liked my fingers and hands. I reconsidered then decided to go ahead and do it. I am a gambler at heart and I felt this bomb was more or less stable. I reached down and slowly removed the pipe bomb from the spindle. I then carried it outside and placed it on the pile of pillows. I then put a pillow over it and tied everything down. I backed away as the firefighter got in the truck and drove off, slowly. The police officer escorted the truck pulling the trailer and the fire chief brought up the rear. I stayed in the parking lot. I listened to the radio traffic and kept looking southward listening for a loud explosion and cloud of dust. It was an uneventful trip. The bomb was left in a locked shed on the Fire Training Grounds.

I went back home in time to gobble down some cold leftovers and clear off the dinner table. I finished my wife/mother duties and sat down. It then occurred to me, my life wasn't normal. I had just experienced a somewhat routine day. I had made repairs to a fire truck, picked up a dead body, faced down the meth head screaming threats against my life, and of course I carried a bomb out of the warehouse. It had been a good day. Everything had gone according to plan. Some days it didn't, but today had gone smoothly.

Tomorrow I would probably meet a woman friend in the grocery store. She will probably ask me "What have you been doing?" What do I tell her? If I was perfectly honest, she would be shocked. I would see her suddenly become uncomfortable. She would stammer some polite comment and try to ignore what I have just said. She may be brave enough to comment on it but probably not. She could no longer identify with me and I would lose her as a friend because she feared I would share more horrible details with her and she wasn't ready for a story that included a severed body part. No, I wouldn't say that. I would keep it light and never transgress on that other side to my life. I lived in two worlds. In one I was a mother who baked cookies, washed clothes and helped with homework. I was a wife who washed my husband's clothes and had dinner cooked when my husband came home. And hardest of all, I acknowledged my husband as the boss of this house.

But in the other world I was boss. I supervised thirty-two type-A employees in situations charged with emotion, tension, stress and danger. I made decisions no one else wanted to make. I was the one they called to make the tough decisions and I made them. But at home, I had to ask my husband's permission to go out of town or to purchase something that cost over a hundred dollars. I had trouble slipping from one identity to another. I was almost a split personality, two people inhabiting the same body. Sometimes they would lap over and that didn't work at all. Neither one of my split personalities belonged in the other's world. I had to see that the two never interfered with the others life. As you could image, it wasn't easy and sometimes I failed.

People think they know me. But most only knew the identity with which they were familiar. Most seldom see the other half. Even if they suspected there was another side, they didn't investigate. My husband was one of the few people that really knew the two Sharon's. He loved one and accepted the other. Other than me, he was probably the next most affected person by my duel rolls. My husband gave me a long leash and allowed me to go out and explore the world. But he still held the end and at times would jerk it and force me to come back. I loved him for the illusion of freedom, but sometimes we clashed. Both lives tugged at me, pulling me in two different directions at the same time.

I grew up in Phoenix Arizona. My parents still lived in Phoenix. My mother never understood my involvement in such a job. She considered it *man's work* and un-lady like. She told her friends I worked for the Fire Department as a secretary. To my knowledge, she never publically acknowledged what I did and didn't want to hear about my adventures. My father on the other hand encouraged me and I can still hear him say, "Go ahead Sis, tell them what you do."

Being married and working in EMS as I did was a hard juggling act that I only barely managed to do. While Rescue Chief being on-call twenty-four hours a day, seven days a week was hard when added to the duties of wife and mother. My husband was left in many restaurants without a dinner partner, checkbook, keys or transportation because my pager went off at a bad time. I once left him standing at a gas station, nozzle in hand no money or checkbook and a perplexed look on his face as I sped to a restaurant one block away where a woman was choking. He learned quickly to not ask, "Hi Honey. What did you do today?" My children also were affected. Most of the time they understood, sometimes they grew tired of my outside activities. Even after the children left the nest, Maurice and I had to adjust to me being gone two to three days a week out of town working. But I have managed to live two separate lives and somehow it managed to work. My life hasn't been "normal" but it has been interesting.

THE PFD TAXI SERVICE

Kee was a "frequent flyer" with the Page Fire Department. I knew his name, date of birth and social security number by heart. I could recite his Post Office Box number, his mother's name and phone number. Kee was an ok guy as long as he stayed sober. But, try as he may, Kee just couldn't resist the siren's song. At thirty-five years of age, Kee lived with his widowed mother about forty miles outside town near the Native American village of Kaibeto, about thirty-five miles east of Page on Highway 98. It is considered normal in the Navajo culture for a son to live with his mother till he marries. She cooked his meals and washed his clothes. Her deceased husband's social security check wasn't large but it was enough for the two of them. Kee helped around the house by chopping firewood and hauling water and he sometimes watched the sheep.

Then, around the third day of every month Kee's disability check would arrive. He was disabled because he was an alcoholic. He was a binge drinker. Your tax dollars supported his habit. His mother wouldn't let him take the family pickup because she knew he would get drunk when he reached town. She also knew he would not return home until his money was gone. It was illegal for anyone to possess alcohol on the reservation, but the border towns provided a convenient watering hole for the thirsty. Kee had figured out how to get to town without a car.

Kee was a little man, barely five feet, four inches tall and around one-hundred and fifteen pounds dripping wet. He had awakened early that morning. He knew his check would be at the post office that day. He got up and dressed in his best Levis, good cowboy boots and new western shirt. He slipped on his leather jacket and combed his coal black hair. He kissed his mother goodbye and walked to the post office, picked up his check and then walked the other mile to the highway. Kee looked up and down Highway 98. He stuck out his thumb as a number of cars drove by. Finally he gave up the hope of hitchin' a ride to Page. It was time for Plan B. He lay down beside the road and waited. Soon a car drove by. Kee began to twitch, shake and flail about. The car didn't stop. Another car came by. Again Kee went into his best interpretation of a full blown seizure. The car pulled over.

I was mowing the lawn when my pager sounded, ". . . unknown medical on Highway 98, mile post 334." That could be anything. I turned off the mower and hurried into the house, grabbed a quick drink of water, quickly washed up and hurried out the front door, keys in hand. At the station I was greeted by another EMT, John. "It's a seizure beside the turnoff to Kaibeto. It's the beginning of the month, want to guess who this is?" He asked as I got in.

"Kee?"

"Probably," he pulled the ambulance out of the bay and onto Navajo Drive. Soon we were on the road. The traffic was fairly light so we made good time. Soon we arrived. Two cars sat beside the road, one with his hazard lights on. Three people stood around a man as he lay on the ground, moving about in unorganized movement. "It's Kee," John said as he kneeled down. Kee's seizure-like movement increased. He began to flail his arms about, arched his back and quivered. He was good. It was exactly the way a seizure should look. Of course, I had to consider this could be real. I briefly considered drug-induced seizures, head trauma, reaction to medication, neurologic problem, etc.

Quickly we had him in the back of the ambulance. Kee had remained still as we lifted the stretcher into the ambulance. He then began to twitch and move his arms and legs about as I set up for an IV. He stopped seizing as I stuck his finger for a drop of blood needed to test his blood sugar. It was normal. I shoved up the sleeve of his leather coat in search of a vein and found one. Just as I was ready to insert the IV catheter, I said "Kee, hold still or I will have to cut your coat." He continued to shake all over but his left arm stopped all movement. He held his arm still. I made the stick, taped the catheter down and started the IV dripping. Then his arm began to shake again. I was now convinced it was all pretend. After a while he stopped. He had to be getting tired by this time. He lay still, not opening his eyes. I applied oxygen and took his vital signs, all normal. I hooked him up to the cardiac monitor, normal sinus rhythm. I decided to not give him an anti-seizure drug because this was obviously not real. I couldn't count the number of times I had done this. I can't imagine the number of times Kee had done this with other medics. Off and on Kee would begin another short "seizure." Then he lay silent again. We arrived at the Page Hospital and rolled the stretcher inside. Just as we moved him to the hospital gurney he opened his eyes. The nurse asked how he felt.

"Good, I want to sign that paper and leave now."

The doctor walked up. "Don't you want to pretend for a while?"

"Pretend?" Kee had an innocent look on his face. "I all well now." He smiled, "paper?" and made a gesture of signing a pretend document in the air.

Sighing, the doctor turned around, "Get him his AMA (against medical advice discharge form)." The doctor then walked away. The nurse brought Kee an AMA form, which he signed. She disconnected the IV and placed a band-aid over the tiny hole. Kee climbed off the gurney, pleasantly said goodbye and then walked outside. He was in town and had ridden in style. He headed toward the park hoping to find some friends there. Kee had no intentions of paying the ambulance or hospital bill because he knew the Indian Health Service and Medicaid would pay any bill he incurred. He wouldn't be billed by the hospital because he checked out before they did anything. He had used the system to get a ride to town and there was nothing anyone could do about it. This happened over and over through the years.

Sometime later, Kee had another idea. The ride into town worked so well, why wouldn't it work in reverse? He went to Circle-K and called 911. "Need ambulance, Circle-K."

"Why," asked the dispatcher

Kee thought for a second, "Heart attack." I remember pulling up beside Circle-K and being met by Kee. Before I could get out, he opened the back door and climbed in. He lay down on the stretcher, folded his arms across his chest and said, "Take me to Kaibeto."

I smiled. "I can't Kee. You said you were having a heart attack. I have to take you to the Page Hospital." We were an eighth of a mile from the hospital and I could see it across the field from where we were parked.

"No, Kaibeto. Medicine Man fix me up."

"Medicine Men make house calls to the hospital. I can't take you to Kaibeto." In Arizona and probably in other states, Medicaid pays for Medicine Men's services.

Kee sat up and looked disgustedly at me, "Then I go nowhere." He got out the back door and walked away. He never tried that again.

Kee wasn't the only one to use the PFD Taxi Service. An Anglo man around fifty years of age lived in Big Water, Utah, about eighteen miles west of Page. His old pickup would break down on a regular basis. He wasn't an alcoholic. But he loved to spend Saturday night at the bar with his friends in Page. If the truck wasn't working he would try to get a ride with a friend or neighbor into town. If that failed, he would fake chest pain. When the ambulance arrived he would say the pain had lessened but he still wanted to be transported to the hospital. En route he would remark how much better he felt. Upon arrival at the hospital he would say he felt fine and would sign an AMA form and walk two blocks to the Windy Mesa Bar. He wasn't charged a hospital bill because he signed an AMA form before they did anything. He didn't have to pay for the ambulance because Medicaid paid the bill. He once asked me to join him at the bar for a drink, but when I asked him if my husband could come along too, he decided to withdraw the invitation. When health care is "free" abuse abounds.

FREQUENT FLYER

To a writer, Kee offers a deep well of never ending stories. This is one of his many adventures. Kee had been drinking at the Windy Mesa, a local cowboy/biker bar in Page. His drinking buddy, Arnold, had not noticed Kee left the bar. Kee crawled into the bed of Arnold's truck with great difficulty. It had taken three tries to get his drunken body off the ground and into the pickup bed. He then curled up in a ball and went to sleep.

Arnold and his other buddy came out of the bar and got in Arnold's truck. Both men could hardly stand so neither had thought to look for Kee. They just drove off. Page lies in a valley on top of a mesa (a flat topped mountain or tall hill). Just outside town is the Little Cut. It is a 6% grade up the side of a mountain and then through a "cut" made in the mountain to allow the road to access to the other side. It is a steep and long climb to the top.

Arnold and his buddy were heading home. They didn't notice when Kee woke up. Kee sat up and yawned. He tried to stand up but ended back in the sitting position. He tried again and this time gained his footing. He staggered and stumbled to the back of the pickup. Kee didn't realize the truck was in motion. In his drunken stupor, he believed he was dizzy and uncoordinated. He didn't realize they were speeding down the highway. Kee staggered and stumbled to the back of the truck, swung a leg over the tail gate and stepped onto the bumper. He then swung his other leg over. He then stepped down onto the roadway at 55 mph. He was surprised as he began to fall.

The driver of the car traveling behind them watched in total disbelief. He said the man just stepped out of the truck and began to roll and tumble down the hill. The car pulled over, missing Kee. The man said Kee continued down the 6% grade, rolling head over heels, head over heels etc. "I didn't think he would ever stop rolling." The witness told me when we arrived. Kee lay in a tattered heap in the middle of the road. He had near terminal road rash. His clothing was shredded and the skin beneath was rubbed off and now glistened with raw exposed tissue. We treated Kee as if he had broken every bone in his body, but later we found out he had no fractures, just soft tissue injury. His mother came and got him and took him back home.

There was just something about a pickup that spelled bad luck for Kee. When Kee came to town, he always could find a "girlfriend." He wasn't picky and they weren't either. As long as he furnished the liquor, the various girls were willing to be his "girlfriend" at least until he ran out of money. This time it was Wanda. Wanda was of average size, only twenty-six years old, but looked forty-six. Someone once said it wasn't the years, it was the miles and in her case they were correct. She liked Kee and together they had a great four days. Then it happened. She decided she wanted to go home. She owned the truck they had been driving around, he didn't. She insisted she was leaving. He insisted she stay in town. An exciting exchange of words then occurred. Then Kee, in his drunken stupor, made a serious mistake, he slapped her. Wanda blew up and just lit into him swinging her fists and unleashing an ungodly string of profanities. Kee covered his face in an attempt to protect himself from her blows. She then turned and hurried to her pickup. Now, Kee was as drunk as she was, probably more. His judgment was all screwed up. As she drove off, for some reason known only to him, he grabbed the tail gate and hung on. She sped off, dragging him behind her. She didn't know he was there and so she didn't stop.

The toes of Kee's boots drug on the pavement as he hung on to the tail gate. He managed to pull himself up into the bed of the truck. Then she saw him in her rear view mirror. Now she was afraid. Kee sometimes could get really mad and this was one of those times. She was afraid of what he would do if he got his hands on her. She whipped the steering wheel to the right and to the left in an attempt to throw him out. He fell to the bed of the pickup but didn't fall out. He then reached through the small rear window and grabbed her hair. She screamed and whipped the wheel again causing him to fall to his right. He almost went over the short side of the truck. He would have managed to say in the bed of the truck if she hadn't jumped the curb and ran up on the sidewalk then hit a fire hydrant. It was a solid crash and Kee went flying out of the truck to the sidewalk. He sat up and reached for the truck just as she put it in reverse and ran over his arm. Before he could do anything, she put the truck in gear and drove forward, running over his arm and lower leg this time. But she couldn't clear the hydrant, so she put it in reverse and drove back over Kee and then she put it in a forward gear and over him again. This time he stayed down. She sped off leaving Kee lying on the sidewalk with tire marks all over his body and water spraying from the damaged hydrant.

Our response time set all records since the accident was less than fifty feet from the Fire Station. Again, we back boarded Kee, pretending he had broken every bone in his body. This time we were close. Not every bone but a fair number of them mostly in his arms and legs. I started two large bore IV's, put him on oxygen and the cardiac monitor. His blood sugar was ok but he was completely unconscious. The woman was stopped by Page Police just as she hit the highway heading south. She told them she couldn't see where he was after she hit the hydrant and she was afraid he would hurt her so she hurried and left the scene. Kee lived to tangle with another pickup a year later. This time the truck was driven by his own mother.

Kee was in town and cold sober. I believe the moon was also blue that night, but I am not certain. Kee's mother saw her son walking down Vista Avenue. She was certain he was heading for Page Tavern. She pulled over. She offered him a ride home. He politely declined. Kee loved his mother and would never talk back to her or show disrespect. He stood beside the pickup at the driver's window and quietly spoke to her for a few minutes. She was disappointed, but understood why he wouldn't go home with her. He still had a few dollars in his pocket. They said their goodbyes and she pulled away.

Her pickup had rails on the pickup bed for moving sheep. Kee's light jacket sleeve hung on the rail and jerked him off balance. He fell forward as his right arm hung in the railing. He fell to the ground, his arm pulled out of the jacket and he rolled beneath the back tire of the pickup. His mother heard him scream and stopped.

When I got there, Kee lay on his back with blood running freely from a large gash on his head. A tire track clearly ran across his chest. He was wearing a bright yellow t-shirt and it was unmistakable where the tire had rolled across his body. His mother stood a few feet away, softly crying. It wasn't her fault; it wasn't even Kee's fault. This was one of the few real "accidents." I had taken care of Kee a number of times but this was possibly the most serious. There was more blood than when he tried to steal that man's truck and he had got the "you know what" kicked out of him. It was even worse than the time he fell off the roof of that U-Haul truck. This time, he could die. The ironic things about this was that it was his own mother and Kee was cold sober.

We took full spinal precautions and kept his airway open and got the high flow oxygen flowing. I started two large bore IV's flowing wide open in an attempt to save his kidneys from the compression injury. I connected him to the cardiac monitor and found his pulse was rapid but normal sinus rhythm. We had him at the hospital in record time. He was flown out to Flagstaff Medical Center and fully recovered. His mother wasn't charged with anything.

It was two months before I received another call involving Kee. The call was paged out for a "man hit by a pickup in front of Taco Bell . . ."

THE CURSE

"It's supposed to be just beyond the pile of boulders. There it is on the left," I said. My EMT partner slowed the ambulance and turned off Highway 98 onto a dirt road. The road was deeply rutted. We crossed one dry sandy wash and came to a fork in the road. "The woman said to turn right." We turned right onto an even more poorly maintained dirt road. Our ambulance was not four wheel drive and several sandy spots were tense. We drove past on Hogan and a trailer. Finally we saw it, a Hogan sitting at the base of a hill just to the left of the road. Four dogs eagerly greeted us. They barked but didn't appear to be dangerous.

We drove up to the hogen and saw the elderly man lying on a thick blanket placed on the dirt a few feet to the side of the front door. "This is a bad sign, they think he is going to die," I said to my driver. Navajo's have to abandon the house if someone dies inside it, so if you arrive and the patient is lying outside, this means they are worried he might die before you arrive. I got out and was met by a man in his fifty's. He was the patient's son. He explained to me his father was feeling ill and needed to go to the hospital. I kneeled beside the patient. He was old as dirt. His arms and body were thin, and frail in appearance. He looked up at me and said, "I am going to die."

"Not yet," I said. I asked a lot of questions, but got very little information in return. We loaded him in the ambulance. His vital signs were normal for a frail elderly man. The cardiac monitor showed a very old and tired heart, but nothing that would kill him right away.

"Thank you for being concerned, but I am going to die."

"Why do you say that?" I asked

He hesitated, and then answered. "I was hit by bones. I will die now."

212

Bones? I began to question him about being *hit by bones*. I pictured him being beaten by a leg bone of a cow. He smiled and in broken English he said he had been cursed and bone powder had been blown on him. His family wasn't rich enough to pay a medicine man to remove the curse, so he would die. He believed he had lived a long, good life and accepted the death sentence imposed on him by the curse.

I told him I could find nothing that would cause him to die and he appeared in reasonable shape. He shook his head and said he was cursed and would die. He thanked me, but made it clear he had given up and had accepted his fate. We arrived at the hospital and I gave the best report I could. I told them I could find nothing wrong with the patient, but he had been cursed and believed he was dying. The doctor was aware of Navajo beliefs and didn't laugh.

The patient faced his impending death with dignity. The nursing staff would take him out into the garden a couple times a day. He liked that. He watched the birds and small lizards with interest. He ate well. He remained in stable condition with normal vital signs. He suddenly died two days later.

MOTORCYCLE ACCIDENT LAKE SHORE DRIVE

The call was a "motorcycle accident on Lake Shore Drive." EMT Mildred Moore got in back and looked at me. "My son just left the house on his motorcycle and he was going to the lake." I understood what she was telling me. She wasn't sure how she would handle it if it was her son.

"There's a good chance it's not him." She shook her head weakly agreeing with me and looked impatiently through the window.

We arrived and Mildred exploded from the still moving ambulance. I got out and rushed up to her. She stood over a man lying on the pavement, his face was gone. She searched him for some form of recognition, then looked at me and shook her head "no". We went to work. The man had no face. He was not wearing a helmet and had ground his face into the blacktop for about seventy-five feet. His eyelid hung loosely from a flap of skin. His mouth wasn't there anymore. Teeth lay scattered about with pieces of flesh. There was a tremendous amount of blood.

NPS Paramedic, Ronald Coffer was there. He was a great Paramedic and never minded sharing a patient. There was enough to go around this time. NPS Ranger Kemper pulled up and ran up to help. He was a tall man, hyper and usually no help whatsoever at an accident scene.

He was not that well-liked by anyone, including his wife and son. I found him mostly irritating. Kemper had the habit at an accident scene of getting in the way. I learned how to solve that problem. He ran up and announced in his loud booming voice, "What can I do?"

I handed him two roller bandages, a large trauma dressing and my blood pressure cuff and stethoscope. "Can you hold these? I am going to need them in a minute."

He was eager to help and said "Sure, just let me know when you need them." Now with both his hands full and his commitment to stand by to assist he couldn't get in the way. He was committed and had to just stand there until needed.

Mildred placed the oxygen mask on the patient. She took her seth and began to listen to the patient's chest. I used the bandages Ranger Kemper was holding but he still had things to hold in his hands. We rapidly put on the MAST suit then log rolled him to the backboard. I then took the equipment from Ranger Kemper and took a quick set of baseline vital signs. He reached down, grabbed one corner of the board and lifted before everyone else was ready. "Hay, wait for the rest of us," Ranger Coffer said in an irritated voice. Four of us then lifted the backboard together and loaded the patient into Rescue-One.

Ronald was a paramedic, but he had temporarily lost his medical control due to a contract dispute between the doctor and NPS. So today he was functioning as a Basic EMT. En route I couldn't get a good airway. Ronald said I should insert a nasal tube down his nose. I had never done that before and hesitated. But the man had no mouth and his wasn't getting enough oxygen so I shoved it in. It stopped. Randy said to "shove as hard" as I had too and get it down. I did, and it was in place. I bagged him (provided artificial respirations using the bag valve mask). I suctioned as necessary. The patient had an airway.

At the hospital the ER went crazy. We EMTs stayed and helped. I continued to suction and manage his airway. Dr. Percy was on call and arrived quickly. He while working on the patient and he asked "What's his name?" I answered, Dale Duncan." The doctor stopped what he was doing and took a step back and stared at the hunk of raw flesh on the table. "Dale Duncan?" he asked in disbelief. "I was talking to him not a half hour ago." He then took a deep breath and went back to work.

Later when the respiratory tech showed up, I backed off. I joined Mildred as she was writing the report. She looked up at me and smiled. "Thanks" she said.

"For what?"

"For that look you gave me, the one that let me know you understood and if it was my son, he would be well cared for."

"Thank goodness it wasn't"

"Yes, but I feel sorry for the patient and his family." I understood what she meant. Sometimes EMT's and paramedics feel guilty when a person dies. Our husband will come home from work, our children from school, and our parents and siblings are doing well. What makes us different from all the families of the patients we treat? Nothing. Why them and not us? I think in some ways that is what bothers those in rural EMS the most. Next time it could be our family member and we might have to treat them. I found myself in that position when I drove up on an auto accident and it involved my husband. I know a woman who crawled into a crushed car, felt for a pulse and announced the driver was dead. It was her brother-in-law and she then had to provide care and treatment for the drunken man who had just killed her sister's husband. Another PFD EMT did CPR on her best friend. A number of EMTs and paramedics I know have run on calls involving their own children. Living in a small community leaves us open to such a possibility and the question isn't "will it happen?" It's "when will it happen?" It haunts us. Whether a volunteer or a paid professional, when faced with an injury or illness of a loved one, I have found they usually charge ahead and do their job, then break down when it's all over.

As we got up to leave, the x-ray tech stepped into the room. "Sharon, could you come look at the x-ray?" That was an unusual request but I followed him down the hall. We stood in front of a x-ray hanging on the lighted viewing screen on the wall. He pointed to a number of black dots in the lungs. "What is that?" he asked.

"Gravel," I answered. I told him of the obstruction I had encountered and that I shoved it down with the nasal airway. He then understood. He told me with the choice I had to make as a Basic-EMT, I had done the right thing. I had caused another problem by forcing the gravel down into the lungs, but the patient had to have an airway or he would have died. The ex-ray tech left in search of the doctor to tell him of this new problem.

I didn't know the patient, but I soon found out that Dale was a heavy drinker and had been drunk that day. He also had attempted suicide a few years ago. He was a wild party animal. He wasn't a good husband and thankfully he and his wife didn't have children. He worked for his father when he felt like it. She had a good steady job and a good reputation.

Not all stories have a happy ending. Real life can be cruel. Dale has come back to haunt me many times. I worked so hard to keep him alive and it worked, but I didn't do him any favors. He

215

spent months in the hospital. Plastic surgery couldn't make him look normal again. Children cried when they saw him. He was sick off and on for a total of eight months, never regaining his prior physical condition. PFD took him to the hospital several more times from his home for a variety of medical complications. Each time I felt guilty that somehow I was partially to blame for his suffering. He never got well. He was found dead in bed eight months after the accident. According to the autopsy it was blood clots that had finally killed him.

I like to think that he had that time to get his life in order. Maybe he used the time to make up for his behavior in the past, a time to set things right with his wife, friends, family and God. I don't know if he used that time constructively. But I hang on to the tiny thread of hope that he did. That is the only reason I can think of, that makes me feel not so guilty for prolonging his death by eight miserable months.

MOM IS ALWAYS RIGHT

I had spent all day working on the new PFD Contagious Exposure policy. I had finally gotten home and was trying to get dinner ready to serve when the phone rang. It was the dispatcher. "Sharon, can you go outside? Detective Parker would like to see you."

I didn't ask any questions. I went outside and found an unmarked police car sitting outside my house. I walked to the driver's door. "What's up?" I asked.

"I wanted you to meet Brice Gibbs." He motioned to the man sitting in the back seat by himself. "He's under cover and will be in Page for the next week." I leaned into the back window and looked at the undercover police officer. I stared at him, looked him up and down, memorizing his features. He was about six foot tall, thin in build. His sandy brown hair hung in his eyes and he needed a haircut. He wore a three day's stubble. His eyes were brown and a small scar could be seen on his left temple. The purpose of this procedure was simple. The man could be injured in the line of duty or just driving from his motel to the restaurant. I responded to most 911 ambulance calls, usually arriving before the ambulance and sometimes before police officers. If the patient was an uncover police office, I would recognize him. I was not to say

216

anything at the scene, to preserve his cover. But I was expected to make sure an officer came to the scene and/or met us at the hospital. I also was to expect him to be armed and perhaps have illegal substances on him. Protocols had been established and I was to follow them.

I continued to stare at him for a few minutes. I then stood up. "It's nice to have met you Mr. Gibbs." He acknowledged me with a nod of the head. They drove off. I went back inside and resumed my duties as wife and mother. It didn't last long. My pager went off.

Soon, I was on Eighth Avenue kneeling in the middle of the road beside a young boy. The area was a quiet residential area. The boy lay silently on the road. Most Anglo children cry, but he didn't. He just lay there, quietly with a sad look on his face. He had ran into the road and was struck by a car going around twenty miles per hour

After a swift exam I asked him why he was sad. "I'm going to die," he said.

"No you're not," His injuries were minor although we were taking spinal immobilization precautions due to the method of injury and children's conditions can change suddenly.

He looked up at me with sad eyes, "I'm going to die."

"Why do you think that?"

"My mom told me if I ran out into the road I would get hit by a car and I would die. I ran out in the road and got hit by a car. My Mom's real smart. I'm going to die." What could I say?

His mother arrived at the scene. I told her what he said. She burst into tears and bent down to kiss her son. "Baby, you're not going to die."

He looked up at her with complete disbelief in his expression, "You lied?"

"Baby, I was trying to protect you. I was afraid you might forget to look both ways and I wanted to make sure you remembered." She started to cry even more.

The boy pondered the fact that his mother had actually lied. Lying is wrong so his mother had done something wrong. This is a lot for a six year old to process. Finally he reached over and took his mother's hand and smiled. "That's ok Mom, I still love you." He was seen in the ER and went home with minor road rash to his knees, elbows and tip of his chin. He was going to be ok.

WHEN A FRIEND SHOOTS HIS SON

The address sounded familiar. I was speeding through the streets of Page in my Assistant Chief vehicle. It was an old blue full size police car with code lights on top and PFD insignias on the door. I had driven my own personal car for years but finally they gave me one to use. It had good points and bad points. The good points were the code lights and I didn't have to put gas in it. The bad points were my family or my dog couldn't ride in it. One other problem I didn't see coming was the fact that every car I got behind when not using the code lights thought I was a police officer and would slow down to a snail's pace. Today I was "first responder" for the Page Fire Department. As Rescue Chief, I would respond directly to the scene and handle the situation until the ambulance arrived. I pulled into "Vermillion" (aka Lake Powell Mobile Home Park.) There were speed bumps and children everywhere so I slowed down. I soon found myself in front of Danny Phillip's home. He was an EMT, Volunteer Firefighter and my friend.

I parked, leaving room for the ambulance that would soon arrive. I grabbed my jump kit and hurried to the front door. Danny stood at the door. "My boy's shot." I didn't wait for the police; I felt I knew Danny enough to enter without police protection. In the dining room, the boy lay on the floor, on his back. I knew the boy well. He was barely sixteen years of age, skinny, black hair, and brown eyes. His eyes were wide. "I didn't move," he said. The boy was named Tim. He had spent a lot of time helping the fire department practice skills. He would pretend to be injured, sometimes lying under a car or tangled in a ladder, etc. He knew what to expect, and had done the right thing. He lay stiff, almost frozen to the spot.

"What happened?" I asked.

"Dad was cleaning his gun; it went off and hit me in the arm." I looked up at Danny. He filled in the blanks. Apparently Danny was sitting in an arm chair in the living room, facing the wide doorway that led to the dining room. He had an antique pistol. It used a "musket ball" type load. The gun went off and the bullet struck the boy as he stood in the doorway. When the police arrived they toyed with the idea that Danny had shot his teenage son. Danny had a temper, drank at times and was a "biker" (tattoos, leather, Harley and everything). He was a bit rough around the edges but, there was no way he would shot his own son. It was an accident. It was obvious to me. After a brief period of uncertainly, the police agreed and accepted the accident for what it was.

"Don't move Tim," I told him. I examined the boy very carefully. The bullet appeared to have entered his left shoulder and on an upward

218

trajectory, struck the left side of his neck. There wasn't a lot of blood. There was no exit wound. I believed the bullet was still in his neck. So was his spinal cord. Musket balls fragment on impact. There was a good chance the soft bullet had shattered into multiple pieces.

"My left hand is numb. Am I going to be paralyzed?" he asked. I looked at his young face. It was full of fear. He knew enough to know that was a distinct possibility.

"Wiggle your toes," I said. He did. I decided to not sugar coat the truth. "I can only see a few drops of blood. There is a small hole, about the size of the tip of your little finger, in your shoulder and left neck, toward the back. The injury doesn't look life threatening. Your hand is numb probably because of a nerve may have been damaged in the shoulder. That's repairable. I know your spinal cord is intact because you can wiggle your toes. I believe the bullet may still be in your neck. It could be near the spinal cord. We are going to take every precaution possible to keep your head, neck and body still so the bullet doesn't move. If it moves, it could cause more damage." The boy understood. He was frightened, but calm. Later he told me that when I talked to him like a grownup, it made him relax and trust what I was saying.

I heard the ambulance pull up. I got on the radio, "It's code-4, bring me an old wooden backboard, duct tape, towels, and a blanket." They knew to not ask questions, they did as ordered. Soon, the crew burst into the room, hands full. They knew Danny and Tim. They were part of our family of EMS. I knew Tim was going to Flagstaff Medical Center or Phoenix and I would never see our backboard and straps again so we used the old wooden backboard and duct tape. The wooden board was easy to x-ray through and additional support was needed to secure him to the board in an extra sturdy manner and duct tape was just the thing we needed.

I explained everything to the crew, Danny and the teenager. "We need to move slowly and carefully. I don't want to use the regular c-collar, because I don't want pressure on the wound. I want him secured in an exaggerated manner to this board. He's going to be on it awhile and I don't want his body to slip or move in any way." Everyone understood. Danny, the EMT's and I kneeled down. I took his head in my hands. "Dear God, please let this work. Don't let this young boy be paralyzed. Please guide us," I prayed silently. I have a feeling the others were saying their own prayers at that time.

"Now, I want you to not move, at all. Stiffen your body like a board. Let us do the work. You've been on a board during drills, so you know how it goes."

"I understand." The boy answered in a voice far older than his years.

The next five minutes were tense. We got him on the board. I held his head so I was in charge. I spoke slowly and concisely. We moved slowly, moving him as a unit, keeping his spine in line, and minimized movement. The boy was brave and did as told. No tears, just a quite serious look on his face. He trusted us but he knew enough to be afraid. After he was on the board, we used the duct tape to secure him. We were careful to not put tape over flesh. He was taped so securely, the joke was "he had to ask permission to blink." After he was secured, I asked him to wiggle his toes. He did. No harm done. The spinal cord was still intact. "Thank you God." I whispered.

The boy smiled. "I can still wiggle my toes, but my hand's still numb."

I checked his fingers. "They are still pink. Capillary refill is good. It's a nerve thing, not blood supply."

"That's a good thing, right?" he asked.

"Yes, no additional harm was done. The nerve thing is important, but blood supply is more important." He said he understood.

He was taken to the hospital. I called on the phone and alerted the doctor and ER staff as to what we had. I told them I strongly believed the bullet was still in there and posed a serious danger to the spinal cord. The doctor was a "rent a doc" and they usually lacked enthusiasm and usually were just barely adequate. He wasn't as impressed as I had hoped, but he understood I was tactfully telling him to keep the boy on the board until x-rays were taken. He reserved the decision about transport to a larger hospital. I knew it was a sure thing.

I turned to Danny, "Danny, before you follow over on your bike, pack a bag, a couple changes of clothing, personal hygiene items, a book to read, and cash, credit card, and insurance info. He's going to Flag or Phoenix. You are going to be gone two or three days. If you go on the airplane, you will need to have your brother, Marvin, drive down and pick you up in a few days." Danny hurried away, and packed a bag. His boy wasn't going to be flown to another town for surgery without him beside him. I left. Danny was detained as police questioned him a little, but I left a firefighter/friend with him and about twenty minutes later, he arrived in the ER.

The doctor didn't see it as serious as I did, but he wasn't brave enough to take him off the board. I had taken Danny aside and told him if the doctor tried to remove the boy from the board, Danny was to step in and refuse to allow it. I couldn't stop the doc but Danny could. The boy was taken to x-ray and it was discovered the soft bullet had shattered into eight tiny sharp pieces. Two were still in his shoulder, six were in his neck, one directly touching the cord and a second one very near. Another piece was near an artery and the other three were scattered about the neck tissue. It was a frightening x-ray.

Danny and I took it and showed it to the boy. He was behaving like a man and deserved the truth. He looked the x-ray over, and then turned his eyes to me "You were right." I smiled.

"Are they going to do surgery on me?"

"Yes. You are going to Flagstaff Medical Center. A Neurologist, a specialist of spinal cords, will do the surgery."

"Am I going to be paralyzed?" he asked me again.

I sighed. "I believe this can be resolved by surgery. I can't promise you. You're old enough to know bad things happen sometimes, but I really believe you are going to be ok."

He smiled. He was a boy this morning, a man this afternoon. He had grown up suddenly and it was obvious he was going to be a strong man, capable of handling the "slings and arrows of outrageous fortune." He was flown to Flagstaff, still taped to the backboard, his father beside him. He went almost immediately into surgery. It was a tough surgery. The doc said the shattered bullet was almost touching the cord and any movement could have severed the cord, rendering the boy paralyzed from the neck down. The surgery took a long time, but was successful.

The young man came to drill with his father around four months later. He still had problems with his left arm, but with rehab and lots of exercise, he said the doc told him it would be as good or very close to the same as it was before the accident. "Thanks for everything," he said with a wide smile to everyone who had had a part in the call.

"You're welcome," he was told. He missed a bit of school but with summer school he caught up. He grew into a nice young man, with complete use of his arms and legs. It could have gone the other way, thank God he survived intact. Years later my good friend Danny died in a horrible accident while visiting Tim in another state. I guess its best we can't see into the future. We might not enjoy the blessings of today if we were worried about what was going to happen tomorrow.

FREE SPIRIT

Susie Otterman was a young high school teacher, EMT and a free spirit. At school she was a strict, unyielding liberal. She tolerated no other political opinion except hers. She gave students low grades if their papers were not politically correct and way to the left. They retaliated by putting Right Wing bumper stickers on her car which would make her go crazy. She was married and had one young son. Years later they moved. It was rumored her husband surprised everyone by coming out of the closet and having a sex change operation. Her liberal "I'm ok, you're ok" belief system must have been seriously strained when that happened.

Susie was a good EMT but many people found her "different." There were a number of issues but this story concerns clothing. She dressed conservatively for work but at home she didn't seem to see the need for clothing. She was a free spirit. She often went about naked. Nudity was *natural and normal* behind the closed doors of her home.

One day, she was on duty and her pager sounded. She looked around and couldn't find her jumpsuit. She then remembered it was in the front seat of her pickup that was parked inside her garage. She ran naked through the house, flung open the door and rushed into the attached garage. She opened the car door and grabbed her jumpsuit. She was slipping it on when she suddenly got the odd feeling she was being watched. She stopped. She slowly turned her head to the side. This was when she discovered, the garage door was standing open.

The neighbor man was standing across the street watering his lawn. He held the hose in his hand as it flowed onto the sidewalk. His eyes were wide with shock and surprise, his mouth hung open. Sue felt embarrassment as she had never felt before. She pulled up the jumpsuit, zipped it and climbed into the car and drove off, not looking toward the still frozen neighbor. Things were awkward at the next parent/teacher meeting.

THE PAGE BOY FIRE

It had been raining most of the day. It was cool but not cold yet. Fall had arrived to Page. The Page Boy Motel was an inexpensive motel located on the corner of the main street of town, Lake Powell Blvd. (previously known as Seventh Avenue) and Bureau Street. It had a two story building and on each side a one story structure that formed a "U". A pool sat in the middle of the complex. The rooms had doors that faced the street and then patio doors opening into the inside courtyard/pool/lawn area. The hotel rented rooms by the day, week, and month. Many out of the town people, mostly off the reservation lived there during the yearly overhaul of Navajo Generating Station.

Room number two was rented to a Navajo man who had a steady job at the Navajo Generating Station. He lived on the reservation just outside town. He and a friend of his came into town early that day, and decided to rent a room and have a little party. They found a willing woman named Vicky and the party was on. Sometime later that day, they lay exhausted from fun and games and lots of alcohol. They were all very drunk. The air conditioner/heater that hung on the wall had been giving the management problems. They said it was fixed. But it made a lot of noise. It isn't clear exactly what happened. The man that rented the room said he had left for work before the fire started. The other man said he had as well. But several people said they saw one man wearing a hard hat run away from the burning motel. Another said she saw two men run away from the room. Anyway, the woman Vicky was left alone.

When the smoke filled the small room, she woke up. Vicky was wearing a black t-shirt. She stood up and pulled on her jeans, but didn't snap or zip them. She staggered to the door, smoke made her eyes sting. She tried to breath, but the black smoke burned as it filled her lungs. She couldn't see as tears filled her red burning eyes. She lost her way and instead of going out the door, she found herself in the bathroom, just to her left before the outside door.

Vicky coughed, gasped for breath. She fell to her knees. She was very intoxicated and the lack of oxygen caused by the thick smoke made her coordination and judgment even worse. The heat in the bathroom was increasing. She fell to the floor, coughing. She tried to think, but her mind was deprived of oxygen and she couldn't figure out what to do. To get out, she would have to turn around, leave the bathroom, turn left and exit the door to the outside. Fresh cool air and safety was only around six to seven feet away. But Vicky would never feel the cool breeze on her face again. She would be dead in a few minutes.

The plastic molding around the ceiling melted and dripped down on the woman as she lay on the floor. She yelled as the melted plastic hit her exposed skin. She tried to move, but there was no place to go. Black suffocating smoke filled the tiny room. The shower curtain and plastic curtain rod began to melt and it dripped down on her legs, but she didn't feel it. She was unconscious. She didn't feel the heat or the flames as they ate away at the thin wall between the bathroom and the main bedroom.

The fire had a big head start when we arrived. As we pulled up, a bystander, who knows why, picked up a brick and broke the sliding patio door. The sudden draft of fresh oxygen caused the fire to suddenly grow in an unbelievable manner.

Day time fire calls were hard. We were often understaffed. Our firefighters work in outside jobs and many were not available during the day. Oh, they usually came, but they couldn't get there until the second or third truck. The first truck that day was manned by Judy Mason, our first official female firefighter, Captain Tanner, Mark Timmons, engineer, the second truck had two firefighters, Brody Smyth and a new guy named Smith that had never even taken out a burn permit to burn weeds before this date. We had a rule that new guys stayed out of the mess and watched until they were trained. But our fire training program wasn't that organized and they were often pulled into working the fire in some capacity. They were hard to tell from other firefighters, they all looked the same and dressed the same. Before the new guy knew what was happening, he was outfitted in a Scott pack and told to get ready to enter the burning room. It surprises me even now, but he did as told.

Firefighter Judy was about five foot eight inches tall and one-hundred and thirty-five pounds. She was around twenty-five years old. Julie had the ax and she knew she better do the job right or it would be blamed on all women in fire service. She had a lot to prove as she walked up to the door that day. She swung the ax back, and then forward. She hit the door frame. She swung again and again. She put everything she had into it. The door gave way and flew open.

Brody Smyth and the new guy entered on their knees with a fire hose. Brody was in front and the new guy had no clue what he was supposed to do, so he just followed Brody. They shot water into the room as they moved about looking for someone. It was hard to see, because the smoke was black and very thick. They could see the bright orange flames in the corner of the room. Brody turned the hose to the fire and let go. It hissed in protest. Brody moved on, the new guy scooted along behind. They searched the room according to protocol but found no one. In the darkness Brody had missed the small door just to the right as he came in the outside door. He had searched the room but forgot the bathroom. He hadn't found Vicky. By that time it didn't matter anyway. They came out.

I had set up medical welfare in the bowling alley parking lot across the street from the fire. It was convenient and we had a great view. Brody and the new guy wandered over and sat down. They were completely exhausted. The new guy didn't look all that good. I took his blood pressure and pulse and both were sky high. He was young, maybe nineteen years old. It was always the young ones that dropped from exhaustion. The older ones paced themselves, the younger ones ran around stuck on fast forward. I gave him something to drink.

I turned to watch as more water was put on the fire. The fire was extinguished. Another crew entered to finish with the smoldering furniture. I left the medical sector with two other EMTs. I was walking around near Engine-Two when I noticed Captain Tanner exit the motel room in a hurry and run up to the Fire Chief. They talked a minute and the Fire Chief then approached. "Sharon, we have found a body. It's in the bathroom. Can you get me a body bag?"

It's hard to explain how I felt at the moment. We all have our fears and mine is burning to death. I know it's not an uncommon fear and most people share that fear with me, any sane person would. I had seen badly burned people before and it's awful. The smell of burnt human flesh is horrible. It gets in your hair your clothing and you can taste it. There are many ways to die, some are better than others. This was a bad way. I didn't say anything. I went and got a body bag. Now our department has really nice heavy vinyl zip body bags but we were never allowed to use them. They were too expensive Chief Nelson always said so I went and got a "shroud". It's a white disposable thing that sort of wraps the victim up. I went and warned my EMTS. They got sheets and followed me to the door. They held the sheets up so the crowd couldn't see the body as it was brought out. I helped wrap the woman's body in the shroud.

"Do you know her?" the detective asked. I looked closely at her soot covered face with singed hair. "No I don't recognize her." Her body was taken to the morgue and the fire scene was guarded by firefighters till the State Fire Marshal got here many hours later.

Now, the rest of the story: It was lawsuit time. Vicky's children had been raised for many years by a sister due to Vicky's lifestyle. But despite the fact that the children hadn't even seen their mother for years they sued the motel for loss of a "mother's love." It was messy. The whole case rested on whether the fire started in the heater/air conditioner or not. Fire Chief Nelson said *yes*. A national acclaimed expert actually wrote an article on it and said *no*. The insurance company finally settled out of court.

Brody was upset at first that they didn't find the body. But he was an experienced firefighter by this time and realized these things happen and in this case it wouldn't have made a difference to the woman. I threw a fit about the untrained firefighter being dragged into a working fire wearing equipment he hadn't been taught to use. Nothing came of it and I threw another fit. "Brody's life and that of the new recruit was put in jeopardy." I suggested a colored band around the newbie's helmet. That way, everyone would know he had not completed his fire training.

Nothing was done. I complained again. I didn't want the next dead body to be that of a firefighter. The fire chief said, "He should have refused."

"He should have never been asked," I countered. This went on for a while. Around two months later Fire Chief Nelson announced he had a great idea. How about us making sure that only trained personnel work within the hazard area? With some help a symbol was designed and all rookies were to wear it on their helmet till they completed training. Great idea, glad he thought of it.

Not long after that the room caught fire again for another entirely different reason. It was strange standing in the same place watching the same room burn. No one died this time. One of the firefighters in jest said "You know that's the room I'm going to book for my mother-in-law the next time she comes for a visit." From then on, we called that room the *Mother-in -law room.*

WHAT RAZOR WIRE?

Will was a twenty-four year old male Anglo. He was six foot, three inches tall, slender and wore his dull brown hair long. He was never seen without his old tattered Coors Beer ball cap. He had been out on his own off and on. He was a master of couch surfing. When he had worn out his welcome with all friends, he would return back home for a while. Will had no ambition whatsoever. He just got up, wandered through life and eventually went to sleep. He worked as seldom as possible. His parents, sister and brother had almost given up on him. The family was sitting in the living room watching television when the front door swung open. Will stood there, minus his hat and covered with blood. His mother jumped up and ran to him, but he pushed her away. "Will! What happened?"

"Nothing," he mumbled. His forearms and hands were slashed as if he had lost a knife fight. Blood flowed and dripped to the floor.

His mother turned around, "William (Will's father), call 911." She tried to attend to his wounds but he just walked past her as if she wasn't even there and staggered down the hallway to the small back bedroom he had been sleeping in for the last five weeks. William called 911.

Fifteen minutes before my pager sounded, Officer De Aquileo was patrolling Vista Avenue in Page. It was a street full of small businesses, storage units, boat repair, etc. After six in the evening the street was almost deserted. He slowed down as he drove past a storage yard of old boats and other vehicles. Page Ice was located in the rear northeast corner of the two acre lot. "Dispatch, 456 will be out at Page Ice for a minute." He turned on his mag light and lit the six foot tall chain link fence. A pool of blood lay on the sidewalk. The beam of light traveled up the fence and a bloody ball cap hung tangled in razor wire that curled along the top of the fence. De Aquileo looked around and found a bloody trail leading off down the sidewalk. He followed the trail. Two blocks down the sidewalk, the trail turned left and he followed it to a well maintained trailer. Just as he started to knock on the door, he heard the ambulance being paged. He looked around and saw the address was the same. He knocked on the door.

I arrived a few minutes in front of the ambulance. As I got out of my car, I was met by Officer De Aquileo. He told me the story. "I think he's higher than a kite. He doesn't even seem to know he's hurt."

"Weapons?"

"No. He cooperated at first so I frisked him. But then he got strange. He's not stable. It's probably Meth. His parents say he has used it in the past. You should consider him dangerous." Over the years I have dealt with alcohol abuse, prescription drugs, over the counter medication and every illegal drug known to man. Crystal Meth is one of the worst. I don't trust a person on Meth. They can be talking to you in non-threatening way and suddenly turn into an enraged madman set on pinching your head off. A Meth addict will become impulsive and exhibit violent outbursts. Meth users will go for weeks with no sleep and next to nothing to eat. They become paranoid and begin to hallucinate. They seldom see pretty butterflies. While working at the Page Hospital as an ER Tech I once sat for hours beside the bed of a young girl who was seeing fifty pound hairy spiders with red glowing eyes. In Santa Barbara, California they did a quick study and discovered that 65% of those in their county jail were meth users. In Anaheim, California in another short study they found 80% of all people arrested tested positive for meth use. They cost the medical community $865 million dollars a year. Because of their addiction, they are not productive citizens and seldom have insurance. The taxpayer picks up the medical bills because of their inability to pay and it costs money to keep them in jail. The sad part is less than 6% of those who go into rehab actually kick the habit (year 2009 figures).

"If he's that bad, why are we here?" I asked the officer as the ambulance pulled up.

"I thought we could give it a try. Maybe he will respond to you guys. I don't know. But before we charge in like the cavalry, I want to give him a chance. He's really hurt bad. He's lost a lot of blood. He really needs you guys."

I didn't like it, but maybe it wasn't Meth. Maybe his disorientation was due to a head injury or low blood sugar or shock. I decided I would go in first to evaluate him and decide if we could transport him safely or not. The back door of the trailer opened onto the rear hallway. The door stood open only three feet from Will's bedroom door. An officer was standing just outside the door and out of sight. I was to walk to Will's door, but not enter the tiny room. I went through the front door and introduced myself to his family and told them we were going to try to help Will. They looked like a nice, hardworking, middle class family. They seemed at a loss as to what to do.

I walked down the hall. Will sat on his bed and looked directly down the hall and saw me coming. I stopped short of his open door. I could see an unmade double bed. It filled the entire room except for a tiny end table and closet door. Officer De Aquileo stood out of the patient's sight to my left just outside the back door. He was a great backup. He was muscle bound and could bench press a Buick. I turned my attention to the patient. Will looked as if he had been wrestling a roll of razor wire. His both arms were slashed with deep gaping wounds. Some of the wounds had clotted but many more wounds still dripped blood. He sat on the edge of the bed with his arms resting on his knees. He was wringing his hands and blood dripped from his fingers. A big pool of blood between his feet and the carpet was soaked. The blood stain was growing bigger. His teeth were rotted. His face had two open sores and one that had scabbed over. He appeared to suffer from coke bugs. I am told it feels like bugs running around just under the skin and Meth users will scratch the skin until it became infected. I noticed his small stereo lay on the end table in pieces. Meth users often take things apart for no known reason and then can't get them re-assembled.

"Hi, my name's Sharon." He looked at me but he didn't seem to focus. He didn't smile or respond. His eyes were rapidly moving back and forth like a trapped animal. He wiggled around wringing his bloody hands. He looked like a piece of popcorn in a hot skillet. "Will, look at me."

He slowly focused and looked me in the eye. "What? I . . . . . I don't . . .Who the hell are you?" he mumbled.

"Your mother called me. You have cut your hands. I am an EMT and I want to help."

Will looked down at his hands and for a brief moment, he seemed surprise to see the blood. He held up one hand and examined it closely. He dropped his hand down onto his lap and seemed to forget it. He appeared more agitated and started repeating over and over again, "Go away, go away, go away, go away. . . . . go . . . . go away."

"Will, you need help."

His voice became louder. "I don't need no help . . . . don't need . . . don't." He lost his train of thought. He became even more restless and tapped his foot. His eyes darted around. It was obvious I wasn't getting through. Lilly Jacobs was on the ambulance. She was pretty and had a gentle manner. Her voice was soft and non-confrontational. I decided to let her try. I backed away. Will didn't seem to notice.

"Lilly, he's dangerous. I don't think it will work, but give it a try. Don't get near him and run to the living room if he makes any move toward you. De Aquileo will step behind you and no one will get past him."

She shook her head in understanding. She entered the hallway and smiled. Will focused on her but didn't seem to understand a word she said. He growled and stood up. Lilly stood her ground. He sat back down and began to rock back and forth. His eyes continued to dart this way and that and he couldn't sit still. He mumbled words that didn't form sentences. He no longer seemed to notice she was there.

"Lilly, that's enough." She backed away. I turned to Officer De Aquileo and two other officers who had arrived as backup. "I'm sorry guys but he's too unstable. If you could take him down and get him restrained we might be able to take him in the ambulance with one of you riding along, but I think he's too high and I'm pulling my crew out."

De Aquileo turned around and addressed his supervisor who was walking up. The four men huddled. I told my crew to stage at the corner to provide a medical backup for the officers, but they were not to transport the patient. The officers decided to overpower him, cuff him and transport in a patrol car. Under the circumstances, I agreed.

The ambulance staged at the corner. I stood on the sidewalk beside it. At my feet I saw the bloody trail De Aquileo had followed. I heard a lot of shouting coming from the trailer and then the officers appeared at the back door escorting Will outside. Will was struggling and putting up quite a fight for a man with his hands tied behind his back and a quart or so low on blood. I phoned the hospital and told them what the officers were bringing in. They needed to have a syringe ready with "kick-a-poo-joy-juice".

This is only one story of the dangers to an ambulance crew when called upon to help a person high on drugs. I have other stories but in many ways they are all the same. The user has lost control and by the time

EMS is called, it's completely out of hand. If drug abuse, legal and illegal, plus alcohol were to disappear off the face of the earth, I would probably be unemployed.

I COULDN'T LET HER DIE

Winter time on the reservation is beautiful. Snow clings to the mountain tops and steep red sandstone cliffs reach silently for the sky. Cedar trees glisten in the sun as they stand decorated with snow and ice. The Navajo are also under siege of respiratory infections. Those over sixty years of age often come down with pneumonia and children under five years of age come down with RSV. RSV is a viral infection that settles in the child's lungs and can kill.

Navajo's family structure contributes to the spread of the disease. It isn't uncommon for four generations to live under the same roof. It's winter so the windows are closed. A cough can travel fifteen feet. Germs on a child's hands are deposited on the door knobs, the fridge door, toys, x-box, and all the other household items around a home. Children sleep several to a bed. When one child brings a bug home from school it soon spreads throughout the household. Older children and healthy adults may get sick, but they fight it off and get better. The babies, the toddlers, the preschoolers and elderly often can't get well by themselves. They need help with medication and at times, hospitalization.

Kayenta, Arizona is on the southern edge of Monument Valley. The area is remote and part of the four corners area. The Kayenta clinic stayed full this time of year. The Monument Valley Hospital had been closed a few years before. The promise of a new hospital had not materialized. The clinic handled emergency and non-emergency medical problems. But the patients requiring hospitalization had to be transported by ground and air to hospitals in Tuba City, Shiprock, Page, Flagstaff, and San Juan Regional. When those hospitals filled up patients were transported by ground ambulance or air to Phoenix, Las Vegas, Dixie Medical Center, and Salt Lake City. I was working for a private ambulance company and we were busy. One call after another and our patients were almost always below five years of age or above sixty-five. I quickly became an expert on RSV.

I had been on duty only five hours and I had already transported one child from Kayenta to the Tuba City Regional Medical Center. I had managed to slip in a quick lunch and I wasn't surprised when I received a page to transport another child to Tuba. My partner and I arrived at the clinic and wheeled our stretcher into the crowded emergency room.

Wanda, a RN, approached us. "Your patient is eighteen months old. She's got RSV. That's her over there. They call her Baby Grace." she pointed across the room to a baby lying in her mother's arms. "I got an IV going. You might want to talk to the doc about her before you leave." She handed me the paperwork and hurried off. I stood watching the mother and child. The child lay limp in her mother's arms. Her mother held a small volume nebulizer (SVN) emitting Ventolin in the form of a white mist that blew into the child's face. The mother looked tired. She obviously had lost a couple nights' sleep caring for this child and possibility other older siblings as well.

I walked over and introduced myself. I touched the child. She didn't open her eyes. I spoke to her. She opened her eyes and glanced at me with eyes that seemed uninterested. "Can I hold her?" I asked. The mother handed her to me. I looked down into the face of an angel. She was beautiful. Her coal black hair framed a face with large black eyes, long dark lashes, and a rose bud mouth. I talked to the child and she didn't smile, she didn't cry, she just lay limply in my arms and didn't wrap her fingers around my finger when I lay it in her hand. Her lips had a slight blue tinge and her skin was pale. She closed her eyes. She was tired, unbelievably tired. Her chest muscles were so tired and sore she now used her shoulders and abdominal muscles to expand her chest. The air made a sound as it moved past swollen and clogged membranes in her airway. She had a low oxygen saturation and was in serious condition. I handed the baby back to her mother. "I have to talk to the doctor and make a phone call. Then we can transport her and you to Tuba." I left the EMT to get a set of baseline set of vitals.

I looked around and found Doctor Norton. The doctor had just walked away from a patient and was standing at the sink washing his hands. I walked up to him. "Doctor?" He turned around. "I'm here to transport the baby to Tuba."

"Yeah, she's not doing well."

"I am surprised she isn't being transported by air."

"Can't get a plane in. It's snowing all around us and it's expected to close in on us within the hour."

"She doesn't appear to be responding to the SVN."

"She did at first, but then her response became less and less. I started giving her an EPI SVN in between Ventolin. It's working for now but it's not going to work for much longer. I can't do anything more. If she stops breathing it's going to be hard to get her started again. The virus has a grip on her. She needs to be on a respirator and heavy antibiotics. I don't have either. "

"What about intubating her here and me bagging her all the way?"

"No, she's still conscious and we would get one try, after that her throat would slam shut and she would die. I think she will make it if you can get your Medical control to approve an Epi SVN." He reached for a paper towel and dried his hands. "Time is slipping away. She'll die here if she isn't transported soon."

"Is it possible a nurse could ride along with us?" The nurse could give the forbidden breathing treatment and my Paramedic Cert. would be safe.

"I can't spare a nurse. We are swamped. I'm sorry." He obviously wanted to help, but if just wasn't possible.

"I'll give my Medical Control a call and see what he says." I walked away and gathered my thoughts. I had a ventilator but couldn't use it on a patient under eight years of age. She was conscious so I couldn't intubate, even if I had the nerve and if her airway swelled shut I probably couldn't get her intubated because of her closed airway. A cric wouldn't work because her bronchial tubes are full of mucus and swelling shut. If she stopped breathing I could bag her for a while, but the throat was going to swell shut and if she was at a hospital they could probably handle this.

Before I transported patients from the clinic to a hospital I was required to call my Medical Control in Flagstaff medical Center. I would give them a patient report, what I plan on doing during transport and where the patient's going. I picked up the phone and dialed FMC. The nurse answered quickly. "1190, this is Paramedic Holbert. May I speak with a doctor?" She went to get the doctor. Usually an RN is fine, but this time I wanted to speak with a physician. He came to the phone. "Doctor, this is Paramedic Holbert. I am at the Kayenta Clinic preparing to transport an eighteen month old female child to Tuba City. She has been diagnosed with RSV. She is seriously ill and would have been flown but because of the snow storm she's being transported by ground. Do you copy?"

"Yes I copy."

"The patient has been ill for two days. She is limp and using accessory muscles to breath. Her respiration is rapid and she is wheezing. Her skin is pale and her lips are a light blue. O2 sats are in the low nineties and high eighties even with oxygen. At first she responded to Ventolin SVN's, but with each treatment she responded less and less. Finally Dr. Norton began alternating Ventolin and Epi SVN's. This proved to be more effective. Doctor Norton expects her to lose her airway and requested I use Epi and Ventolin."

"I copy. Then continue the SVN's."

"Doctor, I am Arizona and New Mexico certified. New Mexico will allow me to administer SVN's of Epi but Arizona won't. I am currently working under Arizona certification and your Arizona Medical Control. I know how and carry the drug but I can't legally give her an Epi SVN. There is no nurse available to ride along with us. I am the only transport available and Doctor Norton believes the child will lose her air way without Epi."

"I give you permission to do so."

"Doctor Miller, you do realize this isn't in my protocols?"

"Yes. Under these circumstances, I give you permission to give her Epi SVN's. Most states allow it."

"Arizona doesn't. Doctor, would you go over possible side effects for the record." He did. "And you fully understand you are ordering me to disregard my protocols and administer Epi SVN if necessary to maintain the patient's airway?"

"Yes. If you get in trouble, I will stand behind you and my orders."

"Thank you Doctor." I hung up. I knew even if he ordered me to give the Epi, I would be in serious trouble. He didn't know it but he didn't have the authority to change my protocols. I was climbing out on a limb. I was trying to cover my tail, but I knew it wouldn't actually do the job, it was just the best I could do. Even if I didn't give the Epi, I would still be in serious trouble for saying I would if necessary. I could lose my certification and never be allowed to be a paramedic again. I had worked so hard to get that certification, but a child's life was far more important. If it came down to a choice, there was no question; I knew what I would do. I just couldn't let her die, regardless of what it might cost me.

I looked across the busy ER. Her mother tried to interest the baby in a bottle. The baby wouldn't take the bottle. Her arms lay limp. She struggled weakly to breathe. She had very little fight left. She was dying unless she got to a higher level of care. I couldn't let her die, regardless what might happen to me. I went to Doctor Norton.

"Doctor, I was given orders for Epi SVN by Dr. Miller in Flagstaff. It's against my protocols and I am going out on the limb about this. I hope you will support me if this becomes an issue with my paramedic license."

"Sharon, I will support you. Now get out of here, she's quickly running out of time. Even Epi won't work for much longer. Good luck."

The EMT had the baby in her car seat and had strapped it to the stretcher. The mother held the Epi SVN to her face. The treatment was completed as I walked up. "Ready to go?" As we stepped outside I looked around. Dark gray clouds covered the sky. Small snowflakes fell. The mild breeze was ice cold. We quickly loaded the stretcher in the ambulance. The mother climbed inside and sat near the end of the bench seat allowing me to sit across from the baby. I found when the baby could see their mother, they usually feel more comfortable with me caring for them. I connected the baby up to our main oxygen tank. I got out the child bag valve mask in case she stopped breathing. I opened my drug box and got out the Ventolin. I set up the SVN in anticipation of her next treatment. I was hoping the Epi SVN she just received would keep her airway open for about half of the trip. Then I could administer the Ventolin and if it worked I might not have to give the forbidden Epi. The only problem was the weather. The snow was falling harder now. I was concerned about the roads. If they became snow covered, our trip would take longer.

The baby whimpered slightly. She was a little more awake due to the Epi SVN. Her mother reached over and spoke softly to her in Navajo. The baby calmed down. I didn't take my eyes off her for the next hour and twenty-two minutes. About fifteen minutes into the trip she stopped breathing. I tapped the bottom of her foot. That irritates babies more than anything. She withdrew her foot and took a ragged breath. She was tired, so very tired and had just stopped breathing. She continued breathing fast and shallow. I could handle a baby who stops breathing due to exhaustion, but if her airway swells shut I feared I could not do much and she would die.

I gave the mother a pillow and she leaned up against the back post of the ambulance and went instantly asleep. I never removed my eyes from the child. I watched each breath. Her oxygen saturation was low so I replaced the nasal cannula with a small mask. Usually a baby will fight the mask, but she was too far gone to notice and accepted it. I turned up the oxygen to fifteen litters a minute. Her oxygen level increased.

When we passed Cow Springs the snow stopped and the ambulance speeded up. The driver and I had worked together a long time and he automatically switched on the lights and sirens. We started to make time. About forty minutes into the transport her respirations became more labored and noisy. I used the SVN of Ventolin. I removed the mask and connected the oxygen tubing to the inhaler portion of the SVN. I held it near her mouth and nose. She inhaled the mist. It caused her bronchial tubes to open up and increase the amount of oxygen that could pass into her lungs. She improved. Her respiration slowed down. She relaxed. Her color improved. When the treatment was over, I replaced the SVN with the oxygen mask. I wondered how long it would last? We were still around a half hour from Tuba. It started to rain. The road was wet. The only good thing was the people living in the area were all snug at home. Traffic was light. We continued to speed toward Tuba. She stopped breathing again. I tried to stimulate her but she didn't take a breath. I took the bag valve mask, removed her oxygen mask and replaced it with the BVM. After three ventilations, she turned her head to the side and took a breath. I put the oxygen mask on again. She began to breathe on her own.

I knew if this didn't last, I had no choice but to administer the Epi SVN. I was in trouble anyway. But I would be in more trouble if I actually gave it to her. I had already decided I would not let her die because of protocol. I was going to administer it if she began to lose the airway. I took the microphone and radioed the hospital with an up- date. "We are ten minutes out, code-three." This alerted them of the critical patient about to hit their back door. Most inter-facility transport patients go straight to their room. This patient wasn't going past the ER until stabilized. I woke up the mother as I continued to stare at the baby, watching her respirations slowly increase. Her breathing became more labored. Her color began to change. Should I give Epi now? Or could she wait another few minutes? Should I intubate? If I got a tube in would she wake up and fight the tube? We drove past McDonalds in Tuba. Just a few more blocks. I watched her closely. The change was slow. I held off on the Epi. I disconnected the oxygen tubing from the main tank and connected it to our portable tank. I began to bag her and inserted a deep breath between her shallow gasps. Her oxygen level was ok, not great, but ok.

We pulled up at the ER entrance and Doctor Keen was standing outside the door waiting for us. She was the accepting doctor and a pediatric specialist. We backed up and stopped. She opened the door. "How's she doing?"

"She's holding her own but she's critical." I hopped out and helped the doctor remove the stretcher. The EMT escorted the mother into the ER. We took the stretcher to a small glassed in room. I unstrapped the car seat and moved her to the exam table. The doctor began checking the baby and questioning the mother. I transferred the oxygen tube to the hospitals main supply. An RN arrived with a hand full of equipment. The EMT and I backed out of the room. I stood watching for a minute. She was so tiny. I left and went to do my paperwork while the EMT cleaned and restocked the ambulance. When I finished the ton of paperwork, I returned to the ER. I found the nurse and she signed the papers.

"How's the baby doing?"

"Doctor Keen got her intubated and on the ventilator. I switched her IV to the good stuff. We won't know anything for a couple of days or so, but I think we got to her soon enough."

The weekend passed. One call after another kept me busy. Although the children were ill, none was as serious as Baby Grace. On my last trip to Tuba I checked up on Grace. Her mother smiled as I walked into the room. "She's going to be alright," the mother said.

"I am so glad." We talked a short while and I left. It was the end of my shift and I drove the hundred miles to Page. I had barely walked in the door when my home phone rang. It was my Medical Control watchdog, Janet.

"Sharon, this is Janet."

"Hi, what's up?" I tried to sound casual but I knew this wasn't a social call.

"You know what's up. You manipulated Dr. Miller into giving you orders to administer an Epi SVN."

"I didn't' manipulate him. I was extremely clear. He completely understood what he was doing and why."

"You know you can't go against protocol even if a doctor orders you to do so."

"She was going to die."

"Don't go there. You broke the rules."

"I didn't give her Epi SVN."

"You would have, wouldn't you?"

"I couldn't let her die. Twenty states including New Mexico allow paramedics to administer Epi SVN's. I am New Mexico Certified. It's in my drug box. I am very familiar with the drug and give it in injections and by IV for other medical conditions."

"Your medical control for this call was Arizona and you are not allowed. You are forbidden to give an Epi SVN in Arizona."

"She could have died. Dr. Miller, Dr. Norton and Dr. Keen agreed the patient should get Epi SVN if necessary. What did you expect me to do? Let her die?"

"You knew better. You shouldn't have even broached the subject with Dr. Miller."

"I did so at Dr. Norton's request. It was the right thing to do and you know it."

"Sharon, I don't care. You have put me in the position of possibly pulling your certification."

"I couldn't let her die. You do what you have to do. But I will fight it and I have three doctors and a grateful mother on my side."

"It won't help. You knowingly broke protocols."

"I never gave her Epi SVN."

She sighed. "I'm through playing verbal tag. You have never had a disciplinary action filed against you. You're a good paramedic but you went too far this time. I am going to let this go as a written warning. I

236

promise you I will pull your certification if you ever do this again. Is that understood?"

"Yes."

"I am having lunch with Dr. Miller today and we are going to discuss protocols."

"Thank you Janet." I hung up and took a deep sigh. I was off the hook. I didn't care if the written reprimand was in my file. I could explain it and anyone with a shred of consciousness wouldn't hold that against me. If they do, I didn't care. I did the right thing. Even if I lost my certification, it would have been worth it if I could have saved that baby's life. Luckily I didn't have to take the final step and actually give her the forbidden medication, but I would have had it became necessary.

Baby Grace went home a week later. She should be starting second grade this fall.

"I DON'T LIKE TO WAIT."

When the private ambulance company (who had lost the Tuba City contract) got the contract for Kayenta, Arizona they called me and offered me a Paramedic job. I had previously worked for them and they were ok so I accepted the job offer. I was on my second day of a forty-eight hour shift. I had just sat down to eat a gourmet meal that I had heated in the microwave when my pager went off. I was partnered with The Flower Child. The Flower Child, commonly known as Tinker Bell behind her back, was covered in tattoos and body piercings. She was a confused person but quite interesting. She was of average size, blond hair cut shoulder length and carried a "carry-on bag" on the ambulance that was huge and weighted almost as much as she did. A personal carry-on bag wasn't uncommon but she took it to an unheard of level. She lived in a small community west of Phoenix and from what I heard, she led a rather odd life. She made up her own religion that involved tiny bits of a dozen different religions. It appeared she choose whatever she liked from each religion and combined it with her crystals and pyramids. It wouldn't have been a problem if she had showed some respect for people who had other beliefs. She loved everyone and everything except organized religion and Christians. She was an unhappy person but harmless. The Navajo's didn't like her. Babies burst into tears when they saw her. Small children ran. I have heard children are a good judge of people. I wonder what she wasn't telling us.

I call dispatch for more details then hurried outside and tossed my drug box into the back of the rig (or "ride" as some medics call an ambulance). The EMT Flower Child had been at McDonalds and it took a couple of minutes for her to arrive. She drove up, leaped out of her SUV and ran to the ambulance. "It's a nine year old girl that was involved in an ATV accident," I told her.

"Where?" She asked.

"Monument Valley."

"Great," she said as she started the rig. I knew what she was thinking. It was dark and we had around thirty miles of hills, curves, and a narrow two lane highway ahead of us (Highway 163). It could be a bad call. ATV accidents can be very serious. It would be about a sixty mile round trip, depending on exactly where in Monument Valley they were located. The roads in the valley aren't paved. There were no street signs, no house numbers and no street lights. I was hopeful the child would be stable when we arrived. If she wasn't, it was going to be a long return trip.

It was a moonless night and early enough to have a fair amount of traffic on the road. Vehicle after vehicle failed to pull over quickly. It wasn't their fault. There were few places where a person could pull over. Most would slow down or pull over a few feet and stop, usually on a hill or curve. We would straddle the yellow line, cross our fingers and continue. "Med-45 dispatch"

My partner was struggling with a semi directly in front of her. It wasn't immediately clear what the semi was going to do. The truck wiggled back and forth, slowed down but still remained a road block to us. I reached for the radio, "Med-45, go ahead."

"Med-45, the patient will be in a black new model Ford pickup. He is traveling in your direction on Highway 163. His flashers will be on."

"Med-45 copies." The ambulance whipped into the oncoming lane and with peddle to the metal we got around. I searched the oncoming traffic for the black pickup. Was it a new black Ford Pickup? A couple of black pickups went past us and I watched in the mirror to see if they applied break lights and pulled over. None did. Car after car, truck after truck, semi after semi drove past us. None seemed interested in us and very few even attempted to pull over.

We were almost to Golding's Trading Post, near the Monument Valley pull off when I saw a dark truck sitting beside the road with its flashers flashing. "There it is, on the right." We pulled over and as I got out I was met by a Navajo man, mid-twenties, dressed in western attire. He smiled and we shook hands according to Navajo custom.

238

"My daughter's in the truck," he began. I listened, not interrupting. Navajo's tell the story in a different manner than Anglos. They usually tell a story in a long wandering manner. I allowed him to talk and I just listened and hoped he would get to the point soon. He did. "She was riding the ATV without shoes and she brushed a bush and a twig ran up under her toenail."

Now it was my turn to talk. "Is there a bleeding problem?"

"No. She cried at first but she's calmed down now."

"Was there any other injuries?"

"No. Just the toe."

"I'll check her out." I walked to the truck. I could see a female sitting in the driver's seat, probably the child's mother. I opened the rear passenger door. A beautiful nine year old girl sat silent and composed in the rear passenger seat. I smiled, "My name's Sharon. I'm a paramedic from Page. Your Dad tells me you hurt your toe."

She was shy and didn't say anything but showed me her toe. A stick disappeared under her toenail and stuck out about an inch. "Does it hurt?" I asked her. She shook her head "yes." "You're very brave." She smiled. Navajo children are taught not to cry and this was the right thing to say. "I'm going to take you to the doctor and get the stick removed. Is that ok?" She smiled and shook her head "yes."

It was decided that her father would carry her to the ambulance. He was going to go with us and his wife would follow in the truck. He was a big man and he carried his young daughter to the ambulance with no effort. He climbed in with her in his arms and gently laid her down on the stretcher. He sat on the bench seat and I strapped her to the stretcher. I sat down beside the father. I took her vital signs and of course they were normal. I chose not to bandage the toe. I took her medical history (uneventful), no meds, and no pre-existing medical problems.

The father and I began to talk. "I'm an EMT. But I'm not working as one right now," the father told me. We talked briefly about EMS and I found out a little about his life and his family. I had one question I wanted to ask but hesitated. After the casual social bonding I decided to ask the question.

"I realize she is injured but as an EMT you know it's not life threatening. Why did you call an ambulance?"

"Oh, I know it's not serious, but if I took her into the ER they would make us wait in the waiting room for hours. If she is brought in by ambulance, we won't have to wait. I don't like to wait."

I had just dodged cars, trucks, semis and livestock, driving code-three on a moonless night. This man had endangered me, my partner and everyone we met on the highway just so he would not have to wait in the lobby. I was mad. But I said nothing. It wouldn't do any good. The ambulance was free to Native Americans and the ER visit was also free. He had nothing to lose and manipulating the system seemed no big deal to him.

We arrived at the ER and brought the girl in on the stretcher. We moved her to the gurney. I gave a quick overview of her injury. I looked at the RN and gave her a nod and walked away. She followed me. Standing out of sight of the father I told her what he had told me. The ER was busy and every bed was full and the waiting room was near capacity. She didn't like abuse of the system either. She smiled and thanked me for the information. She walked to the back door and got a wheelchair and walked toward the patient and her father. I started my paperwork as the father wheeled the girl out into the waiting room for a long wait. I smiled. All is well.

WHAT'S THE WORST THAT COULD HAPPEN?

Mrs. Tso (pronounced "so") was a traditional Navajo woman. Her husband had passed away two years ago. She lived alone in a Hogan just west of Cow Springs. Her oldest daughter lived in a trailer that was parked nearby with her husband and four children. Just before dawn, Mrs. Tso was awakened by a sound outside. She slept fully dressed as most older traditional Navajo women do, so she rose quickly. She grabbed her rifle and went outside. It was dark as the moon had set and the sun wasn't visible yet. Her attention was drawn to the sheep pen. Coyotes wandered the area and they loved nothing more than to kill and eat sheep. Each sheep was worth at least two-hundred and fifty dollars so losing one sheep to coyotes was a noticeable loss to the family's worth. She walked around the pen checking the fencing. She then stood looking into the dark desert. She could see movement in the darkness and knew that coyotes were nearby. She bent down and picked up two rocks and tossed them into the darkness. The coyotes hurried away.

Mrs. Tso walked back to her home. She picked her way through the desert. About twenty feet from her front door she stepped on a rock. Her body shifted awkwardly to the right. Off balance, she fell to the ground. Her right hip struck a rock about the size of a baseball. Pain shot through her hip. She lay still for a minute and then attempted to get up. The pain was intense. She lay back down and waited to be found. She lay on the cool desert sand. She listened carefully, fearful the coyotes may come back or worse, wild dogs. She was helpless as her gun lay seven feet away and she couldn't move from the spot where she lay. The sun slowly peaked over the red sandstone cliffs. Mrs. Tso saw her daughter open the front door to her trailer. Mrs. Tso yelled "Help! Help me!" Her daughter ran to her mother. She yelled to her husband to call an ambulance.

The Tuba City Regional Medical Center (TCRMC) was completely full. There wasn't a single bed empty in the entire hospital. The clinic portion had no empty chairs and people lined up and out the door. The ER was also full. People filled the ER waiting room and out in the hall people sat on the floor with crying children sitting in their laps. It was respiratory infection season and it was running wild on the reservation.

We were called to transport Mrs. Tso. X-rays showed she had fractured her right hip. My partner Rick Stone and I were to take her to Flagstaff Medical Center for further treatment. Mrs. Tso was in a small enclosed glass exam room. It would help shield her from the respiratory illness that plagued the majority of ER patients. I listened to a quick report from the nurse. Rick took her vital signs. I could see she was in a lot of pain. I have pain medication in my drug box but in this case the drug of choice was Demerol. "Can I get you to give her some Demerol before we leave?" I asked Jewel, a RN.

"Sure." She hurried off. I waited beside my patient. I examined the patient as her daughter stood nearby translating my questions into Navajo. She was a small woman, around eighty pounds dripping wet. She lay quietly, not moving because of the pain. She was dressed in traditional Navajo attire, long pleated skirt and a dark blue velvet tunic top. Her black hair was streaked with gray and held by a strand of wool, secured in an oblong bun at the nape of her neck. She was alert and cooperative. After I completed my examination, I left and made my call to Medical Control. On non-emergency transports (from one medical facility to another) it was protocol to notify Medical Control of the transport. I walked back to the small glass room.

I looked through the glass wall into the ER. Every bed was occupied and two people in wheel chairs sat near the nursing station waiting their turn. Most of the people were ill with respiratory problems. The room sounded with coughs, moans and crying children. The ER Staff hurried from one patient to another. Things were getting done, but to the casual observer, it appeared unorganized chaos. I watched the RN that had promised Demerol for my patient. She was busy with an elderly man in the corner. I wanted to get out on the road, but I couldn't until my patient had pain medication onboard.

241

"Let's get her on the stretcher then we can just leave if she ever comes back with the shot," Rick, an EMT went in search of a slide board. It's a thin plastic, flexible board used mostly in the x-ray department. The ER used one to slide the patient from a gurney to a bed or stretcher to gurney. He returned with the plastic board. The patient didn't speak English but she seemed to understand what we were doing and cooperated as best she could. We slipped the board under her good hip and used it to bridge the space between the gurney and the stretcher. Using the sheet to drag her over, we slowly moved her to our stretcher. It obviously caused her some pain, but she bravely handled it. I took a sheet and folded it over for padding and slipped it between her injured hip and the metal rail of the stretcher. I looked up and saw the nurse checking in a new patient. She had completely forgotten about us.

"Rick, stay with her. I'm going to see if I can't get pain meds for her. Don't leave this room till she gets her meds." I wandered off and chased down Jewel. She was taking a patient's temp in their ear. I learned a long time ago that telling someone how they are inconveniencing you doesn't work to get them to do something for you. You have to make it worth their while. "Jewel, If I could just get Demerol for my patient, you could have the room."

Jewel looked up at me. "Just wheel her over by the door, I'll get the med." I had no intention of moving her from the room till she got her shot. Possession of the room was my only Ace in the hole and I wasn't going to give it up until I got what I wanted. I wandered back to the room. The ER remained chaotic and Jewel continued to hurry here and there. I was getting tired of just standing around and my patient was very uncomfortable. Just as I was losing my patience, Jewel ran in. She was running in hyper drive. She lifted the woman's skirt and gave her an injection in her hip. "There, seventy-five milligrams of Demerol on board. Have a good trip." The nurse rushed out.

Seventy-five milligrams of Demerol? Is that what she said? Seventy-five milligrams of Demerol for an eighty pound woman? I would have been happy with twelve-and a half milligrams. Seventy-five was going to put her in respiratory arrest. I looked around the ER. I had a decision to make. "Let's get out of here."

Her daughter said good-by and asked us to tell the receiving nurse, she would be driving to Flagstaff tomorrow morning. She gave me her cell phone number and asked I give it to the nurse. I said I would make sure the nurse got her cell number. We quickly wheeled the stretcher out and loaded her in the ambulance. Rick pulled out of the parking lot and moved down the pothole maze of Main street. I connected her to oxygen with a non-rebreather mask and turned it up to fifteen litters. She didn't need it yet but she would soon. I wanted her oxygenated when she went into respiratory arrest. Rick slowed down and went around a large brown cow walking down the middle of the Main Street. We turned right onto Highway 160 and headed west. I took out the bag valve mask and sat it on the bench seat. I looked through the small window to the driver's compartment, Rick was watching me and it was obvious he was surprised I had got that piece of equipment out and set up.

"Everything ok?" he asked.

"Yeah." I slipped on cardiac leads and an oxygen sensor on her finger. Rick continued to glance in his rear view mirror. He was trying to figure out why I was doing this. It looked as if I was engaging in "over kill". He would know in a few minutes. I decided to surprise him.

We were about nine miles from the Highway 160 and 89 Junction when she stopped breathing. I reached over and raised her feet up. I removed the oxygen mask and moved it to her forehead. I tipped her head back to open her airway. I took the hose and connected it to the BVM and fitted the mask over her face and gave it a squeeze. Air from the bag was forced into her airway and into her lungs. Her chest rose. I began to count silently, giving her a breath every five seconds.

Rick saw I was now bagging the patient. "What's going on?" He understood she had stopped breathing but was at a loss as to why she had quite breathing. "Do you want me to turn around?"

"No, don't turn around. They gave her three times the prescribed dose of Demerol and she's in respiratory arrest. It will wear off in fifteen minutes or so."

"What?"

"She OD (over dosed) on Demerol. It will self-correct in a few minutes. Code-three would be good."

"Oh, yeah." He flipped on the lights and siren, stepped down on the accelerator and we were off and running. I continued to bag her. Her oxygen saturation stayed acceptable. I hit the automatic blood pressure cuff and it pumped up then deflated slowly. Her blood pressure was a bit low. I reached down and raised her feet even more. Five minutes later I took another blood pressure and it was now acceptable. She lay there unable to breath. The Demerol had killed her respiratory drive and without my breathing for her, she would die from the over dose.

Twenty minutes passed and then twenty-five minutes. She began to breath, slowly and too shallow. I continued to use the BVM and gave her a breath between her normal breaths. Soon she began to breathe at a normal rate and opened her eyes. I took another blood pressure and discovered it was back to normal. I lowered her legs and put the oxygen mask back in place with eight litters a minute. She was no longer in danger and the rest of the trip should be fine.

I moved up to the small window. "Rick, she's back to normal now. You can shut down the code three."

"You knew she was going to do this, didn't you?"

I smiled, "Sure. A woman that size, who normally didn't take pain meds couldn't process that much Demerol. Respiratory arrest was a sure thing."

"Why did we take her?"

"It would have delayed transport for an hour or more. This way we got out of there and the patient did alright in the long run. Rick, when you were in my EMT class, didn't I tell you if you can handle it, it's not an emergency?"

"Well, yeah, but you could have warned me."

"It was more fun to watch your expression when she stopped breathing." The rest of the trip was uneventful. The patient had been kept well oxygenated and she rested comfortably. We arrived at the hospital and took her to her room. I gave a report to the accepting nurse.

"Was she allergic to Demerol?" the nurse asked.

"No. She just quit breathing because seventy-five milligrams of pain med was too much."

"So Tuba over dosed her?"

"Not intentionally. The patient isn't any worse for wear. I just wanted you to know about it so you can lower her dose of pain meds. I wouldn't want you to think she tolerated such a high dose."

The next day, the ER was far less busy. I took Jewel aside and told her what happened. She was upset. I'm sure she never did that again. A few weeks later I got my paperwork back after medical control had gone over the report. I was commended for my actions. A "good job commendation," is hard to come by. It made my day.

DRIVE SHAFT PROBLEM

It had been cold all day. After the sun went down the rain started to fall. It was payday and the dirt parking lot across from the bar, the Windy Mesa was full. Jim was off the reservation and didn't have a warm dry bed to sleep in when in town. He was cold and didn't want to get wet. After drinking all day, his judgment wasn't as good as it could have been.

He crawled under a pickup to give him some protection from the rain and went to sleep.

Joe had drunk and played pool at the Windy Mesa, but it was now time to go home. He wasn't drunk so driving home shouldn't be a problem. He quickly walked to his pickup through the rain and jumped in, started the engine and put it in gear. Suddenly he heard something. "What was that?" he said out loud. He stopped. He could still hear something strange. He turned off the motor and listened, he could hear better now and it sounded like a man yelling. He got out to investigate.

Joe bent down and under his pickup he could see a man. "Get out from under there." No answer was heard, just moaning and unintelligible words. A buddy walked up.

"What's up?"

"Some drunken Indian is under my truck." Both men bent down and tried to drag Jim out from under the truck. "I think he's hung up," Joe commented.

"Yeah. . . let's call the police and let them handle this."

I was watching TV when the call came in. I left my warm, dry house and headed to the fire department for an "unconscious man." The rain beat on the windshield as my car traveled down the street a small stream formed in the gutter. Doug and I plus another EMT who's name I can't remember were on the crew. We got in the ambulance and drove the few feet across the intersection to the scene. A number of people were standing around a pickup. The police told us about Jim and how he had apparently gone to sleep under the truck and when Joe started the engine, Jim became entangled in the drive shaft.

I got down in the mud and crawled under the truck on my belly. Not my first choice, but it was the only way to evaluate the patient. Jim had long, thick black hair. The hair was twisted around the drive shaft. His coat and shirt was also twisted around the shaft. I tried to tug the hair, but it was tight. Doug appeared at my side. "Can we jack the truck up?" I asked. "NO, I don't think so, the grounds to soft and muddy."

Doug bellied down in the soggy mud to help. We took scissors and began to cut the clothing away. It was harder than expected with no light, cold mud, water seeping into our clothing. It was cold. We cut away, more and more. The man was unconscious, moaning, moving a little, but obviously not aware of his predicament.

We got most of his clothing cut away from the drive shift, but now his hair trapped him. I began cutting his hair. I didn't want too; I knew he would be very angry when he sobered up, but how else to extricate him? The patient was lucky. This type of incident often results in the patient's hair being ripped from the skull, a kind of "scalping." The driver had turned off the motor soon enough to save Jim that fate. I snipped and cut his long black hair, until his head suddenly dropped into the mud, splash.

I dropped the scissors and took his head in my hands and lifted his face out of the muddy water. We then, as carefully as possible slid him out from under the truck. He moaned. We put him on a backboard. I was shivering and so was Doug. We loaded the patient into the warm ambulance. We all felt the warmth and were happy to be out from under the truck.

The man had soft tissue injuries to his hands, and some of his hair had been ripped out, and his body temp was a bit low but other than that, he appeared to be uninjured. His altered level of consciousness appeared to be due to alcohol. We transported him. At the hospital, we quickly turned him over to the staff, wrote a quick report and hurried home.

The rain was steadily falling. When I walked in my husband asked, "What in the world have you been doing?" He laughed at me, covered in mud. ". . . . playing in the mud with a local." He laughed as I hurried off to a hot shower and a clean change of clothing.

"WHO KILLED THE DUCK?"

One evening, I sat at home and listened on my scanner as the ambulance handled a one car rollover a long way out on the highway. I wasn't on call and so I just sat and listened. After the ambulance had dropped off their three patients and returned to the station, I couldn't take it any longer. I had to know the details.

EMTs are by nature nosey. If after a call they want to know more about what "really happened," they would often go down to the station and listen as the EMTs would tell the story. Now, like most things in this world, it would cost you, but most were willing to pay. The price was you had to help clean.

This night I had nothing to do and craved a little excitement even second-hand excitement, so I went down to the station and started to help the cleanup and listen to the story unfold. But it didn't unfold, not exactly. There were four EMTs on the call and three seemed a bit unhappy with Doug Alton, the fourth EMT.

Now Doug is easy to run with. He is a good EMT. I listened to what they didn't say and tried to figure out what on earth he had done to make them give him the cold shoulder. The call involved three drunken

246

Native American men. It was winter and a cold night. On their way back home the driver had some problems keeping the car on the road. Finally he lost control and the vehicle left the road and rolled. All three men were unconscious when the ambulance arrived. How much of their unresponsiveness was due to alcohol and how much to the accident?

All three were placed on backboards and strapped down, using good spinal precautions. The desert was wet and mud clung to their shoes. Mud caked their knees as they knelled beside their patients. The cold dampness seeped through to their skin.

By the time they had got back to the station, both EMTs and ambulance looked like they had played in a mud bog. I carried a jump kit over to the sink and opened it. It was a mess. Mud was clinging to many of the instruments. Some bandaging was ruined. I emptied it completely and started to wipe the goo off the tray inside. Then I notice something. I picked through the mud and drew out an object. I couldn't identify it. I tossed it aside and continued to clean. It became apparent there was a foreign substance mixed up in the mud. I examined another sample closer. It was a feather.

Now what on earth were feathers doing in a jump kit? Doug walked by about that time. I held up one of the feathers, "Who killed the duck?"

I wasn't ready for his reaction. His back stiffened. He got an expression of rigorous anger. His eyes turned to slits and his mouth clamped shut in an angry expression. "I guess I did." He turned around and huffed off. The other EMTS laughed.

"What's going on?" I asked.

"Doug waited until we got the three men loaded in the ambulance and then he cut off one of the patient's coats."

They all laughed. "Yeah and it was a down jacket."

"It exploded. Feathers flew everywhere!"

"They fussed about it all the way in...." said Doug.

"It was a regular snow storm with all the tiny feathers flying around in the ambulance. I couldn't take a breath without sucking a damn feather down my throat."

"That's an exaggeration." Doug said.

"NO IT"S NOT!" they all said in unison It took a long time to get the mud and feathers cleaned up. Doug took a bit of teasing. He didn't know a down jacket would explode if cut or ripped open. He found out the hard way.

Later that evening two of the men were released. But the third was going to the Indian hospital in Tuba City for observation. He hadn't regained consciousness. They believed he wasn't seriously injured but they didn't want to take a chance. I was called to do the transfer from the hospital to the airport. I remember walking down the hall and entering the x-ray room were the man lay. He lay still, on his back. His breathing was normal. Then I saw them. Feathers, feathers in his hair, in his ears and from my angle I could see one stuck up his nose.

I burst into laughter. The nurse looked strangely at me. I rushed from the room and tried to calm down, but the laughter kept coming. The other two EMTs went inside and came out laughing too. We were glad he was unconscious because to laugh at patients isn't acceptable. But sometimes you can't help it. We transferred him and later we found out he wasn't badly injured and went home two days later. For years poor Doug suffered the torment of having to put up with us teasing him about "killing the duck." It was a tender spot for quite a while.

THEY WATCHED MY BACK

I hurried out of the Tuba City KFC with a box of chicken to go. I climbed behind the wheel of the ambulance and opened the box. I took a chicken strip out and began to enjoy the delightful flavor. The radio came to life. "Officer Tso to Med Unit 42."

I hesitated answering but put the chicken down and answered. "Med Unit 42."

"Can you come over here? I have a man I want you to check out."

"I'm by myself, Tate is back at quarters." I looked around and saw the officer's car about two-hundred yards to my left. I could see Tso standing a few feet away from another man.

"I need you over here."

"76" (en route) I put the chicken back in the box, wiped off my hands and started the ambulance. It was a short trip. I got out and took in the scene. I could see the officer wasn't comfortable with this man. I sensed tenseness in the air. The patient sat on a stump about ten feet to the north side of the quit residential road. I didn't recognize him. He was tall, slender and wore his graying hair long. He was Native American but had a lot of Anglo blood in him as well. He sat with his head down.

I approached to within six feet in front of him. "Hi, my name's Sharon. I'm a paramedic. Do you need help?"

He slowly raised his head and looked me in the eye, "Hell no." His expression was one of anger and his tone was confrontational. The look in his eyes was cold.

248

"I see blood. What's the matter with your side?" On his left side, just above his belt his shirt was bloody. I believed he may have been stabbed.

"Get the hell away %#@!*&^$%." His voice became louder. He gestured with his right arm as he spoke.

Out of the corner of my eye I saw my EMS partner, Tate pull into the KFC parking lot, got out and slowly walked toward us. He apparently heard over the radio my conversation with the officer. He approached from behind at an angle so the man could not see him. The officer saw him. No words were spoken, but all of us knew what we were probably going to be forced to do. I started talking to the man again, keeping his attention as the two men moved into position.

The officer and the EMT positioned themselves just behind the man on each side, slightly to the rear, just out of his peripheral vision. They were about three foot, away. One step forward and they could grab him. I had been in this position many times before. Violent situations were far too common in EMS. I often was the bait in front of the violent patient. I would keep the patient's attention on me as I tried to calm him/her and get them to cooperate. My life and limb was in the hands of my fellow team mates. If the violent patient lunged at me, I was depending on my team mates to grab him/her before he reached me. If he/her did get to me I had to be ready to defend myself until my partner reached us.

I trusted Officer Tso and EMT Tate. We three had done this a number of times before. I continued to talk to the man and he got louder and more threatening. I was careful to keep my distance but his growing hostility concerned me. He was bleeding from what appeared to be a stab wound. I couldn't just leave him. Without warning his right arm dropped to his boot and he withdrew a long butcher knife, sprung to his feet, and lunged at me screaming "I'll kill you Bitch!"

I took a giant step back as the two men leaped forward and the EMT grabbed his left arm and the officer grabbed the one with the knife. I backed away further. The men continued forward and slam dunked the attacker to the ground face first. I hurried around and pounced on his legs around the knees and held on. The struggle continued for a couple of minutes, dust was flying and obscenities filled the air. The officer wrestled the knife out of the man's hand and cuffed him. I let go of his legs as the men lifted him to his feet. I looked at the knife, it was long and deadly. The officer and EMT were mad. Bright red blood flowed from the attacker's side. "Hold him and I'll bandage his wound," I said.

"No," answered Officer Tso. He and the EMT roughly drug the prisoner to the patrol car and unceremoniously threw him in the back seat and slammed the door. The officer turned to the EMT and me, "Thanks guys." He drove off toward the hospital.

I used my cell phone and called the hospital ER to notify them of Officer Tso's pending arrival. I told them the patient was bleeding from a possible stab wound in his left side. I warned them he was dangerous.

"You ok?" Tate asked.

"Yeah, I'm ok. I was sure glad to see you."

"I heard the radio traffic and drove over."

"Thanks," I said. I walked over to the ambulance and he returned to his car. We met at quarters. I parked the ambulance, turned the key off and sat still for a minute. I had just had a man lunge at me with a big knife. Tso and Tate had my back and worked as a team and brought him down before he reached me. That's good team work.

This story was repeated many times in my career. I have worked in offices where I wouldn't trust the person at the next desk with my stapler, but law enforcement officers, firefighters, and EMS personnel learn to trust their very lives to their partners and co-workers. Team work is a matter of life and death EMS.

RELIGIOUS FREEDOM

Religious Freedom is a priceless freedom granted by the Declaration of Independence and Bill of Rights. I am a Christian. But, I know not everyone shares my beliefs. I know and accept that there are many ways to worship God, false gods or no god at all. I respect a person's right to choose their own way in this world. In my work, I try not to step on other's beliefs, in the hope that they will not step on mine. But, at times, religious beliefs complicate my efforts to provide emergency care. Difficult decisions sometimes had to be made.

It was a beautiful summer day at Wahweap Marina on Lake Powell. I was on the ambulance, responding to the launch ramp for a report of a boy with a fractured leg. We drove up and saw a small ski boat with people around it. I walked up and introduced myself. The patient was eight years old. His leg was obviously fractured midway between the knee and ankle. It didn't look like a bad break, but bad enough. At least no growth plates were involved. His mother, an average woman about thirty years of age was obviously upset. She made a few comments about us hurrying up and nervously glanced at her watch and scanned the lake, as if

250

looking for someone. Finally, I took her aside as the other crew members splinted the boy's leg.

"There's more to this, isn't there?"

She hung her head and answered softly, "Yes."

"What's going on?"

She took a deep breath and told me her husband and she belonged to a church that didn't believe in doctors. She said her husband was driving another, slower boat and would get here soon. She was certain he would refuse medical treatment for her son and she realized her son's leg would grow crooked if not casted properly.

"Are you his birth mother?" I asked. All I needed was one parent's permission.

"Yes."

"And, if we can get him to the hospital and his leg splinted before his father arrives, what would happen?"

"I am certain he would be mad at me, but he would allow the cast to stay."

I turned and yelled at the crew to get the boy in the ambulance at once. I was driving and with the mother in the front seat, I drove code three (lights and sirens) to the hospital in a wild race. I phoned the hospital and explained the situation. Doctor Birch was waiting for us when we arrived. We carried the boy in the room that was all set up with portable x-ray and everything we would need for a cast. We moved like a tape on fast forward.

An x-ray was taken (simple fracture) cast was applied by the doc with me and another EMT assisting. We flung plaster all over the walls, ceiling, floor and us. But we got the cast on the boy by the time the father stormed into the room. He looked at us all covered in plaster. He looked at the boy's leg, anger on his face. Then it softened, he turned to his wife. She met his gaze with eyes filled with pain and silently begging for forgiveness. She and he stood there looking at each other for a minute and he walked out. She followed him. They talked softly in the hallway. The father came back in.

"I understand what you did and why you did it. I believe my wife committed a sin by allowing you to treat my son. She is weak. But......... it's done. The cast can stay and in six weeks we will have a local doctor remove it." He went to his son and picked him up and the three of them went to check out. Legally, the child's mother gave us permission to treat so we had not broken any law. But what about a parent's right to make medical decisions for their child? When one agrees and one disagrees it becomes a gray area. I had a decision to make that day that isn't covered in a text book. I believe my decision was a good one. The boy will have a sturdy, straight leg to walk on as he grows up. Someday he may choose to walk in his father's footsteps, maybe not, but his options are open for whatever he decides as an adult.

This story happened a few years ago. But this issue is still causing emergency personnel difficulties. Fire, Police and EMS walk a fine line between respect of a person's religious freedom and doing their job. In my area the LDS Church members (Mormon) wear sacred under garments. They believe they protect the person wearing the clothing. We try to respect them by not cutting the garments if at all possible. I have stood by waiting for a Navajo Healing Ceremony to be performed before I could transport a patient. Another time I had to wait for "lying on of the hands" of a mainstream Christian Church. I try to not judge, but at times religion interferes in timely transport and standard of care.

In 2010 frustrated Saudi Arabia firefighters were not allowed to rescue twelve young girls who burned to death because they were not wearing their burkas when they tried to escape their burning school. They were dressed in their nightgowns and therefore it was against civil and religious law for male non-family members to see them unless they were dressed in the heavy robe and hood of the burka. Since the firefighters were not family members and the girls were dressed in nightgowns, the girls burned to death while the firefighters stood by, unable to help.

In Canada in October 2009, while arresting two dangerous radical Islamic men, to render the scene safe, they pat searched the wife of one of the men for weapons. They were doing their job and securing scene safety. The two police officers were forced to apologize to the Islamic community for offending their religious beliefs.

In September 2009 a private Australian ambulance happened upon an accident and offered to assist an Ambulance Victoria (AV) crew already on the scene. Problems began when private operator Rian Holden checked the blood pressure and pulse of one of the victims, a "Muslim woman in traditional dress." Alert to the insult of a male medic touching her, members of the AV unit "abused" Holden and his partner and ordered them to depart. Police were called to assure the departure of Holden from the area. (This is his real name since it has been published in a newspaper.)

Where is the line drawn? We in emergency services are still struggling with that question. Educating EMS responders on cultural and religious differences help, but one size does not fit all situations and not all people of the same ethnic group worship in the same way. It's an ongoing issue with few answers.

THE ONE IN A ONE HUNDRED

I was a paramedic for Page Fire and responded from Station One on Coppermine Road to the back of what had once been Thrifty Drugs. It bordered the City Park where the "Park People" hang out. The Park People were the result of unrealistic laws of the Navajo Nation. In an attempt to keep alcohol off the reservation, the Navajo government made it illegal to possess alcohol on your person, in your vehicle or your home on the reservation. So the Navajo's who want to drink come to border towns such as Page and drink. They visit family or become temporary "homeless" people. Not all, but many are binge drinkers and will drink until the alcohol and their money are gone. They drink in secret, hiding the bottles or drinking elsewhere and then going to the park. It's a lovely park with soft green grass and lots of trees that provide precious shade. PFD gets lots of calls to the park.

The First Responder was a Fire Captain for the PFD, Rick Stone. I knew him well since he also worked part time in Tuba for a private ambulance company and was often my partner while on duty in Tuba. He was a good EMT and I trusted him and his judgment. He was standing by a Navajo couple, both in their late thirties. I got out of the ambulance and walked over. He gave me a report. "She's complaining of not feeling well and being dizzy."

The woman was of average height with about an extra fifty pounds. Her black hair was cut short. She was wearing a red t-shirt and shorts. I began to question her. She said she had eaten an hour ago (could rule out low blood sugar). She complained of a headache and being dizzy. Rick cut in, "Sharon, she can walk to the ambulance."

"No, not yet," I said. Rick wasn't happy. He was functioning in the fire Captain Mode and when wearing that hat his word was law. But, this was medical and I was a paramedic and he was an EMT basic, so weather he liked it or not, I was in charge. He backed down, but didn't like it. I then noticed her knees, elbows and the palms of her hands. They were scratched. "Did you fall recently?" I asked while indicating her injuries.

"Yesterday we were at the Chains (at the lake) and she tripped and fell," her male friend said.

"Did you black out?" I asked.

"No," she answered.

I then saw her reach up with her right hand and rub her neck. "Does your neck hurt?" I asked.

"Yeah, I think I hurt it yesterday."

"And it still hurts?"

"Worse," she said.

253

I reached up and removed her hand from her neck then took hold of her head.

"Stand still and don't move your head," I told her. "J.T. go get the spinal immobilization." My partner spun around and hurried to the ambulance.

"Is this absolutely necessary? She's been walking around for twenty-four hours." Rick obviously didn't agree with my decision. I knew that few people break their neck from a standing fall, but it can happen. I didn't know this woman's history, but people who overindulge in alcohol often have brittle bones and she might. A fall equals spinal precautions in EMS. It's common knowledge that ninety-nine out of a hundred don't have a broken neck. But one in a hundred has a fractured or broken neck and is in danger of being paralyzed. She also had a bad headache and was dizzy. I knew she had been walking around, but that doesn't matter, she may be in serious danger of living her life in a wheelchair and on a ventilator. I wasn't about to gamble with this woman's future. I began to treat her as if her neck was broken and unstable.

I looked at Rick, he was completely convinced this was nothing and the woman should walk to the ambulance. "Rick, its protocol." He shook his head in disgust, but didn't say anything else. J.T. arrived. As I held her head, Rick slipped on the c-collar to help stabilize her neck. J.T. slipped the backboard behind her. Her male friend held her ankles, Rick and J.T. were on either side as I held the head. The backboard and she were lowered to the ground. She was strapped down. I checked and she could wiggle her toes and didn't have any numbness in her extremities. I slipped a pillow under her right knee because it hurt when straightened out. We transported her to the hospital.

At the hospital they saw she was on the backboard and so the doctor had her neck and knee x-rayed. Her knee was just badly bruised but her neck wasn't. Her neck was fractured at c-3. It appeared to be stable (cracked, but not completely broken into two pieces). The injury wasn't as bad as I had suspected, but she was dizzy and if she had fallen again it could have snapped and resulted in her being paralyzed. Rick learned something that day and my belief in protocols was reinforced. She was the reason we put one hundred people on a backboard knowing ninety-nine people don't need it. She was the one in one hundred.

BOY VS MOTOR HOME (not all stories end happily)

Tommy was six years old. That morning he had carefully dressed himself in his new school clothes. Black pants with pleats, black tennis shoes, black t-shirt and to top off the ensemble, a camo backpack for his books. He was Navajo, with brown skin, black eyes and lots of thick black hair. He liked school and was looking forward to the new school year that had just started a few short weeks before. Tommy lived on the Navajo Reservation about twelve miles outside town just north of Highway 98. He rode the school bus every morning and again that afternoon as it returned him home. The bus stop was on the south side of Highway 98. He and his brothers plus various neighbors and friends would board the bus for school. In the afternoon the process was reversed. He was doing well in school and his parents had high hopes for his future.

That September day in the fall of 1991 was to be the last day Tommy had on this earth. His mother didn't know it when she kissed him goodbye that morning. He didn't know it when he attended school and worked hard to learn his lessons, lessons that he would never need again. He waved goodbye to his friend and boarded the school bus for the ride home. He smiled a wide friendly grin at the bus driver as he exited the bus.

The bus had stopped as close to the south side of the highway as possible. The driver swung out the "Stop" sign on the side of the bus. The road was only two lanes with a tiny strip of asphalt along the edge, leaving the bus halfway in the lane of traffic. Motor home number one saw the bus and stopped in his lane. Motor home number two didn't and all the driver saw was a motor home stopped in the middle of the road. The driver didn't take time to consider why, they were in a hurry. The driver wasn't going that fast when he (or she) swung the motor home into the on-coming lane to go around.

Tommy and his two young cousins walked in front of the bus while the driver watched the rear view mirror. The driver's view was blocked by motor home number one and the bus driver didn't see the second motor home until it emerged into her view as it came around motor home number one. It was only a few feet from the children.

The driver, in complete terror, screamed and beat on the window. She stood up and yelled as did the other children. Tommy was in front of his two cousins. He looked and saw the first motor home had stopped. He looked and didn't see any traffic coming in the west bound lane. He walked into the west bound lane directly into the path of the second motor home.

Tommy's tiny body was struck with a dull thud, the bumper snapping and breaking bones. He was stuck to the front of the motor

255

home and carried about thirty feet and then fell to the side of the road as the vehicle braked to a stop. The driver, in complete panic, drove off. Witnesses were traumatized; some screamed, some cried, some just sat staring at the horrible scene. The bus driver's hands trembled as she reached the microphone and screamed hysterically into the radio for an ambulance. The message didn't make a lot of sense to the dispatcher. The words were jumbled and the sentences fragmented, but the main idea was conveyed.

The report I got was a five year old boy had been hit by the school bus. I was in the back of the ambulance that day, filling in for an empty slot. When the pager sounded I immediately realized this could be a bad one and checked who I was on with that day. Lupe and Gordon formed my team. Gordon was a great EMT. Lupe was experienced and reasonably good. I was satisfied with the crew. Gordon was one of the best EMT's the Fire Department had. He would do anything asked of him. He was an excellent driver and I liked running with him. Lupe was quickly approaching a hundred pounds overweight. Her black hair was worn long and often got in her eyes on a call. She was always hyper and talked ninety miles a minute whether on an emergency or causally discussing the weather. I suspected that diet pills helped to fuel the hyper state, but I could never be sure. I was PFD Rescue Chief and Lupe was a "butt-kisser" so no matter how I tried to avoid it, we became well acquainted. Gordon drove faster than he should have, but we didn't say anything. The distance was eating up time, precious time.

A helicopter company had just recently gotten an Arizona license to operate in the area. It was a God send to patients and medics. But the Page bureaucracy didn't like anyone playing with their own little empire and had fought it all the way. City Hall, at the urging of Chief Nelson, feared a decrease in revenue. For every patient transported by helicopter, Page Fire lost the ability to bill for the call. So, the Fire Chief had made it very clear we didn't call the helicopter unless we had two or more patients, thus allowing us at least one patient to bill for the call. To assure this happened, only the Fire Chief could request the helicopter to respond within PFD's area of service. Unfortunately for Tommy, only he had been hit by the motor home. Of course outside agencies such as a law enforcement agency could dispatch without anyone's approval.

En route I expected to be turned around at any time. It made logical sense to use the helicopter. They were paramedics and we were basics. They could be at the scene in five minutes, we took twenty. They could take him directly to a trauma center, we had to stop at Page Hospital and after exam and x-rays, the doctor had to arrange air transport, an accepting doctor had to be found, a hospital room had to be reserved, and of course the ton of paperwork had to filled out, faxed and photocopied over and over. Time plays an important part in the survival of a trauma victim and Tommy didn't have a lot of time. Damn the protocol that would not allow us to request the helicopter. I knew I was dead meat if I made the "suggestion" on the radio. This protocol went against common sense. It had been developed by Fire Chief Nelson, to protect his turf. In private conservations, he had expressed his resentment at intrusion into "his" area by an outsider (the helicopter company). I had tried in vain to change his mind.

In anticipation of the call, the helicopter crew hurried to their helicopter and started to warm it up. They sat there listening to the radio, waiting. Again protocol demanded they wait to be invited. No invitation came. No officer from the scene requested them, even after being reminded of the helicopter by the PD dispatcher. The Fire Chief was monitoring the radio traffic, but didn't intercede and request the helicopter. As we got closer, I began to realize we were actually going to be the ones. The ambulance rolled code three . . . a very fast code three. We hung on and made our plans on who would do what. We all knew this was a load and go, scoop and run. I silently damned the Fire Chief and his protocol that wouldn't let me pick up the radio and shout "Send the damn helicopter!"

It wasn't that I didn't know what to do for the child. I had handled many such trauma cases. It was just that for the first time we had advanced life support and a helicopter waiting on the pad, ready to go and for some mysterious reason, they were never asked to take the call by the officer at the scene or the Grand-Poo-Paw of the Page Fire Department. I have never gotten a good reason why. I believe the officer at the scene was too involved in patient care. His own child was this boy's age and it touched him too personally. He knew the PFD was good and the new helicopter was "new" and an unknown. I think he forgot how important the time element could be in such a situation and decided instead to go with the known. I know the reason why the Fire Chief didn't request the helicopter was because there was only one patient involved and the city would lose money.

The ambulance stopped and Lupe and I jumped out, our hands full of equipment and the big bulky orange and white jump kit. The scene was charged with electricity. The tension was tangible. I could almost reach out and touch it. People stood around with eyes that spoke of some unspeakable horror they had just seen. "Which bus hit him?" I asked as I looked around. I could see a very large motor home and a school bus.

"The motor home. . . ." answered a school big wig that had descended upon the scene the second he had heard a school bus had been involved. I didn't realize until hours later that the motor home I saw wasn't the one that hit him. "He's bad," was about the most detailed medical description I could get.

We walked up to the boy. My eyes were scanning his body assessing his condition before I even reached him. It didn't look good. The boy was lying face down in the sand and weeds just a few feet from the side of the road. He was whimpering and trying to move. I kneeled down beside him and cut his clothes off down to his shorts and checked his injuries. They were bad. He was dying. His legs were broken and lay in unnatural angles. The left leg was folded up onto his back with the foot turned completely around the wrong way and up by his head. A huge avulsion (a large chunk of skin held on by a flap of skin) was located in his thick black hair. Blood was in evidence, but not as much blood as you would expect.

The police officer kneeled at the boy's head. He stroked his hair and talked quietly to the young boy, trying to quite him as a father would quite his restless child under very different circumstances. Anyone that says police are cold and hard should have been there. They feel just like anyone else. I honestly believe that at that moment, he would have traded places with that little boy if it had been possible.

The entire operation took only a few minutes. We took full spinal precautions by holding his head and supporting his body. He was log rolled to his back, onto the backboard. Lupe unfolded his leg and put it in as natural a position as possible during the roll. The boy's immediate life threatening injuries appeared to be mostly confined to below the waist. I ordinarily don't straighten angulated fractures, but the boy was dying. He was bleeding inside. I had to try and slow down the bleeding so I had decided to use the MAST suit. We would use it to increase his blood pressure and splint the lower extremities at the same time. In the big city the MAST suit isn't used much, but in rural settings where long transport times are common, it is. I personally have seen the suit buy precious time for patients.

We quickly loaded him into the ambulance. Lupe and Gordon Taylor put on the mast suit and pumped it up. I sat at the boy's head and put on an oxygen non-rebreather mask and turned it up high. I got low blood pressure and that was a bad sign. Children are new and everything works well. When injured, they compensate for blood loss and do it well. If there is a noticeable lowering of the blood pressure in a child, that is a bad sign. They can no longer compensate and it's downhill from there on. I looked down and saw his right foot at an odd angle. It wasn't broken.

Something was strange with the leg. I ruled out the Hare Traction Splint because I suspected the hip and/or pelvis was broken, causing the foot to fall in an unnatural way. The boy responded to the slight rise in blood pressure brought about by the MAST suit and splinting. The added oxygen helped as well. He began to try and move. His whimpering and moaning increased, but he never actually responded to us. He didn't know where he was and what had happened. Maybe that was a blessing for the little boy.

Lupe got two pedal pulses which surprised me. I was fairly sure the straitening of the leg would have interfered in blood flow if it had blood flow in the first place. But he had blood to his toes. I looked down at him. He was so young. He was in pain and his tiny body had been mangled beyond belief. Even if he lived, which I doubted, he would never walk normally again, if he walked at all.

The driver drove like a bat out of hell to the hospital and we didn't care. I didn't expect to deliver a live little boy. No one was more surprised than me when we pulled up at the hospital and he was still breathing, labored, but still breathing. Edgar El Terra (a nurse practitioner) was the first face I saw when the back door opened. He quickly jerked the stretcher out and I jumped out to assist. "What do we have?" he asked.

"He hurt bad and going downhill. Everything's broken from the waist down."

We wheeled the stretcher up the rear entrance (the regular ER entrance had a trench dug across it.) We lifted the boy and backboard off our stretcher and onto the waiting hospital gurney just inside the back door of the pediatric entrance. Edgar and the crew pushed the gurney fast down the hall. We were running. I was running alongside giving a verbal status report. "His left leg, tib/fib and femur are badly fractured as well as his ankle. The right leg is fracture too. There is something wrong with the right hip. I think the pelvis is fractured. Vital signs were going down. We couldn't get a blood pressure just before we arrived here. We reached the emergency room and found a large group of hospital staff waiting. They were all wearing gowns and were holding their sterile gloved hands in the air. They sprang into action. You could see it in their eyes. They too thought he was dying.

I walked out into the hall and stood still for a moment collecting my thoughts. Damn it. No one should die that young. It was such a waste, such a loss. He wasn't the first child I had watched die, but it hurt just as bad as the first time. This was something I never got use too. I'm glad I didn't. To coldly accept the death of a child is to isolate one's self too much, to go beyond and to become less than human. I hurt but I would never show it, not to anyone on the crew or at the hospital. Only later would I cry for Tommy.

At last someone remembered the helicopter. A nurse ran to call for it to transport the boy to Flagstaff Medical Center. The boy needed surgery. His mother came in with the child's grandmother and aunt. I went into the ER room. "Dr. Sager, the child's mother is here and wants to talk to someone." He looked up, "Then go talk to her, Sharon." He turned his attention back to the child. I sighed and left the room. I had been given this assignment too many times before. I find talking to the next of kin harder than caring for the injured themselves.

I opened the door and the three women turned and looked up at me with eyes that begged for good news. The mother's eyes were filled with tears as she twisted a handkerchief. The aunt tried to comfort her sister and had an arm on her shoulder. The grandmother sat in quiet dignity. She was a strong woman and had prepared herself for the worst. Her sad eyes told of other times and of other losses.

I pulled up a chair and sat down. They leaned toward me. I guess everyone develops their own style when it comes to this sort of thing. My style is patterned after the style I would like others to use if the situation were reversed. I give the facts, the injuries, avoid any real details of how it happened if possible because of police investigation and then what is being done now, where he was being sent, and then sum it up with "condition of patient report".

"My name is Sharon. I was on the ambulance that picked up your son. Dr. Sager has asked me to talk to you. How much do you know?"

"Only that a motor home hit my son. His cousins came running home screaming he had been hit."

"That part appears to be true. I don't have all the details; I was very busy caring for your son. But he was hit and thrown to the side of the road." I waited for a second and let it sink in. I then continued. "His legs are badly broken. There is a large cut on the back of his head. He isn't awake. They are going to fly him to Flagstaff Medical Center."

"Why?"

"His broken legs will require surgery to repair. Your son is in critical condition. He was hurt very badly. The doctors are working hard to stabilize him. He is young and strong but this is very serious." I stopped again as the aunt talked to the grandmother in Navajo. The woman shook her head in sad understanding. The mother asked again what happened and I told her I had no other information. She then was quite. Her thoughts appeared to be raw anger focused on the unknown driver that had done this to her son. The aunt had a few more questions. She avoided the word death. To say "your son may die," is to will it, according to Navajo beliefs, and may cause it to happen. So I tried to get that point across in other ways more acceptable to the Navajo culture. I am afraid

260

most people hear only what they want to hear and I don't think they heard the negative side of the report. But I tried and that's all I could do.

I stood up. "Thank you," the boy's mother said. I took them to the chapel/waiting room where they could wait in private. I expected the doctor to come in later and tell them the boy had died.

We went back to the station. The ambulance was a mess. We cleaned and replaced used supplies. We also talked over the call among ourselves. This is a very informal defusing and it helps to release the stress of the situation. Everyone I know in EMS would rather walk on hot coals than treat a seriously injured child. We spoke freely about our feelings and opinions. Nothing is written down, nothing left the fire station and none of what was said during that defusing has been reveled in this book.

The story gets complicated at this point. Dr. Sager, for only reasons only he understands, took off the MAST suit. He wanted to splint the boy's legs with two hair tractions splints. The hospital didn't own pediatric hare tractions splints. The helicopter service didn't own any. The Nursing Supervisor called me at the fire station. I realized, to give them our two pediatric splints would mean we wouldn't have needed equipment for weeks. Flagstaff was very slow retiring equipment. And sometimes they didn't return it at all. We had used the Ped splints (sized to fit children) twice in the past two weeks. They are required equipment on our ambulance as dictated by the State. What about the next child that needs a splint?

I usually am the one to grant or deny such requests, but this was a hot potato. I gave the phone to the Fire Chief. It was his fault the boy wasn't already in Flagstaff. The hospital was saying the boy was stable and they thought "he would make it." I had never been so surprised. Were we talking about the same little boy? I also was mad that the doctor had removed the MAST suit. It was the perfect splint for his legs, hips and gave some help in his blood pressure. I know altitude and air pressure would be an issue with helicopter transport, but it was manageable.

The doctors said the boy was stable. Chief Nelson told them "no." He used the fact that the doctors believed the child to be stable to refuse their request. He told them all ambulances in Arizona were required by law to have an adult and child Hare traction splint on the ambulances. He reminded them that only last week we used one on a girl hit by a car. To give them away would possibly short someone else that might need it and would leave us in an awkward legal situation. I knew the law, I knew we used the splint a lot and if we sent it to Flagstaff, we would never see it again, but I probably would have given it to them.

The Nursing Supervisor was mad. Then Doctor Ledman called. He made the same argument, but this time louder. The Fire Chief didn't like his judgment being questioned. The two doctors didn't like their judgment being questioned either. "It isn't our fault you don't have the equipment you think you need," the Chief pointed out to the angry doctor. "And why yell at us, the company you are using to transport him should have that equipment." It got nasty. Doctor Ledman slammed down the phone and called the acting city manager and got the same answer. After thinking a little, the Fire Chief called them and said they could have one, but not both. Doctor Sager hung up on him.

The boy's shattered legs were splinted another way and was loaded on the helicopter. The doctors were still optimistic. The mother took off in the family car toward Flagstaff. The helicopter took off. Half way to Flagstaff, Tommy died. His mother drove to Flagstaff thinking everything was going to be alright. She arrived at the hospital two and a half hours after her son died and was told he never made it alive to Flagstaff.

Doctors Sager and Doctor Ledman wrote nasty letters to the Fire Chief protesting the "heartless decision" to not share needed equipment. A copy went to the acting city manager, but he politically decided not to pass it on to the city council. No one outside the three of them and the crew and some of the hospital staff know of the letter or the controversy. Both doctors blamed the Fire Chief for the boy's death and never forgave him. In a small town that became an awkward problem. The Page Fire Department ordered a backup pediatric Hare traction splint the next day and the hospital did also. The boy was buried. His parents sued the school and the driver of the motor home.

The driver of the motor home had left the scene of the accident and was picked up in the next town. The man said he was driving, but witnesses say the woman was driving. The man was tried and convicted and got less than two years in jail. With parole, I doubt he served even a year. Most people believed he was taking the rap for his wife. I don't know. The school bus driver knows she did all she could and followed all the rules, but she still blames herself for the boy dying and for months she had nightmares that forced her to relive the moment of terror when she realized the boy was going to be hit. She took a few weeks off work. Finally she returned to her job as school bus driver but she told me it wasn't the same.

As I write this story, I realize a number of wrong decisions were made that day. But, no matter how hard we wish we could, no one can go back and change what happened. I'm not surprised the boy died. But his death cost so many people so much and they are still paying today. I just wish all of the stories could end happily, but real life it isn't always like that.

I am the type of person that learns from their mistakes. Part of my anger about that day is my own lack of guts. I should have called the helicopter and lived with the consequences. I didn't and I regret that. I was a coward. It probably wouldn't have made a difference in the outcome, but the two hours delay in getting the boy to a trauma center was not in the patient's best interest. Everything wasn't done for the boy and I was partly to blame.

Many years later I found myself in a similar situation. It was a different Fire Chief but the same policy with minor changes had been brought back to life. The call was around forty-five miles east of town on Highway 98. It was a reported one car rollover with on seriously injured female. "She's having trouble breathing," was the report from helpful bystanders. I know bystanders reports are not always correct, but what if they were right? By PFD procedures I could not request a helicopter for one patient on a bystander's report alone. I remembered the boy and I had vowed to not make that mistake twice. I called for the helicopter.

I remember arriving and found a Navajo Police Officer on the scene. A woman lay on the edge of the highway. She was eagerly sucking on the oxygen tank provided by the officer. I looked out into the desert and saw the car. The officer said the small car had left the roadway at highway speeds and sailed through the air and landed head-on into a rocky area. I opened her blouse and discovered a bright red mark indicating she hit the steering wheel with her chest. It's called a "DORF" injury, "FORD" written backwards. She was gasping for breath and was in respiratory distress. I suspected numerous fractured ribs and/or sternum. Before I could do more, the sky lit up with the helicopter's landing lights. It landed in the middle of the highway. The crew came over and I gave them a report. They took the patient directly to Flagstaff Medical Center.

When I got back into town I was greeted by the Fire Chief. He was mad. "She didn't sound that bad. You could have handled the situation without the helicopter!" the Chief loudly proclaimed. I was guilty of not bringing a patient back in the ambulance and this entire incident resulted in PFD not being able to bill anyone. His voice was elevated and he was very mad that I had ignored PFD protocols. I agreed with him that I knew better but I had called for the helicopter anyway.

This time I did the right thing even if it went against the rules. Another difference from the last time, I was a paramedic this time. I began to sling my weight around. I reminded him "I was required to error on the side of the patient and I believed the patient needed a higher level of care than Page Hospital was able to provide". I remembered the small boy lying in the sand and remembered my vow to never be a coward again and do the right thing regardless of protocols based on money. I quit backing up and went on the attack. "How dare you question my professional opinion? She was badly injured and needed a trauma center not our small town hospital. If you push this, I will get my Medical control involved and you will lose." He backed down. I wish I had had the nerve to stand up so many years ago to the other fire chief, but I couldn't go back and change what happened. But this time I stood up and did what was right. It felt good and it soothed my guilty conscious a little.

"SHARON.........HE'S DEAD".

It was a cold day in early December. I was at home when the pager sounded. I recognized the address. The man who lived there attended the same church I attended. He was elderly and in poor health. I had already been on a number of calls because of his cardiac and other health problems. I rushed out the door. He lived only a block away. I beat the ambulance and rushed to the front door.

I was met at the door by his daughter. I knew her well. "Sharon. . . . . he's dead." She was obviously emotionally upset and crying.

"Stay here," I said. I hurried down the hall. I entered his bedroom and found him lying in bed. He was dressed in PJ's, lying on his back. A sheet and blanket was pulled up to mid torso and his hands were folded on his chest. His skin was grayish and there was no obvious rise and fall of his chest. I didn't doubt he was dead. I reached over and with my cold fingers I felt for a carotid pulse on his neck. As I touched his neck, his eyes suddenly popped wide open. He looked up at me and screamed. I screamed. His daughter screamed from the living room and rushed down the hall.

He looked into my eyes and saw surprise. "Sharon?" Then his face changed, he understood, "You thought I was dead, didn't you?"

"Well, you looked dead."

"Daddy? You're not dead!" his daughter yelled.

"No honey, I'm not dead," he answered as he sat up.

"I'm sorry, you were so . . . . . still. . . . . ." I was trying to explain why I was there.

He then burst out laughing. I started laughing and his daughter joined us. "Oh, Daddy. . . . .I'm so glad you're not dead," she hugged her father.

I looked up as the police arrived with the ambulance crew on their heels. "It was a false alarm." We all left the man and his daughter alone. I am so glad he wasn't dead.

SET MEDIC

In this book I am trying to give a well-rounded taste of the various aspects of working in EMS. One area I haven't covered yet is that of a movie medic. One winter I worked as the set medic for a California production company. The movie is now a cult classic, "Motorama." Someday I may write more of my adventures with this movie and others, but for now this one story will have to do.

This story begins when we were shooting down at Lee's Ferry. It was December, cold and overcast. Small patches of snow lay here and there. No tourists, no fishermen, no river trips, just a small deserted boat launch ramp on the Colorado River. We were set up to film a scene on the banks of the river. A female NPS ranger wandered around with an annoyed look on her face. The movie company almost had to leave a hostage at ranger headquarters before they were given permission to film on the banks of the river. Most of the parking lot near the river was cluttered with cameras, vehicles and trailers.

Part of the shot would be filmed here and the rest would be filmed off a house boat on Lake Powell later. I found a spot out of everyone's way and sat my folding chair in the large, empty portion of the parking lot, and lay my kit beside me. The ranger walked over to me and announced in an arrogant, condescending tone, "You will have to move." I asked why. She said, "You are in the driveway and could hinder traffic flow."

"What traffic? I asked. "I haven't seen a single vehicle all morning."

"Well, one may come and you are in the way."

I reminded her that "All traffic was blocked for the filming, wasn't it?"

She hesitated then told me, "You can't sit in the driveway. It's against the rules."

I really didn't care where I sat, but I was bored and had nothing else to do so, I went along and played the game. "Isn't the law written so someone would not be injured if a vehicle were to pull into this parking lot?" She shook her head "yes". "But the road is blocked and no vehicles can access this lot, so the danger of me being run over by a vehicle is non-existent. Therefore there is no traffic to block and I am not in any danger if I sit here."

She digested what I said. Independent thought was something of which she did not appear to be capable. She went back to her rule book, "It's against the rules for you to sit here. You have to move or I may have to arrest you."

I sighed. "You live in Page, don't you?" She shook her head, "yes". "People in Page treat rangers like lepers, and this is why." I moved my chair over three feet and she stomped off. Over the next six hours no car appeared, no foot traffic, no nothing. A light snow began to fall. The ranger didn't come near me again. If she had approached me differently, I would have moved without comment. It really wasn't that big a deal. She just worded it the worst possible way to enlist the most negative response possible from me. As much of the movie as possible was shot outside the boundary of the Recreation area for obvious reasons.

A few days later we were getting set up to film in the same area. The shot involved two young men attacking an older man and killing him. They were to drag his body to a shallow stream and throw his body into the water. While lying there face down in the water, he would pump a small pump he had in the palm of his hand. Red dye (fake blood) would flow into the water and drift downstream. End of shot. Sounds simple enough, doesn't it. There were a number of things to consider when setting up this shot.

I remember sitting and watching the three men practice the fight. It was like a dance. At first it was in slow motion and finally it grew to look real. Hours upon hours was spent setting up the track the camera would glide upon as it followed the men dragging their victim. Three days after we had arrived, they were ready. The sun didn't cooperate so the shot was delayed. Finally the cameras rolled. I watched them shove and hit the older man. He fell to the ground and was kicked. Then one man picked up a board and hit him repeatedly with it. It did look real. He lay still as the two men talked about what to do with his body. They then each grabbed an arm and began to drag his limp body toward the stream that was out of the shot. The camera was rolled along the track, carefully following them as they moved across the desert floor. Then it was "cut." The shot was over.

We picked up everything and moved to the stream about a half mile away. It was overcast and cold. Patches of snow were scattered about on both banks of the small stream. The water was about six to ten inches deep. Little rocks littered the stream bed. Shooting began at sun up and lasted till sun down. We had no protection from the breeze that would come up most afternoons. It blew over snow and even though I was dressed warmly, I never felt warm.

I was setting up my medical area when the older stunt man walked up to me. He was in his mid-sixties. He appeared to be in good shape for his age, but he definitely was nearing the end of his career. "Excuse me," he said. "I think I need to talk with you a minute about this stunt." He had been a stunt man for years and had been in a number of movies I remembered. His most recent had him fishing and he dove off the small fishing boat just before it was cut in half by a big power boat.

"What is it?"

"This is confidential isn't it?"

"Sure."

He cleared his throat. "I wouldn't want anyone to think I can't do my job. I can, but I wanted you to know about my slight medical condition."

He had my attention now. "What medical condition?"

"I have had a couple of scares with my heart over this past year. I am supposed to be tossed into ice cold water and I wondered if it might cause a problem, you know, with my heart."

"I'm not sure. Did you have a heart attack?"

"No just funny little beats that cleared up on their own. I feel great. I'm not really worried but I wanted you to be aware."

It was clear he was going to do the stunt one way or the other. I had dealt with stuntmen before and they are a stubborn lot. His problem was probably a run of A-Fib that self-converted. It's not an uncommon problem, but at his age it could be a problem and cause a serious stroke or not convert back to normal and leave him in chronic A-Fib. I told him, "This might not be a problem, but it could." I explained the possible problems. "As long as you know this and still are determined to do it, I will try to minimize the possibility of a problem. But I will be prepared for the worst. I won't mention it to anyone." He seemed relieved.

"Thanks," he said as he left.

I had two days to prepare. I decided there was no way I could get around the fact that he was going to be tossed in ice cold water. We were in the middle of nowhere and no dry suit was available. My second best plan would be to do my best to limit his expose for an extended period of time. I decided to see he was warmed up immediately after the shot. I got a salamander heater, a tent, dry clothes and lots of fluffy towels. Hot coffee would be available and lots of hot packs.

I also had others to deal with. The lowest on the totem pole were sent into the water to pick up rocks. The area where he would be tossed was to be rock free so he landed only in mud. They were young and eager to get into film making and although it was obviously not their idea of fun, they rolled up their pants, took off their shoes and waded out into the icy water and picked up the small and medium rocks. They were careful to leave the rocks on both banks. Their fingers and toes turned red quickly and I had to restrict their exposure to the water. It took a number of dips and warming up periods before the job was done. They were very careful to do it right because if they missed a rock it might hurt the stunt man. I would time them in the water and then call them out. They would dry off their feet and put on warm socks and sit near the heater drinking hot coffee till they stopped shivering and the color returned to their phalanges (fingers and toes).

The day came for the shot. The sky was still gray and a light snow fell off and on. I went up to the older stunt man and asked how he was doing. He said he was fine. I watched as he was outfitted with a small clear tube that ran from and bag of fake blood taped to his chest. The tube ran under his arm and to the pump in the palm of his hand. The cameraman and director came over and explained to him what close ups they wanted to get. They explained how he should count slowly to ten before he pumped the fake blood into the water and how he had to lay there as long as possible partially submerged in the water. He said he understood.

I had a medium sized tent set up out of the shot. Inside were his dry clothes. Hot coffee lay heating on a camp stove nearby. The heater was pumping hot air aimed at a folding chair where he would sit. I also had my medical bag and equipment discreetly nearby if he were to have a problem.

"Quite on the set!" Everyone shut up. The two stunt men came dragging the older stunt man from the right hand edge of the shot. He lay limp as they stopped at the spot beside the creek. Each man took an arm and leg and swung him a couple of times and then let go. He hit the water with a loud splash. He lay there, face down, not moving. I held my breath. Then I saw the red fake blood drift to the surface and float down the stream. He still lay. I was beginning to worry. One camera moved in for a close up of him face down in the water and the second camera followed the red blood flow down the stream. Then he got up, gasping for air. Applause erupted from those around. It had been perfect. It looked great and definitely real.

I hurried forward with a warm blanket and tossed it on his shoulders. He was led to the lawn chair and sat down in front of the heater. Someone took off his boots and socks and put hot packs on the soles of his feet. I dried his hair and exposed skin with a towel. I bent down and whispered in his ear, "Are you ok?" He nodded his head "yes." He warmed his feet and hands at the heater for a few minutes. He then got up and hurried to the tent and took off his wet clothing and dried himself off. He dressed in dry warm clothing and returned to the lawn chair where I handed him a cup of hot coffee. He gratefully accepted the hot liquid. He stopped shivering and relaxed. There was no cardiac involvement as a result of the stunt. It was our secret.

After the movie was "in the can," I received a job offer. They wanted me to come with them to California. Hollywood people are a strange lot and I think they liked me because I didn't judge them. I just did my job and tried to not be too shocked at their strange behavior. I would be working for a major movie studio as movie medic. I would work with various production companies on sound stages and on location. The pay was great and I loved working as a movie medic. I was quite honored to be asked. If I had been single I would have packed up immediately and followed them to California. But I was married with children. My husband had a good job and our home was in Page. I had to decline the offer. Months later I received an engraved invitation to the premier showing of the movie in Hollywood and a pen with the emblem of a dragon used in the movie. I wanted to go so bad, but the timing was all off and I missed the premier. I rented the movie about a year later and when the icy stream shot came on I watched closely. It still looked great. My name is on the credits as set medic. I really had fun.

THE FBI, ATF AND ME

April 11, 1956 initiated the construction of the Glen Canyon Dam. It is located on the Colorado River just south of the Utah Border in Arizona. It was built to provide vital water storage for Utah, Colorado, Wyoming, New Mexico, Nevada, California and Arizona. The dam is a concrete arch type and was finished in 1964. It stands today five-hundred and eighty-three feet above the river channel. Behind the dam is Lake Powell, two-hundred and sixty square miles of water storage and recreational area. Its deepest point is around five-hundred and sixty feet and it is one-hundred and eighty-six miles long. It has one-thousand, nine-hundred and sixty miles of shoreline, more than the shoreline of the Pacific Ocean on the west coast of the United States. The power plant has eight generating units and provides 1,296,000 KW of power to New Mexico, Utah, Phoenix Arizona and southern California. Over three million people visit Lake Powell Recreation Area every year.

Page Arizona sits on top of a Manson Mesa (a flat topped mountain) almost a thousand feet tall overlooking the lake. The high desert provides few trees, lots of sand and beautiful sandstone rock formations. Highway 89 is the lifeline to the rest of the world. It's a narrow, two lane highway with few passing zones. It winds its way through northern Arizona and southern Utah. The entire area is sparsely populated. Page went from a construction housing area in 1959 to around 6,500 people today. The nearest larger cities (40-50,000 population) are Flagstaff Arizona and St. George Utah, both at about a three-hundred mile round trip. The nearest big cities are Las Vegas, Nevada and Phoenix Arizona, both about a six-hundred mile round trip. As you can see, the community is isolated. In the winter, Page seldom has significant snow, but just drive ten miles out of town and the roads can be impassible, sometimes for three days or more.

I am giving you a "tour" of the area so you can appreciate the problems involved when a VIP arrives in the area. In the year 1983 the lake reached full capacity. A ceremony was planned. In 1966 Lady Bird Johnson came for dedication ceremonies. This time it was First Lady Nancy Reagan. She was going to speak at the ceremony to mark the project's completion with the filling of the "water storage reservoir" also known as Lake Powell.

Weeks before Mrs. Reagan was due to arrive in Page, the town, the nearby resort and the dam were swarming with FBI, ATF and untold other agencies. They would arrive at a spot that seems completely non-important and leap from a black SUV with tented windows and begin taking pictures and snooping around. They wandered behind restaurants and motels, drove the residential streets looking for what, I haven't a clue. Most were "men in black" types except the undercover agents. The undercover agents were easy to spot; they tried to look like locals or tourists, but most failed miserably.

Two weeks before the ceremonies, a meeting of all the involved agencies was called. I represented the medical response for the event. I had attended similar meeting in the past as PFD Rescue Chief, but this was different. I walked into the room and found I was the only woman in attendance. It was full of men dressed in uniforms identifying the agencies, Coconino County Sheriff's Department, Page Police, Navajo Police, Arizona Department of Public Safety (Highway Patrol), FBI, ATF, National Park Service, The Bureau of Land management, Fish and Game, Utah Highway Patrol, Cane County Sheriff, and Utah's Glen Canyon City's (now known as Big Water) one and only police Officer. I am certain I have missed some agency, sorry. I found a seat at the large table and sat down. I knew many of those present, but there were unfamiliar faces in the group.

Usually when there was a meeting of the local law enforcement it was a jovial atmosphere. Unfortunately the Federal agents had managed to kill that. The Federal agents were an intimidating and humorless group. No smiles, no casual conversation, and no respect whatsoever to rural or local law enforcement agencies.

The Federal agents strutted around like peacocks, filled with self-importance that crossed over into arrogance. It was clear after the Federal agent in charge had uttered his first sentence, this meeting wasn't a brainstorming session, it was a meeting designed to tell the stupid hayseeds what to do and how to do it. No room for discussion, no room for local input. The officers in the room knew this and sat quietly, but not happily in silence.

The ceremonies were to take place on the dam. The top of the dam had a wide roadway and a stage was going to be constructed. VIP's from a number of states and local dignitaries would sit on the stage. Speeches would be made and First Lady Nancy Reagan would be the keynote speaker. The general public would be allowed to fill the rest of the space on a first come basis. The local, state and national news media would cover the event.

It was very clear that the Federal Agent viewed the general public with disgust. He spoke about controlling them like one might speak about herding cattle or mindless sheep. I knew many of the "general public" that planned on attending. They were good hard working people. Their tax dollars paid this man's salary. They were my friends, family, co-workers and neighbors. They would have been insulted if they had heard the things he said or implied in that meeting. I was offended and didn't like the Fed's attitude or the look of contempt on his face. His deity complex was wearing thin.

After some general condescending remarks, the presentation became serious. An environmentalist group that had plagued the area for a number of years was now making threats about disrupting the ceremony. This group of militant environmentalists didn't care who they hurt, as long as their environmental and political issues were publicized in the news and written media. The building of the dam many years ago had been rather controversial. The environmentalists had objected to the Central Arizona Project that included the dam and the resulting flooding of the Glen Canyon to form the "reservoir" to be named "Lake Powell".

A little background might help at this point. There were a number of concerns that were presented, sometimes very loudly. One of the most promenade arguments was that to cover this beautiful canyon with water was immoral. There are always two sides to a controversy. The other side said the water storage project was vital to the survival of the southwestern

United States. The area didn't even have a road to it so few people had ever even saw the canyon. It was uninhabited by humans. The water would rise slowly, giving wildlife plenty of time to relocate. Also, those in favor said the construction of the dam would result in a road being built and that would offer access for people and the lake would offer recreational opportunities. The other side continued with "People are bad and undeserving, leave it undisturbed for the lizards and coyotes." For the record, fifty years later, the lake is enjoyed by many people and there are still many lizards and coyotes in the area.

The project was approved in 1957 and work began in 1959. In 1983, the year of this meeting, the dam received three to eight bomb threats a day, an average of 2,007 a year. The violent environmentalists group had recently been concentrating on the north Kaibab. There was logging in the area. Some bird watcher reported he "thought he may have heard the call of a spotted owl." The environmentalists were protesting and called for logging to be shut down. This industry employed several hundred people in an area that didn't have many employment opportunities. This group of tree huggers would drive long thick nails into the trees and when the logger's chain saw would hit the nail, the chain would break and whip up and strike the logger in the face, tearing large chucks of flesh from his face, arms and shoulders. Eyes and fingers were lost. These were men working to feed their wives and children. The logging was supervised by Land Management and the Forest Service. The trees were cut down in a scattered, random pattern. It thinned the forest but still left it with a natural look.

Vehicles were vandalized with spray paint announcing "PIG" on law enforcement, Park Service, Forest Service and Bureau of Land Management vehicles. Head lights were smashed, tires punctured, and windows broken. Even civilians who had permits to harvest the fallen timber that had fallen naturally (for their fireplaces), had their vehicles damaged severely if they happened to be in the wrong place at the wrong time. This group had no problem with violent acts. They believed the *ends justified the means*. I always believed what you did on the journey to your goal also counted. They didn't. Achieving the goal was all that mattered. They had recently turned their attention away from saving trees and had made threats about the ceremony on the dam and doing "something to be on the six o'clock news." Law enforcement had a right to be concerned.

"Now, we will address the medical sector. Who handles the ambulance around here?" I raised my hand. He appeared unimpressed. Pointing to a drawing of the dam, bridge and visitor's center on the white board he said "You will have three medics on the dam. You will stage an ambulance here," indicating the west side of the bridge across the highway from the Visitor's Center.

I looked at the diagram. I calmly looked him in the eyes and said, "No . . . . I will not stage an ambulance there." There was an audible intake of breath in the room. I had just shocked everyone. I had said *no* to a federal agent.

The agent looked as shocked as everyone else. This was the first display of emotion he had shown since arriving in northern Arizona. He hesitated. The room was quite. I sat there silently, waiting for a response. Finally he gained composure. "Why?"

"I am not a bomb expert. But if I wanted to make a spectacular statement that would give me my fifteen minutes of fame on the nightly news, I wouldn't bother with the dam, it's too heavily guarded. I would put a few plastic milk jugs full of gasoline in my back seat, drive my car onto the bridge, get out and set it on fire and just walk away." Complete silence engulfed the room. Visions of a burning car filled their heads. It was obvious no one in that room had considered that. They had been concentrating on the dam. I continued. "The bridge is in full view of the speaker's platform and the cameras would just swivel around and film the flaming car for the six o'clock news. The burning car would block access to Page and the nearest hospital. My ambulance would be trapped on the wrong side. It's a two-hundred mile trip from the west side of the bridge to the east side if the bridge isn't usable."

Again, silence. Then they all began to talk at once. The FBI agent called for order. He then looked at me and said, "You have a point. Would parking on the east side of the bridge be acceptable?"

"Yes," I answered. The topic was changed and around a half hour later, the agent concluded the meeting. The day of the ceremony I had to smile when I saw the Park Service ambulance on the west end of the bridge sitting beside a large bulldozer. The PFD ambulance pulled up beside a second bulldozer sitting beside the road on the east side of the bridge. Apparently the FBI had decided the best way to clear the bridge would be to use a bulldozer. A bit crude, but effective. The ceremony went well and there were no disturbances noted.

Logging on the North Kaibab was shut down for twenty years even though no spotted owl was ever seen in the area before or after the "possible bird call" was reported by the hiker. Hundreds of men lost their jobs and the lumber mill was closed. A year later the environmentalists snuck away from a tour of the dam and dropped a long zig-zagged black paper almost four hundred foot long down the face of the dam. From the bridge it looked like a crack in the dam. A member of the group took pictures that circulated among the more radical environmentalists. Authorities took it as a threat and beefed up security.

The dam still stands today. It continues to hold back the lake that provides recreation for the general public, the highway now provides access to one of the most beautiful areas in the northwest and provides a more convenient route to and from Phoenix and Las Vegas. The small construction housing area became the town of Page, and the Navajo's living in the area now have schools, shopping, churches and highway access off the northwestern section of the reservation. Many of the original radical environmentalists have evolved into the average working class who have found ways to legally work non-violently to help the environment. Some of the more radical have died or are in nursing homes today, but they have been replaced by others who believe the *end justifies the means*. The dam still receives many bomb threats every day.

THE WICKED WITCH OF THE WEST

Anna Marie was six years old and the proud owner of a new bright red bicycle. Page is a small town and children are granted more freedom than those living in a large city. Anna Marie had been given permission to ride her bicycle up and down the block in front of her house. That day she got brave and without permission road to the corner of the next block, then the next. She found herself on the corner of a busy street near the post office. She stopped and looked around. She saw someone she knew across the wide street and decided to ride across to show them her new bicycle.

Anna Marie looked to her right and started across. She never saw the small blue car coming from her left. He didn't expect her step into the street and hit his breaks only seconds before he struck her. The impact hit her left side. The bumper struck her femur and snapped it. She and her bicycle were thrown ten feet to the pavement. She wasn't wearing a helmet and her head hit the hard roadway with a thud. She lay motionless.

I was at the airport with Rescue-One. Beside me sat a new ambulance driver. I was attempting to teach her how to parallel park. "Just a little bit more, that's it, now turn the wheel." She did as told and the rig slipped between the cones. "That was great. Now, you do it and I'll keep quite." The pager sounded. The training lesson was over.

I let her drive to the station then had her scoot over to let the third crew member take over driving. We arrived quickly at the scene. I hurried to the little patient. The girl was lying on her back with her left leg badly

274

angled. She was moaning and moving around a little, but not fully conscious. The bystander attending her was known to me. He was an EMT but didn't run with PFD.

"What do we have?" I asked.

"Six year old girl was riding her bike and was hit by that blue car. Her left femur is fractured. Her left arm may also be broken. She hit her head and is in and out of consciousness." This was serious. The femur can cause massive blood loss and children didn't have that much blood volume to lose. The head injury was also of serious concern. I called for the Hare traction splint. My partner put her on high flow oxygen and took hold of her head. I slipped on a c-collar. The driver arrived with the Hare traction splint and sat it up. The little girl woke up and began to scream. She was looking directly at me with terror filled eyes. She was in the most pain she had ever felt in her short life. I was a still a basic so no pain meds were available but if I could get it splinted it would lessen her pain. I took her shoe off and then grasped her foot in my hands and slowly pulled on it. She screamed as the driver applied the splint. The splint was designed for a fractured femur. The splint was designed for a fractured femur. A Hare traction splint is a device made of hollow tubing and elastic straps with Velcro snaps. It is placed up under the pelvic bone and the leg lies on the adjustable straps that run the length of the splint. The femur bone when broken will overlap. The sharp ends of the bones cut and tear soft tissue including blood vessels. There is always serious blood loss with a femur fracture. The rescuer pulls the foot and stretches the leg and the overlapping bones fall back in place and the damage from the sharp bone ends is lessened and pain level decreases. After it was applied her pain level decreased and she stopped screaming and lay there crying. We quickly got her log rolled onto the backboard and secured her to the board. As my two partners loaded her into the ambulance I called the ER. I gave them a report. Our ETA was only two minutes. I could see the hospital from where I stood.

En route to the hospital I got a set of vital signs. She drifted off into unconsciousness as we pulled up to the ER entrance. She didn't wake up again until days later. She was more or less stabilized and flown to Phoenix Children's Hospital. She underwent surgery and months of painful rehab.

Anna Marie was a tough little girl. With her family's help she regained her strength and began to walk again. Her mother moved in with her sister who lived in Phoenix so Anna could go to rehab. The thing that bothered Anna the most was the fact she had to drop out of first grade. She spent her summer in Phoenix in and out of the hospital.

Finally fall came and Anna Marie and her mother returned to Page. Anna was thrilled to be home with her family. She was allowed to go back to school that fall. Anna still walked with a sever limp but in time that was expected to improve. She loved school and tried to keep up with the other children. She did a pretty good job. She grew stronger each day. But as children sometimes do, she over did it. Her leg was still weak and as she and her classmates were walking down a hall in a straight line behind their teacher her leg folded up and she fell to the carpet.

We pulled up in Rescue-One five minutes later. I carried the big bulky orange and white jump kit as my partner carried oxygen and suction. We were met by a man in a suit who led us to the girl. She lay on the floor softly crying and rolling back and forth. She was in extreme distress. Her teacher told us she had broken her leg six months ago and had just returned to school. I kneeled beside the child and she looked up at me and burst out with a blood curdling scream that echoed through the halls. It was as if the Wicked Witch of the West had come for her. I was surprised. Children usually like me. I backed away. I let my partner, Charlotte take over. She was the mother of five and with a motherly approach she calmed the child. The little girl remained calm as long as she didn't see me. The very sight of me caused her to go into a screaming fit. At the time I had no idea why.

She didn't appear injured in any way. But she insisted her leg hurt and remained emotionally distraught. We loaded her in the ambulance, but I had to ride up front because my presence only caused her to scream. At the hospital her mother managed to calm her down.
The doctor said her leg had folded up because she had been over using it and it simply gave out. She wasn't really injured.

The ambulance was cleaned and restocked and reports were written. I handed my report to the doctor and he explained why the girl had acted as she had and why she was so frightened of me. "She's the little girl that was hit while riding her bicycle up near the post office six months ago." Now I remember her. "She has just got home after a number of surgeries and extensive rehab. It was traumatic for her. She was told to be careful and go easy on the leg. When it folded she thought it was starting all over again. Then she saw you. You are the only one she remembers and she associates you with the horror and pain of that day. When she saw you she was reliving that day in her mind."

I now understood. I felt bad that I had caused her additional emotional pain. No one wants to be remembered that way by a beautiful little girl. A few months later I saw her and her mother in the store. The little girl was walking with only a slight limp. I went the other way and avoided them. I didn't what to chance causing her anymore distress.

276

FOUR WHEELING, EMS STYLE

Lone Rock Beach was an exciting place during the summer. It's a large wide sandy beach with access by lake and road. I remember as I stood on Waikiki Beach in Hawaii and thinking, "Is this it?" It was so small! This 911 story involved a house boat full of old friends tied up to the beach. The houseboat was anchored to shore improperly and drifted in a half circle over the water at the rear of the boat. Hugh had been drinking on and off all day. He wasn't drunk but he was buzzed and his judgment was impaired. He had been diving off the back of the houseboat all day. What he failed to understand was the boat moved back and forth, sometimes to the left, then center then right, then center again and back left, so on and so on. To him, he was driving off one stationary point, the back of the boat. But in reality, the water looked the same but the depth varied as the boat drifted back and forth. That hot summer day he dove into the water one too many times. He hit what we call "hard water," (rocks).

Pagers were set off, a three person EMT crew responded, Roger, Doug and I. We arrived at the turn off and traveled down the sandy road as far as we could go. We stopped and considered our options. The boat was about a quarter mile on down the beach. Our vehicle could not go any further due to the deep sand. A pickup truck drove over and offered to take us to the patient. We accepted and loaded our equipment into the back of the pickup. Roger climbed into the passenger seat, and Doug and I climbed into the truck bed. I sat down and held on tightly. We took off fast. Because of the deep sand, a vehicle had to use speed to move forward. "Keep your foot in it," is the advice of those who travel through deep sand. It was a rough ride, but short.

We arrived and were met by some of the patient's friends. They explained the situation and helped us carry our equipment to the patient. Most of the bystanders had been drinking, but no one appeared drunk. As I approached the patient I saw a man in his mid-thirties. He was of average build and weight. He had dark brown hair and was dressed in swimming trunks. He lay on his back on the sandy beach with his legs still in the water. His head was held still by his childhood friend named Garth. His friend looked up at me, "I'm an EMT, I think he may have injured his neck." I understood what he was saying. He didn't want to upset his friend, but he believed the bones were broken and he was worried that the sharp broken bones could at any moment sever the delicate spinal cord. One false move and this man could die or live the rest of his life as a quadriplegic (paralyzed from the neck down).

"Keep holding his head still." I directed Garth. "Hi, my name is Sharon. I'm an EMT with the Page Fire Department. Can you wiggle your toes?" He did. "Can you squeeze my hand?" I slipped my index finger into his hand and he squeezed them. "Do you have any numbness or tingling in your hands or feet?"

"Yeah, my feet and hands kind of tingle." This told me some damage may have already occurred and/or the cord was swelling.

Roger took over holding the head absolutely still. Whoever holds the head is usually in charge. Roger was the type that always insisted on being in charge. He was now the leader and it was obvious he also had no intention of getting wet. I applied a c-collar around Hugh's neck. Then Doug and I took the shoulders and hips and Garth took the lower legs. The driver of the pickup took the backboard. The patient was log rolled as a unit to his left side as the backboard was slipped under him. He was secured to the backboard with straps. We moved him up on dry land. My shoes were filled with water and fine sand and one small pebble. My jumpsuit from the knees down was wet and covered in damp sand. We dried off the backboard as best we could using towels offered by bystanders and then applied a generous amount of duct tape. He was securely secured to the board that would act as a splint for his possible neck and/or back fracture(s).

We loaded him into the back of the pickup. Roger again climbed into the passenger seat. Doug, Garth and I climbed into the back of the pickup truck. We lay over him to keep the backboard from bouncing around. The ride was rough, very rough. We spun out in the deep sand, lunged forward, throwing a sandy rooster tail behind the pickup. I hoped we had done enough to stabilize his neck.

In a cloud of dust and sand, we slid up to where we had parked. Doug, Roger, Garth and I reached in and removed the backboard. The pebble in my shoe caused a shot of pain as I walked carrying my share of the backboard to the ambulance. Garth said he would meet us at the hospital. We didn't speed. It was more important to take our time and pick our way around pot holes and negotiate dips slowly. I called the hospital to give them a report. "We are transporting a 35 year old man who dove off the back of a houseboat and hit the lake bottom. He has neck pain and is in full spinal immobilization. The patient has movement in all extremities and reports tingling in his hands and feet. Vital signs are normal and there is no significant medical history. Our ETA (estimated time of arrival) is twenty minutes." They said they would be waiting for us.

At the hospital, the doctor immediately told the nurse to arrange air transport to Dixie Medical Center in St. George, Utah. He kept the man on the board and sent him to x-ray. The x-ray made it obvious that the

278

man had broken his back around T-3. His spinal cord was still intact but he was in serious danger of becoming a quadriplegic.

I limped into the bathroom and took off my jumpsuit and shoes. I was wet and covered in gritty sand and coated in a light layer of dust. I washed the legs of the jumpsuit off, rinsing the sandy mess down the sink. I removed the pebble then took a paper towel and cleaned my tennis shoes. I took off my jeans and washed the muddy sand off. I rinsed the ton of sand out of my socks and redressed. The clothing was wet, but it was summer so everything should dry quickly.

Garth and his wife arrived at the hospital. Hugh now understood why everyone was so worried about him and thanked Garth for his help. When Air Evac arrived Hugh asked that Garth be allowed to fly with him. He had no family here and he had performed as an EMT in such a way the patient just might make it through this problem intact. They decided to allow Garth to fly with Hugh even though they were not family.

A couple of months later a thank you note arrived. The man was up walking and healing well. Its times like this that make me feel that it's all worth it.

I WAS AFRAID HE WOULD STOP BREATHING

"The pager hasn't gone off while I've been on duty for two weeks," Mildred Moore complained as she browsed through the meat counter at the grocery store.

"Well God only gives you what you can handle." I smiled. It was an old joke with the volunteers.

Mildred laughed, "I guess so." No EMT wants bad things to happen but they like to go on calls and during slow times they get restless. The way we keep from feeling like vultures sitting on a fence waiting for someone to break a leg is to say, "I don't want something bad to happen but if it is going too I wish it would happen on my shift."

Mildred was a new EMT. She was a tall, rather large woman. She had grown up poor in a mining community in southern Arizona. Mildred struggled trying to give the impression that she was "high class." One example was when she spent a lot of money putting up a hand carved front door with gold plated door knocker and knob. Her home was her "proof" of her "upper class status." The funny part of it all was no one particularly cared one way or the other. She was well liked for who she was not her social status or bloodline. She was pleasant, a team player and a good

EMT. I liked working with her.

"I have found a great way to get it to go off," I said as I tossed a roast in my basket.

"How?"

"Just invite guests over for dinner and it's a sure thing you will get a call."

She laughed. "Well we will see. Aren't your friends from California coming over to your house for dinner tonight?"

"Yes they should be in around five or so." The friends were the Oakland's. They vacationed often at the lake and planed on coming in from their camp spot and having dinner with us that evening. By this time I was an old pro at juggling guests and the pager I wore on my belt. I went home and got dinner started a bit early. I set the oven very low to cook the pot roast. I sat the table, got out the rolls and placed them in a conspicuous place. I left a note with steps on it for my husband "just in case."

Just like clockwork at four forty-five the pager sounded. I kissed my husband goodbye and gave him the note. "It's an accident with multiple patients at Waterholes Canyon a few miles outside town. Go ahead and eat without me. I'll get back as soon as I can."

When I arrived at the station the driver, Gus Garnett was loading Rescue two. I slipped on PFD's ugly yellow jumpsuit over my clothing and climbed in the front. "Who's our third crew member?" I asked through the tiny window.

"Bonnie." She was the wife of PFD's first Fire Chief, Jude Owens. She was a pretty woman that everyone liked. Her husband wasn't as well liked. We sat impatiently waiting for her. There was no officer at the scene yet.

"Let's roll without her," I said. We pulled out of the station. When we reached the stoplight the driver yelled that he could see her car approaching the intersection. We pulled into the gas station on the corner. Bonnie also pulled into the parking lot and parked. She jumped out dumping her purse, stethoscope and jumpsuit on the ground. She franticly bent down and picked them up and ran for the ambulance. Half the town was watching. Then I heard my name being called. I looked up and saw the family from California getting gas. I yelled, "Go on over to the house. Maurice is there. I'll get back as soon as I can." They smiled and waved. Friends of an EMT had to learn to go with the flow. These were good friends and took the incident in stride. Bonnie climbed into the back.

We arrived at the accident located a few miles south of town a few minutes later. The road dips down and crosses a bridge over a narrow and deep canyon named Waterholes Canyon. On the other side the road goes up a hill. At the top of the hill to the east was a wide flat area. The pickup was totaled. It had "end-doed," gone end over end. The truck went nose first into the deep sand and rolled over onto its top, crushing the roof inward. The momentum then caused the truck to stand up on the tailgate. At that point as it started to flip onto its wheels the force of the rotation caused the unrestrained female driver to take the windshield out with her body. Her restrained six year old son followed his mother through the opening. The pickup then continued back onto its wheels.

I got out and stood still for a second and looked over the scene. Tunnel vision can kill and I had learned to survey the entire area before wading into a mess. The woman lay fifty feet from where the truck rested on its wheels. The boy lay about thirty feet beyond, over a slight hill. Bystanders that had stopped were with the injured.

The woman looked the most seriously injured. Bonnie was a gentle and sweet person that got along well with children so I told her, "Bonnie you go to the boy. I'll take the woman." Bonnie's eyes grew large. She had been an EMT for some time but had only a small number of calls under her belt. She was a lot better than she gave herself credit for. Years of being told by her husband that she was dumb and useless had brainwashed her into believing him.

Not allowing Bonnie time to argue I hurried to the woman. She lay on her back on top of the crushed windshield. If she had been wearing a seat belt she would probably be walking around with only cuts and burses right now. I knelled down. The bystander was in his early sixties. He held her hand and looked at me concerned. "She goes in and out. She starts to moan and thrash around and then gets quite." Just then she began to moan. She moved her head back and forth. Her arms flung around. Then she grew quite. I noticed she didn't move her legs.

"Have you seen her move her legs?"

The man gave it serious thought. "No."

"OK." I got a second willing bystander to hold her head still. I got out the BP cuff and slipped it on her arm. Her BP was good. I began a secondary exam. When she hit the windshield it "scalped" her. Her scalp lay peeled back and the white of the skull showed. Hair clung to her scalp. This is a horrible looking injury but in reality it can be fixed fairly easily and usually leaves few scars that are usually hidden in the hairline or creases in the forehead. I cut off her dirty pink tank top. She had red marks and the beginning of deep bruises all over her body. She was wearing shorts so exam of her legs were easy. I took her tennis shoes off and ran my pen up the sole of her foot. No movement was noted. I pinched the toe and still noting. I was beginning to suspect the woman had broken her back and would never move her legs again. I hoped I was wrong. I looked down at her as I slipped on the oxygen mask. She was around twenty-seven years old. She was an attractive woman with thick black hair cut to shoulder length. I tore myself away from visions of her spending the rest of her life in a wheelchair. I applied a dressing and bandaged the open wound on her head.

I got up. With 2,500 square miles to handle we were often on our own. I had learned to use bystanders. If controlled and given jobs they could handle they were a great help. Urban EMS providers didn't like helpful bystanders. But I relied on them. The older man had taken her pulse before I arrived so I knew he knew how. "I have to go check the other patient. Could you watch her? If her breathing or pulse gets faster or slower, or if there is any change, just yell. I'm only over the hill." He shook his head in agreement.

I hurried over the hill. Bonnie wasn't having as good a relationship with her bystanders. They were pushy and the three men were all telling her what to do. Bonnie was flustered. I slipped into my most authoritative manner.

"What do we have Bonnie?" She looked up with pleading eyes.

"His femur is broken."

"Vital signs?"

"They are ok."

"Ok. Get the pediatric hare traction on him. Then backboard him. I'll find Gus to help you." I looked up at the three men. They started talking at once. Each had his own idea of what should be done. After allowing them to talk for a minute I interrupted. "Look I know you want to help. But we are trained EMTs. Bonnie is doing exactly what she is supposed to do. You mean well but you are in the way. Now if you want to watch that's ok but don't talk to her and let her do her job." Gus walked over, and I told him what I had told Bonnie. I walked with the driver to the ambulance. "Don't let the bystanders get in your way."

"I won't," he said as he pulled out the traction splint. I got the equipment I needed and went back to the woman. The police had arrived. Together with help from the officer and bystanders we carefully log rolled her onto the backboard and tied her down. She went in and out of consciousness but never fully came around enough to answer a question.

Soon both patients were in the ambulance. We hurried to the hospital. I didn't trust the little boy. Children can look great one moment and be dead the next. Femurs bleed and a six year old doesn't have a lot of blood. He looked great. He was in pain and whimpered and had tears in his eyes but he didn't cry. He was a brave little boy. I radioed in to the hospital a report. At the hospital we unloaded the woman first because she was on the stretcher. We left Bonnie with the boy and rushed his mother into the ER. "Her vitals are low. She's unconscious and hasn't moved her legs since the accident." The doctor looked her over and went to work.

I went back and Bonnie and I got the boy on a gurney. As we rolled him into the other ER room he looked up at the nurse and with wide eyes filled with pain and pleading he said, "Can I have a leg pill?"

"A what?"

"A leg pill. My leg hurts so bad." Tears formed in his eyes. Tears formed in the nurse's eyes.

"I'll get you one soon. I promise," the nurse said.

Bonnie and I went back to the ambulance. "I was so afraid when you left me alone with the boy."

"Why?" I asked.

"What if he had stopped breathing?"

"Do you know what to do if he had stopped breathing?"

"Yes."

"Then you didn't have a problem. You are a good EMT. You are a lot better than you think." All the years of her husband telling her she was stupid had given her doubts. She needed encouragement (or a new husband).

She smiled. "Yeah I guess you are right. I could have handled it."

The woman was flown to a trauma center. She lived. The boy healed beautifully. But the mother was stuck in a wheelchair paralyzed from the waist down. Five years later I went to another accident and she was a passenger this time. She wasn't injured that seriously. She was sitting in her wheelchair in the back of a pickup that left the road at sixty miles per hour and flipped on its side. She and the wheelchair went for a brief flight and landed in soft sand. We transported the driver of the vehicle, her and the wheelchair to the hospital. If only she had been wearing a seat belt at the first accident everything might have been different.

PINK HAIR ROLLERS AND THE CAT

I had washed my long dark hair and rolled it up in pink hair rollers. I had been under the hair drier for about twenty minutes when the pager clipped to my collar went off. I jumped up and grabbed the comb and put it in my teeth and hurried to the door. I was flinging pink hair rollers out of my hair as I ran for the car. I jumped in and started the car and backed out into the street. I put the car into drive and suddenly I heard the most horrible blood curdling scream I had ever heard. It was coming from the back seat. Suddenly my large black cat jumped up on the seat screaming. I didn't know he had snuck into the car for a nap. He didn't like cars and he was horrified. I pulled up at the stop sign still ripping pink hair rollers out my hair and flinging them over my shoulder, my comb was in my teeth as my cat was running laps around the inside of my car screaming in complete hysteria.

A car slowly tuned in front of me and pulled aside me. It was a woman I only vaguely knew. She smiled and indicated she wanted me to roll down my window. I have no idea why, but she wanted to tell me something or talk. Time was ticking away and I had a limited time to respond to the station. I also thought of my cat. If I let him out now he would never stop running. I shook my head "no" and drove off. I know from the look on her face she was shocked at my unfriendly failure to take time and be social. I arrived at the station as the last hair roller bit the dirt. I got out as my cat lapped through the back seat and slammed the door before he got back up front. I ran into the station with cat hairs all over my jump suit and combing my long damp hair.

I can't remember the call so it must have been routine. After the call was completed I returned to my car. The cat lay asleep under the front seat. I got in and started the car. The cat made strange noises but stayed hidden for the trip home. I left the window down on the car so the cat could escape when she came out from under the seat. I found a trail of pink hair rollers leading all the way into the house. That woman never attempted to speak to me again. I am certain she thinks I am a complete nut.

DISIGNATED DRIVER

Nothing is ever simple. I was a brand new "newbie" EMT. I had never been to a serious emergency. I sat in the back of Rescue-2 with a big excited grin on my face. We had been dispatched to an accident at Black Mesa. That was about eighty-five miles east of Page on the Navajo Reservation. The "Rez" as it is called, is the largest Indian reservation in the United States. They had an EMS system, but they just didn't have enough ambulances or EMTs so they sometimes had to call neighboring EMS agencies. The report was a woman had driven off the winding road leading to the top of Black Mesa. We sped through the night, flashing lights lighting up the desert.

We were only six or so miles outside of Page when the report of a second vehicle accident was broadcast. There was not another ambulance within over an hour's drive. The second accident was supposed to be a car off the road and possibly one man injured. It was located about thirty miles out and we would come to it before the first call.

EMT Nelson was driving and Doug was riding shotgun. Doug was an experienced EMT. He was around five foot nine inches tall, average build and weight. He wore his sandy blond hair cut short and wore glasses. He was a manager of a local store and usually dressed in dress pants, dress shirt and tie. I liked running with him. He taught me a lot and built my confidence as an EMT.

It was a moonless night. Roger said, "We will stop and quickly check it out. Hopefully he is just drunk and pulled off the road to sleep it off. If not, we will backboard him quickly, put him in the ambulance and keep heading to the first accident." That's against all the rules, but in rural EMS you do what you have to do and we were the only game in town. It would be his problem documenting the fracturing of the rules.

The dispatcher called us and reported she had an ambulance heading for the Black Mesa (1st accident) but wasn't sure of their ETA (estimated time of arrival.) She seemed to think we would get there first even with the second accident. Roger considered telling the Navajo Nation ambulance heading to Black Mesa the call was all theirs, but he decided to wait and see what developed with the second call. Then just when you think it can't get any worse it does. "Rescue-Two, we have a report of third accident at MP 310 with multiple patients."

"We can't save the entire world," I said.

"You can't trust the public's reports," Doug said. I soon found the following week how right he was after rushing code-three eighteen miles on curvy mountain roads, down a 6 % grade to a reported two car head on to find two pickups with their hoods up and battery jumper cables strung between them.

Just about that time the dispatcher called back. "An officer has arrived at the second reported accident and says the car is gone. . .... Cancel." Roger passed a semi-truck loaded with hay as Doug keyed the radio and answered, "Rescue- Two copies, we are cancelled on the second call." Now there were only two, but the third call had reported multiple patients. Roger gave it some thought and decided if the third accident was really bad, he was going to call dispatch and tell her to notify Kayenta that the Black Mesa accident was all theirs.

We were eight miles from Page and only two miles from the third accident. Then I saw it up ahead. Four cars had stopped and people were running here and there. It was hard to see exactly what had happened. We pulled up and hopped out. I heard Doug radio the dispatcher that we would handle this accident, but the other responding ambulance would have to handle the Black Mesa call.

Doug and I were met by an excited woman. She babbled on and on, not finishing sentences and making very little since. I looked at the four cars that had stopped and none of them looked damaged. I could see flashlights bobbing around in the desert north of Highway 98. The woman then pointed into the blackness, toward the bobbing points of light. Doug took off and I followed. Fifty feet later we come upon the boundary fence, a barbed wire fence strung along the side of the highway to keep livestock off the road. The fence wasn't damaged but I could see a pickup on the other side. How did he get from the highway to the other side of the fence and not damage the fence?

I looked around as Doug struggled with climbing through the fence with the jump kit. Now I could see how it happened. The truck was driving away from Page, heading east at a high rate of speed. The road curved sharply to the right but the truck had continued straight. It then went up a slight sandy hill that acted as a ramp and the truck was launched into the air and had cleared the boundary fence to land on the other side.

What I didn't know at the time, Mr. Young had come to town and bought lots of alcohol. He then did what any alcoholic father would do, he shared the liquor with his two teen age sons, age fifteen and seventeen. After running out of money and alcohol, he had tossed the truck keys to the designated driver, the fifteen year old because he appeared to be the least drunk of the three. The teen had missed the curve and had launched the pickup into the air in great stuntman form. When the pickup landed nose first then rolled over on its top and rolled again, coming to rest on its wheels. The three had been ejected from the vehicle and it now lay scattered about the sandy desert.

Doug was hung up in the fence when the other EMT arrived with wire cutters. He cut the fence and the three of us passed through without incident. We branched out, looking for patients. The Roger found the oldest son, very dead, lying beside his new black cowboy hat. I glanced at him as I hurried past. I was trying to keep up with Doug. He found the youngest son, alive but seriously hurt.

I kept looking around for more patients and I noticed a line of blood running down a sandstone rock that sat on a sandy hill. The desert was dark with no moon showing that night. I glanced around and thought

I saw movement in the darkness. Coyotes? I thought. I wasn't afraid of coyotes, but a pack of wild Rez dogs scared the bee-gibbies out of me. I took a deep breath and followed the blood trail and found the father. He was wearing cowboy boots, jeans and a red western shirt, the Navajo uniform. He had landed on hard sandstone rock. He was lying on his back, unconscious and very seriously injured. His respirations were irregular and shallow. His pulse was beating so fast, I couldn't count it. Blood was everywhere. I was a new EMT but I had no doubt this man was going to die. Suddenly and blond woman came up. She was obviously excited and held a gallon of water in her hand.

"Please, may I baptize this man?" she pleaded with me.

Now, I personally believe whatever forgiveness we receive from God is between God and the person. I don't believe in third party intervention. But, some religions do, and she was right, this man needed all the help he could get. I could see no harm, so I told her, "Sure, go ahead, but make it quick." I began my exam.   She sprinkled water on his head and said a quick prayer, smiled and backed away. Roger joined me. He went to the man's head and began to check it for injuries. His hand hit wet hair. He pulled his hand up and looked, expecting to see blood. There was no blood. He touched his hair again and looked at his hand in confusion. "His head is wet!"

"He's just been baptized," I explained. He looked at me with a very confused look on his face and turned back to his work. It was over an hour later before I could explain how an unconscious man lying on the dry desert sand got baptized.   The father and his fifteen year old son were examined, back boarded and loaded into the ambulance. As I climbed in I heard the Kayenta ambulance call in and report they had arrived at the scene of the first accident. On the return trip the EMT drove and Doug cared for the father. I ended up with the fifteen year old. I remember as I was taking his vital signs he looked up at me and in a weak voice asked, "Where's my brother?"

I remembered the dead young man. "Was he wearing a black cowboy hat?

"Yeah," he answered with slurred speech.

"He's being cared for. I don't know his condition." OK, so I lied.

He was quite for a couple of minutes then asked, "Why isn't he in here?"

"There isn't room. Now relax, your brother is being cared for." I began to ask him questions about what had happened. He answered slowly and with slurred speech, but I found out the details. We sped through the moonless night with red, blue and white overhead lights lighting up the desert. We arrived quickly at the hospital. We took the boy and his father into the ER and gave the doctors the report.

After the ambulance was cleaned and back in service and all the paperwork had been completed, we picked up our equipment and started to leave. We passed by the police standing in the hall. We had already told them what the boy had told us. The Department of Public Safety (Highway Patrol) officer and Navajo Police officer stood in the hallway outside the father's room. One told me that Mr. Young would rot in jail if he lived. "No man has the right to do that to his children." Mr. Young died soon after arriving at the ER. Little did we know that he not only killed one son that night, he killed the second son as well. It would just take longer for him to stop breathing.

Sam, the youngest son went on to follow his father's example. Over the following years I went on call after call involving his drinking and driving, his drinking and walking, his drinking and fighting. I remember I once picking him up at school where he was drunk and in a fight. He was crying about his dead brother and told me the story of the accident. I didn't tell him I was there.

Over the next twenty years he never held a job that I knew of. He never owned a car or a house. He continued to live with his mother and younger siblings. He never married and never had children. He spent time in jail for petty crimes such as shoplifting and panhandling. When his disability check would arrive at the beginning of the month (he was disabled because he was an alcoholic), he would drink until he passed out. We would sometimes be called to the park and find him unconscious, lying in vomit and urine soaked jeans. By the middle of the month, money was getting short and fights would erupt among the park people. He had only a little money left to buy liquor so he would drink Lysol or mix wood alcohol (rubbing alcohol) and Listerine to drink. By the end of the month we would pick him up in DT's (withdrawals from alcohol) He worked hard on slowly drinking himself to death.

Twenty years of hard drinking and he finally managed to kill himself. I was called to LeChee (Leche-e), a small Native American community on the southern border of Page. I remember entering and finding him lying on his sister's couch where he had passed out drunk the night before. He was found by his family, not breathing. Janet (a paramedic), Sarah (an RN) and I were on the call. We worked the full code on the living room floor, trying to give him every chance we could to live, even though it seemed he didn't want too. His mother and his younger siblings wanted him to live. Also, if we didn't work him, the family would have to abandon their house because he would have died in the house. By working him we were giving him a chance, however so small and saving

288

the family home. We pumped him full of every drug we carried that could remotely help. We intubated him, started IV's, CPR and everything we could think of.

We continued CPR and placed him on the stretcher. I was doing compressions and Sarah was bagging him (using the bag-valve mask to provide oxygen) while Janet pushed the stretcher to the ambulance. We all knew he wasn't going to make it. This was considered "PR CPR" (public relations) or a skills workshop. It didn't hurt him and regardless of why we worked him, it gave him a chance no matter how remote the chance for success. We loaded the stretcher. Sarah had stopped bagging him to load. I jumped in and hurried to bag him. I expected one of the women to jump in and take over compression. But much to my surprise, they were talking to each other and closed the door. I was alone. "Hay guys! I need help!" The door opened as both apologized. Sarah jumped in and started compressions as I continued respirations. We continued all the way to the hospital. At the hospital they gave it a brief try and called it. We couldn't resuscitate him. He was thirty-five years old. It took twenty years, but his father finally killed him too.

ESP AND THE EMT

People who serve in Emergency Medical Service form a close knit group. We see each other under the worse kind of stress. We know each other's strengths and weaknesses. We know each other in a way few other people know their fellow workers. Words aren't even necessary at times; each knows what the other is thinking and responds accordingly. We learn to read subtle body language, tones and choice of words. We can read the real meanings. The communication between working team members is unique to emergency work. This closeness may be the only way to explain what happened early in my career.

I was talking on the phone to Janet Marley, a fellow EMT. She and I had moved from Phoenix around the same time and had gone through the EMT class together. We were good friends. Suddenly I had the overwhelming feeling that my pager was going to go off and soon. This overpowering certainty left no doubts; it was a sure thing. "Janet, I have to go. The pager's going to go off."

"What? I didn't hear anything on the scanner?"

"I can't explain it, but I have to go, goodbye." I hung up. I then hurried around the kitchen and quickly laid out lunch for my two sons that were due home from school any minute. As I finished I hurried to the front door and picked up my keys and slipped on my shoes. My pager sounded. I wasn't surprised.

I didn't know it but strange things were happening to two other people also. Rene was an EMT and on call that day. She got out of her car to go get her mail at the post office and the same strange premonition hit her. She knew beyond any doubt that she was going on a call. She hurried into the post office and withdrew her mail. She hurried outside and almost made it to the car when her pager sounded.

At the fire station Roger Nelson had just completed a vehicle check and was preparing to go home. As he opened the door to leave, he stopped. He too experienced the oddest undeniable feeling that somewhere in town, someone needed the ambulance and his pager was going off any second now. Roger shut the office door and walked into the ambulance bay and hit the button raising the door and started the ambulance. His pager sounded as he drove it out front to await the rest of the crew. The secretary ran from the office out into the bay and handed the driver the address. "It's a baby not breathing, CPR in progress."

The driver looked at the paper and then looked up at the secretary. "It's Lynn's address." Lynn Jesse was an EMT. She had experienced more tragedy than anyone should ever have to experience. She buried her first husband while she was still in her early twenties. Their son died a few months later from SIDS (Sudden Infant Death Syndrome). She later remarried and their son also died from SIDS. Her new baby was a girl. She and her second husband had sighed with relief. SIDS affects mostly boys and now there were monitors available.

Now her last remaining child's heart had also stopped beating. Life isn't fair. If I learned one thing on the ambulance, it's that. Rene and I made it in record time. The ambulance raced to the address only two blocks away. We all knew her and we silently went over infant CPR in our minds while en route.

The ambulance came to a screeching halt and Rene and I flew up to the front door and flung it open. Lynn stood in the living room holding her daughter. The look on her face made you want to go hug her. She had tears running down her cheeks and complete raw panic in her eyes. She rushed up to me and shoved Terra into my arms. I looked down, expecting the worst. Terra looked up at me and smiled. The driver came in and with his arm around the now sobbing Lynn, led her out to the ambulance. "Go get the baby's monitor," I told Rene. I held the baby up near my face where I could feel her breath against my cheek. I kept her there, carefully watching her. I didn't trust her. Lynn had sobbed that the baby had stopped breathing and her tiny heart had stopped beating three times. Each time Lynn had performed CPR and her tiny baby had responded.

Rene and I walked out the door and to the ambulance. Lynn, by choice, rode in the front seat. She had done the right thing and had saved her baby's life by restarting her heart three times, but she wanted no more of it. She relinquished responsibility by handing the baby to me. I have never been so complimented in my life. She gave me the most precious possession she had, her baby daughter, and trusted me to do the right thing. How did I feel? Honored, but frightened. I kept my eyes on this baby. She was beautiful. Her coal black hair framed her angelic face with ringlets. She stared back at me with wide blue eyes. I knew how important it was that this baby live. After Lynn buried two others, she couldn't stand to lose this one too. The baby kept breathing all the way to the hospital. At the hospital, the doctor took over. I walked into the hall. Lynn had regained some of her composure. She thanked us. We stayed around till her husband arrived. Back at the station, while doing reports we each admitted to the advance warning. It was spooky.

Later, after Terra recovered, I was talking to Lynn and told her about how the entire crew knew something was wrong. She told me that from the moment the monitor went off until we rushed through the door she was thinking how she wished the EMTs were there. She said she knew who was on that day and franticly wished it was us and not her doing CPR on her daughter. "Next time instead of sending us panic signals, throw in the address too." She laughed. Thank God there was never a next time involving Terra. The girl is a healthy, beautiful eleven-year-old at the time of this writing. Sometimes there are happy ending.

WHEN THE PATIENT IS YOUR HUSBAND

In the rural setting, those in EMS realize the next patient could be a good friend or their loved one. It isn't a matter of "*if*" it's really "*when.*" It is a fact of life in rural EMS that EMTs and Paramedics will eventually have to handle a 911 involving a friend, co-worker, neighbor or close family member. I personally had to handle a number of emergencies involving close friends and twice was called to emergencies involving my loved ones. It's hard, but it has to be done and I did what I had to do, like other EMTs and Paramedics faced with the same situation.

The day I was tested, I had just completed an ambulance call involving an injured child at the elementary school's playground.

Thankfully the child wasn't badly injured and the call went well. I was driving back home when I noticed two vehicles stopped at a stop sign two and a half blocks from my house. One of the vehicles was my husband Maurice's truck. As I neared the scene it was obviously a car accident. I got out and saw my husband's truck had been hit from behind at thirty-five to forty miles per hour. His truck sustained some damage but the car that hit him from the rear was totaled. I could see my husband standing beside the passenger door to the vehicle that hit him. As I approached I could see he was brushing glass off a six month old baby in a car seat strapped in the front passenger seat. The child's mother was very upset but appeared uninjured. "I was looking for something in my purse on the floorboard. I didn't see him (indicating Maurice)."

My husband was an EMT and he looked up to give me a report. "She hit me from behind, hard. I think I got most of the glass off the baby. She doesn't look hurt." I looked down at the baby. She wasn't crying and there were no obvious injuries. The mother took her baby out of the car seat and held her.

I got on the radio. "F-3 – Page," (PFD Rescue Chief to Dispatch).

"F-3, go ahead."

"I drove upon a MVA (motor vehicle accident) involving two vehicles and three people. I am at the corner of Elm and North Navajo, by the school. Please send a police officer and page an ambulance. Patients are code-four (stable)."

"Officer is en route and I will page the ambulance." Officer Freddy Carver arrived quickly. Maurice worked with his father out at the plane (Navajo Generating Station) and Freddy was a friend. The woman was driving a company car. The company was owned by her and her husband. She had a current license and registration but no insurance. She was visibly upset. She insisted she and her baby weren't injured and didn't need an ambulance. It was her right to refuse and this time it appeared that might be the right decision.

I had called the ambulance for Maurice. He was doing exactly as I told him too. He continued to talk and talk and talk. Neither behavior was normal for him. He told me he had stopped for the stop sign and she hit him. He described how his head whipped back and struck the rear window. He described seeing *stars*. This is a text book case of concussion and a serious chance of spinal injuries in the neck area. I asked him if his neck hurt. He said it did, but he was alright. I heard the ambulance radio they were en route. They would be here in a couple of minutes. I sat him down on the curb. He continued to talk nonsense and appear somewhat confused. I saw the ambulance drive up. "Stay here," I told him. He smiled a blank smile and I think he agreed.

292

On my way to the ambulance the officer stopped me. "Sharon, Mo doesn't have both ores in the water."

"Yes, I know. That's why I called the ambulance. If the woman changes her mind, page a second ambulance." I turned and walked away. I met the crew, all well known to me. Lilly Jacobs, Ola Hawkins and Tom Hankins. I gave them a report. I ended with "I want you to take exceptional care in spinal stabilization. I have a gut feeling something is really wrong with his neck. He is also confused, so he probably has a concussion as well." The crew and I walked over to Maurice, who was still setting on the curb. He was pleasant and cooperative but not firing on all cylinders. I backed away and let the three person crew care for my husband. I trusted them. I love my husband and I felt comfortable leaving him in their care.

As I approached the officer he asked, "How is Mo?" He was the only person we knew who called him Mo but my husband didn't care so he continued to refer to him in that manner.

"He has a concussion and may have neck injuries. But for now he's ok."

"What about the truck? Should I call a tow truck?"

"It appears drivable. I have to get to the hospital, Dr. Birch is on and he needs guidance."

The officer laughed. "Look, have dispatch call Yellow Front. My son is working there. Have him walk over and drive the truck home." The officer assured me he would. I left and hurried to the hospital.

I arrived just as the doctor walked up to him. He too knew my husband and they had been fishing together. He immediately realized Maurice wasn't his usual self. He took me aside. "I think the concussion isn't a serious problem, at least not right now. I am more worried about his neck. I am going to order x-rays."

"Make sure you order a swimmer's view."

"I don't think that's needed." It was an awkward shot to do and he knew it.

"I have a gut feeling there's something wrong with his neck and it's possible it's around C-8." The cervical spine consists of seven vertebras. C-8 actually describes a location, not a spinal vertebra. It's where the cervical spine attaches to the thoracic spine, around the knot you can feel where your neck attaches to your body. It can only be x-rayed with the patients arm extended over their head, similar to a swimmer taking a stroke. The x-ray is taken from the arm pit view angled toward the neck.

"Ok, swimmer's view it is." He walked off and wrote the orders.

293

I went in and saw Maurice. He was strapped solidly to the backboard with a cervical collar around his neck. He was in good spirits. "Don't move your head. Do you understand? It's very important." He smiled and indicated he understood. I wasn't sure. It was obvious he didn't know how close he was to being paralyzed from the neck down. If I was right, and I prayed I wasn't, he was only a centimeter away from having the dislocation or fracture severing the cord. The cord was only the texture and strength of an almost cooked piece of spaghetti and it would only take the slightest movement. He was wheeled to x-ray. I followed and waited outside. After the x-rays he was taken back to his room. I went in with the doctor and x-ray tech to view the x-rays.

The room was dark; the x-rays glowed on the screen. I am not an expert, but immediately I could see the problem. Maurice had dislocated C-7. It protruded outward. He was in trouble. The doctor turned to me, "I am calling Air Evac and they will fly him to Phoenix." I shook my head in approval. His and my family was in Phoenix so that's the best place to take him. I was familiar with the hospitals in Phoenix and the one Maurice was going to for treatment.

I walked back in and Maurice still lay on the backboard. "Don't move your neck."

"Yeah, everyone tells me that."

"Honey, there's something wrong with your neck and you shouldn't move your neck, at all." I worried that he didn't completely understand how important it was for him to lay still. He wasn't all there and appeared to not retain information. His short term memory was affected by the concussion which is to be expected. "Air Evac is coming to take you to Phoenix." Before I could continue, he moved.

He looked surprised. "Something's different."

My heart stopped. "What do you mean?" I was near panic.

"I don't know exactly, but it doesn't hurt now."

"Wiggle your toes," I told him. If he couldn't move his toes my husband had just became a quadriplegic, paralyzed from the neck down. He wiggled his toes. "Stay here. Don't move." I hurried off and found the doctor and told him what had just happened.

He yelled to the nurse, "Get him back to x-ray!"

In record time x-rays were done. As the Doctor, x-ray tech and I stood staring at the new x-rays I laughed out loud. "Look at that!"

"Yeah, that's great!" The dislocated vertebra had slipped back in place. We hurried down the hallway and into Maurice's room. The doctor did a detailed exam on movement and sensation. Maurice appeared back to normal except for some pain in his neck, a headache and a mild concussion.

I looked up and my youngest son, Stephen had arrived. I left the room and met him in the hallway. His employer was Doug, a PFD EMT and when the police called, he drove Stephen to the accident. Stephen drove the truck home. Then Doug drove Stephen to the ER to check on how his father was doing. "How's Dad?" he asked. I happily gave Stephen and Doug the good news.

I got to take Maurice home. He missed a week's work. His concussion resolved and he returned to normal. His neck continued to hurt off and on. We considered suing but what good would it do. The woman who hit him didn't have insurance. Her husband and her house were mortgaged to the hilt and their business was failing. They had no car insurance and the home insurance didn't cover car accidents. They didn't have two pennies to rub together. Suing them would be a waste of time. All we would end up with was our lawyer's bill. Maurice's neck improved but sometimes still hurts even today.

Later the EMTs and I discussed the call. They told me they had never been so complimented that I would back off and allow them to care for my husband without me interceding. "How did you stay so calm?" one of the EMTs asked me.

"I wasn't calm. I was jello inside. I just managed to look calm. I walked away because my hands had started to shake and I need to back away. I trusted you. All of you are highly skilled and I knew you would give him the best of care." I meant every word. They were humble but felt good that they had been there to help me through an emotionally trying experience. That day I had personally been tested and I guess I passed. I still would rather walk across hot coals than do that again.

DISASTER DRILLS and TRAINING EXERICES

When I was Rescue Chief of the PFD, only the staff was full time, the rest of the personnel were volunteers. Sometimes an EMT might go months and never use a Hare Traction Splint or some other piece of equipment. They may go on a fairly good number of calls but not a heart attack. Unlike the large city, practice was about the only way to guarantee that the EMTs were ready for whatever their next call might be. In order to maintain a high skill level, it was necessary to have weekly drills. They were two hours a week where the volunteers would be introduced to new equipment, updates, news and were given the opportunity to practice skills.

295

Volunteers are a strange breed. Managing volunteers is like herding cats. They are usually type-A personalities, intelligent, completive and bore very easily. I was responsible for keeping them awake and interested during the drills. I devised drills that stayed away from dull lectures whenever possible and video's just put them to sleep. I tapped my theatrical side and started staging accidents and situations that would allow them to try out new equipment and apply their skills in a setting that mirrored as closely as possible real life. I often added a completive edge to the drill and they quickly accepted the challenge.

One Wednesday night I got three volunteer patients, my oldest son (around 11 years old at the time) the wife of a firefighter and the husband of an EMT. In the big city garage that was attached to the fire station I set up three stations. Station one was a pickup with a bicycle stuffed under it and my son tangled in the mess. Station two was a car with a woman sitting behind the steering wheel complaining of neck pain after a collision with another car. Station three was an intoxicated man outside a bar who had been stabbed.

The thirty-two EMT's were divided into teams of three and were to handle each incident as if it were real. We had practice bandages and they used equipment off the ambulances. Vital signs were to be taken and written down along with the time and they questioned the "patient" as if it was real and the patient would respond as if it were real. When they completed the station the patient would give them the patient's view and I or another staff member would offer comments on where they did well and where they could have done better.

At each station there was often a hidden problem, something they should possibly expect, but usually something they didn't expect in a drill. Station One was interesting. When the EMT crawled under the car to extricate the "boy patient" he found a cooperative patient. The first time they moved him he screamed a blood curdling scream and almost every one of the EMTs tried to stand up with the car on their shoulders. The patient then didn't cooperate and my son was a great actor and behaved like a very frightened child in serious pain. The EMTs discovered the station wasn't really about extrication from under the vehicle. It was more about soothing a frightened patient to obtain cooperation.

Station two went smoothly. A KED was used to remove the woman from the car. It's a green vinyl covered device designed to splint a seated conscious person. It works well but is time consuming and takes team work to apply. One of the crew members has to position themselves in the back seat behind the driver's seat and hold the patient's head still as the device is applied. The zinger to this station was the baby bottle on the back seat and a teddy bear. The mother asked, "Where's Timmy?" She was

296

basically ignored most of the time or her question was misunderstood. After they got her out, I would remove the baby blanket on the driver's side floor board of the back seat and there lay a baby (our CPR baby). The EMT who had held the head had stomped all over the "baby" during the mother's rescue. This reinforced the important issue of being sure of how many patients are there.

Station three involved an intoxicated patient who had been stabbed. I had taken a rubber knife and taped it so it appeared to be protruding from his left side, just above his belt. At first he was cooperative, but while the EMT was bandaging him he got more and more insistent that he wanted to get up and find his attacker. He used bad language, became aggressive, and shoved the EMT. Finally he withdrew a toy gun and stuck it in the ribs of the EMT and said "bang, bang." The lesson to be learned is all patients should be searched, especially one that shows aggression.

This is only one example of what we did to help keep our EMTs on their toes, ready for anything. Disaster drills was another way to expand the system to include the various agencies in the area. They were held once a year. They involved multiple patients and the Rescue, Fire, police agencies and the hospital participated. In our area children are bussed great distances off the reservation into town to school and during the summer tour buses are everywhere so the possibility of fifty or so patients is real.

There are two ways to view a disaster drill. One way was to completely surprise the department. This can cause serious problems with confusion as to if it's real or not and the EMTs and Firefighters are set up to fail. PFD has had a couple of fire chiefs that liked to do this and then would humiliate individual rescuers when they made a mistake. It made the chief appear "all knowing" and the EMT as "stupid." I chose the second method. I liked to set them up to succeed. I would offer a drill on managing a disaster. Then I would tell them we were going to have a drill in two weeks on a Saturday. I didn't tell them the time, place or type of disaster. When it was paged out the dispatcher said, "This is a drill, this is a drill . . . . we have a report of _____. This is a drill." By setting them up to succeed they went away feeling good and ready for the real thing.

I would get volunteer victims, young, old and everything in between. I would lay out cards with patient description of injuries on the table and they would choose what they wanted to be. One time a rather large man chose to be a "laying down patient," and the firefighters who carried the three hundred pound man complained. I told them I didn't assign him to do that, he chose it. I also reminded them, three-hundred pound people can be involved in any disaster and they just had to deal with it.

Make up was applied. One time I put a t-shirt on the sidewalk and burned holes in it. I put it on the patient. I applied red makeup where there were holes and then rubber cement. I took a pin and plucked the center of the rubber cement and the red showed through. It looked so much like second degree burns it fooled the doctor until he touched it and the red makeup came off. Usually there was between twenty to thirty victims, sometimes fewer, sometimes more. I let my imagination fly away.

I once planned a disaster drill involving a bus load of children. The isles of a school bus are very narrow and restrict an adult in full turnouts. Access is also limited. I found lots of children of firefighters and EMTs that loved to be patients for our drills. My younger son, Stephen was the one pictured on the front page of the local newspaper with serious eye injuries. All victims were well prepared and knew what to expect. They were very good actors and they helped our department stay well trained. We never had a problem using children, friends and family. I want to take this opportunity to thank them.

Another drill involved a building that was slated to be torn down. I set pepper fog to look like smoke and red lights that resembled flames. The inside had been partially demolished and there was lumber, sheetrock and other debris lying around. It was dark inside. The zinger to this drill was the first arriving captain was grabbed by a hysterical woman that wouldn't let him go and his men entered without him. She was good and precious minutes passed before he could get away from her.

I also had hidden a baby beside a young woman padded to appear about six months pregnant. She kept mumbling "My baby, my baby." They thought she was talking about her unborn baby not the doll that lay just beside her in the darkness under a piece of cardboard. The note pinned to the baby said, "If found within the first twenty minutes, I am alive. If not, I am dead." When the firefighters carried the mother out of the building to the treatment center, she waited and five minutes before the deadline she told the EMT her baby was still inside. I like to design the drill so the people succeed, not fail. I still remember the fireman running with the baby in his outstretched arm. He was running as fast as he could, the expression on his face was sheer panic. He seemed to forget it was a drill. He ran up to me, "Did I make it?" Yes, he did. A cheer went up from the other firemen as he placed the "baby" into the arms of the "mother."

Another drill was at the airport and it involved twenty people (the average number on a sightseeing airplane). We used a far corner of the airport and the firemen hosed down a pretend plane as EMS managed twenty patients and transported them to the hospital where they called in

298

staff and went along with the drill. The one problem involved two men handcuffed together. One was unconscious. The conscious one had a badge and identified himself as an air marshal transporting the criminal to Phoenix. The question was, was he really the marshal? Both men sort of looked like the picture. One man needed immediate attention but it was awkward because he was handcuffed to the other. The keys to the handcuffs and gun was lying about twenty feet away. "Toss me the key and I'll get the cuffs off. And bring me my gun," the air marshal asked. What would the firefighters or EMT's do? They handled it right. They checked both men for weapons and then moved the two men to a treatment center where a police officer came over and sorted out the mess. This also gave police a situation to deal with out of the ordinary. By the way, the conscious man was the criminal. If he had been allowed to get free he was to flee on foot.

I once set up a water truck and put a chemical placard on it that was highly toxic and deadly. The water leaking from it was supposed to be the chemical. The truck had hit a tour bus with thirty people on it. The tour bus was an old school bus with a paper sign saying "Desert Tours". The first EMT on the scene ran up to the bus and was declared "dead" from toxic fumes. Lupe had to set out the entire drill because she was dead. Oh, another thing, some of the passengers didn't speak English and that complicated matters. Thank goodness for the Spanish Club and the father of a doctor at the Page Hospital.

Another disaster involved me making a realistic looking bomb. It involved a tour group at the water treatment plant. A bomb went off. I made a second bomb. Terrorists often will set two bombs, one to do the initial damage and a second designed to get those responding to help the victims. I took three flares and duct taped them together. I took a small clock and taped it to the flares and took a loop of colored wires and taped them to the clock and flares. It looked very real. I then placed it in a reasonably obvious place. If it wasn't discovered, it would "go off" in ten minutes after the first arriving truck. They found it.

An interesting side note: Many years later, two firefighters were in a second story storage area at the new fire station. They were cleaning it out and throwing away stuff we no longer needed. A firefighter, who joined sometime after the bomb drill, reached into a large cardboard box and withdrew the "bomb." He freaked out. The other firefighter also freaked out. They called the captain who remembered the drill and he laughed, "Oh, that's Sharon's bomb." Police were called to verify it was indeed harmless and then it was dismantled.

MR. & MRS. KELLY, A LOVE STORY

Ken Kelly was a big man. The years had not caused him to bend with age. His stride was long and confident. His wife Jill could walk under his outstretched arm. He had been a school principal and she had been a school teacher. Together they had spent most of their life teaching children on the Navajo Reservation. They retired but stayed active. My husband and I met Ken and Jill when we joined the Civil Air Patrol. Although there was a large age difference we became good friends. I enjoyed Ken's quick wit and Jill's friendly outgoing manner. They were by far two of the most intelligent people with whom I had come in contact in a long time. The one thing that you would notice about Ken and Jill was their love for each other. It seemed to just radiate from them. They were totally devoted to one another. I felt comfortable around them and enjoyed listening to their many stories of places they had been and things they had done. They had lived an interesting life. The CAP (Civil Air Patrol) branch in Page disbanded after struggling with problems in leadership and territorial disputes with the Flagstaff Branch. The Kelly's went in search of other stimulating pursuits. My husband and I concentrated on the Fire Department. We began running in different circles and lost touch with them.

A handful of years passed. Ken stayed healthy but Jill started to forget simple things. Her once sharp mind turned to a dull confused state of disjointed thoughts and actions. Alzheimers slowly turned her into an empty shell that went about her life almost like a kindly smiling zombie. Alzheimers had stolen the mind of Ken's wife but in his blind devotion he refused time and time again to send her to a rest home. He took care of the woman, with whom he had shared his life. He bathed and dressed her. He cooked for her and waited on her. She would look up with empty eyes that showed none of the sparkling intelligence that had once been there. Ken continued to love the woman even though they could not share that special bond that had once been theirs. I remember driving by their home and seeing him raking leaves and her standing there, holding a large garbage bag and staring straight ahead with blank eyes as he put leaves in the bag. I felt sorrow for the loss of her quick and brilliant intelligence, but most of all I felt admiration to Ken's devotion to his wife.

I had just arrived at work. An unusual man walked in and looked around. He was about forty-five years of age, five foot, five inches tall. His hair was graying at the temples. He was dressed in a trench coat, suit, dress shoes and a hat. He looked like he had stepped out of a 1940's movie. He spoke like Dick Tracy in a monotone that showed only dead seriousness. I almost laughed. The office of Page Fire was small and had

300

just enough room for desks for the secretary, the Fire Chief, and the Assistant Fire Chief and Rescue Chief. The secretary was in the middle of a phone call when the man entered. I asked him, "What can I do for you?"

"I want copies of the reports involving a two vehicle accident at the intersection of North Navajo and Eighth Street on October fourth of this year."

"And who are you?"

He looked insulted that I didn't recognize him. "I am Detective Carlton Combs of Baker, Baxter and Brown." He was so serious the secretary was having problems not laughing out loud. She struggled at suppressing her laughter.

So he was a private investigator for a law firm. "Who do you represent?"

He hesitated. "The poor unfortunate woman involved in the collision of course."

"Of course." I opened my desk drawer and handed him a release form. "Just have her fill out this form, sign it and have it notarized."

He leaned forward, both hands on my desk. "I haven't time for all this. Its public record and I want copies now."

"They are not public record, they are medical records. I cannot release them without her written authorization."

"You don't understand." His voice was getting louder. I think this was his attempt to intimidate. He was wasting his time. "I MUST have the records. I have driven from Salt Lake City and it is of upmost importance that I return with the Fire Department's account of the accident."

"Mr. Combs," I began.

"I prefer Detective Combs" he said in a condescending tone.

"Detective Combs, this is a legal issue and I will not provide the requested documents without her permission."

He straightened up and took a deep breath. "I am going to City Hall and report your unreasonable attitude. You should have the report waiting for me when I return."

"Go ahead and report me. But be aware that even if the City Manager or Mayor orders me to give you a copy, I will not give you one until you return that form."

He spun around and stomped from the office, slamming the door behind him. Vickie and I both burst out laughing. "He has seen entirely too many movies," she said.

"I completely agree." Just then my pager sounded. The address was just a block and a half down from my home. It was the Kelly's house. "Officer requests ambulance to 5342 Pine Street." No hint of what was wrong was broadcast and that made me uncomfortable. As first responding EMT, I hurried to my car. The Fire Department Secretary Vickie came with me. She was a new EMT. We were there in record time. As I pulled up in front of the house I noticed three things. The Sunday paper was still lying on the doorstep along with the Monday morning paper. The police officer that stood six feet away from the front door and did not appear to have any intentions of going inside. The third thing was Jill standing just inside the screen door, stake naked.

I walked past the officer and confronted Jill. "Jill, do you remember me? My name is Sharon. . . ." I babbled on in a friendly manner smiling and talking gently. I could see she didn't understand a single word I said but she smiled. I opened the screen door slowly and entered. She moved back still smiling and a blank look on her face. The Saturday newspaper lay beside the chair unread. The phone lay on the floor with the receiver off the hook. The kitchen had milk sitting on the counter no other food in sight. Where was Ken? Jill smiled.

"Vickie, take care of her." I turned and ran down the hall calling out Ken's name. "Ken! Ken!" I was coiled tight and emotionally involved. I knew Ken would never leave her alone and he was in this house somewhere. I was afraid of what I would find but I had to find him. I stormed into their bedroom and stopped. Lying on the floor was Ken. He was on his left side. He was dressed in a white t-shirt and dress pants and socks. The smell of urine was everywhere. He had urinated on himself and the red carpet had died his clothing red. He looked dead. I didn't want him to be dead. He was my friend. I kneeled beside him and touched his neck, searching for a pulse. His eyes popped open. "Ken?" I said as I rolled him over. "It's me, Sharon." I could see that he understood. I could see his eyes filled with a question. I smiled. "Jill's all right."

He closed his eyes in grateful prayer. I did a quick exam. He had suffered an obvious stroke and had laid there for forty eight hours or so unable to move. He must have listened as she wandered from room to room in confused disjointed activity. He must have feared she would hurt herself or wander away without him to care for her. The two days must have been a hell for him. I hooked up the oxygen and turned it up. He tried to smile as I talked to him reassuring him that Jill was well and being cared for. The ambulance was still a few minutes away. "Can you stay with him a minute?" I asked the officer.

"Sure." he answered.

"Ken I'm going to go check Jill." I could see he understood. I went to the dresser and found a pair of flannel pajamas and a pair of slippers for Jill. I carried them back to the living room. Jill was sitting in a chair. Vickie was kneeling beside her talking in a gentle, comforting manner. Jill looked up at me with eyes that for a brief second seemed to form a question.

"Ken has had a stroke. He is alive and we are going to take him to the hospital," I told her while hoping something would make since to her. She smiled again that vacant smile. "Here Vickie get her dressed." I handed the clothing to her. I remembered the proud woman Jill use to be and I wanted to restore some of that dignity by getting her dressed before the entire world descended upon her home.

"F-3, Rescue One?"

I keyed my radio "This is F-3 go ahead."

"We are one block away."

"Good. We have a CVA (stroke) patient. Bring another oxygen bottle mine's about empty." I hurried back to Ken. He lay where I had left him. His color was better. I took his pulse again. He had diminished pulse on his right side. He was dehydrated. His paralysis was pronounced on his right side. His left side wasn't functioning well but then he had laid on that arm and leg for two days and nights. I backed off and let the crew load him onto the stretcher. I walked back into the living room. EMTs Sarah and Vickie were caring for Jill. "Sarah, she has Alzheimers and she probably hasn't had anything to eat or drink for at least forty-eight hours. She may be taking medication and if she is she hasn't had that either. Be sure the hospital knows she's a patient also."

"I will." Sarah turned back to Jill. Compassion for this woman showed in everything Sarah and Vickie did for her. Jill was now dressed and wearing a nice robe. They had combed her hair and slipped on her house shoes. The crew with the stretcher came back up the hall with Ken laying on it. Jill jumped up and when she saw Ken. She let out a little whimper and covered her mouth with her hand. Her frightened eyes stared at Ken. Sarah put her arm around Jill and tried to comfort her. Vickie led Jill over to the stretcher and took her hand and moved it out to touch Ken. Ken smiled a lopsided smile. Jill whimpered again and tears formed in her eyes.

They were both taken to the hospital. The crew left them in the hospital's care. Later after the paperwork was done Sarah decided to go back to the hospital and check on them. She was gone longer than I expected. When she returned she was mad. ". . . .There she sat over an hour later still tied to the wheelchair and sitting in the hall!"

"They hadn't done anything for her?"

"Nothing. Not a thing. They hadn't even looked at her. Well I stormed up to the nurse's station madder than I have been in a long time. I guess I got a little loud. A doctor came up. I explained that Mrs. Kelly was a patient too. He said he hadn't realized she was. I demanded he immediately check her out. He walked with me back down the hall. That poor woman just sat there staring ahead not realizing the great injustice that had been done to her. After checking her out the doctor proclaimed she was slightly dehydrated, but generally she was in good health and not ill or injured."

"Well, what now? You can't leave her sitting in the hall."

"We aren't a nursing home. Can't someone come get her?"

"Their daughter lives in Flagstaff and she can't be here until tomorrow."

"Well I don't know what we can do with her," said the doctor.

"How about putting her in the empty bed in her husband's room?" Sarah suggested.

"Well I suppose in this case we could make an exception." EMTs develop a mother hen attitude toward their patients and they protect them as they would their own family. Sarah didn't trust the hospital and she stayed till Jill had been safely tucked away in bed.

Ken and Jill were taken to Flagstaff and shared a room at a nursing home. Their daughter visited often. Ken regained his ability to walk and speak. But after a second and then third stroke he finally passed away. Jill's body continued to live even though it was now an empty shell. She just existed with no obvious purpose, just waiting to die. Within a year of her husband's death, she was released from her earthly bonds and went to join her beloved husband, Ken. It's hard when your patient is a friend.

WELL, NOBODY'S PERFECT

Page tavern was a hole in the wall, a real dive located down Vista Avenue. It was an old wooden building that needed to be torn down. It sat beside a tree that offered shade to those too drunk to walk or drive home. Deb was the owner and bouncer. She was Anglo, dressed in a flowered mumu and usually had ugly pink rollers in her dyed straw blond hair. She was three-hundred pounds and stood an imposing six foot, one inch. She was as tough as they came. Bikers and brawlers alike would back away if she got involved.

Inside the tavern was small, with only six bar stools at a wobbly wooden bar. The floor was never mopped or swept out so it appeared at first glance to be bare dirt. There were four small tables and some mismatched chairs over in the corner. The one and only bathroom was outside and in the back. Most of the patrons would just urinate on the tree outside rather than go into the disgusting bathroom. I didn't blame them.

Most of the customers were Navajo Indians on disability (because they were alcoholics). Around the third of the month they got their disability checks and headed to the Page Tavern. The check would usually last a couple of weeks and during that time, business boomed.

Page Fire was called to this location often. It was said Deb would continue to serve anyone until they ran out of money and I believed it. She also appeared to seldom check ID. I lost count of the number of FDGB (fall down, go boom) calls. Backwards off the bar stool usually resulted in injury to the back of the head. Fights were common, but by the time we arrived, Deb had forced the fighters outside into the parking lot. Unconscious with or without seizures also occurred more times than I cared to count. It was job security.

I had been an EMT for a while, but had just recently become a driver. I had never driven on a real emergency. I pulled up outside in the parking lot. Most of Deb's customers didn't own a car or had just wrecked it, so there were plenty of parking spots. The man lay face down on the asphalt. The two other EMT's walked over to him and began to examine him. I was met by the victim's "buddy," a well-known alcoholic.

"He drank too much and threw up on Deb. She threw him out." He told me. I had seen Deb throw someone out, usually she would grab them and heave them out the door with great speed and force. They would be launched into space, flaying their arms and legs about, attempting to fly. Their body would make a graceful arch then land unceremoniously in a wadded up heap in the parking lot. From the looks of things, this time was no different. "Did he get up?"

"No, he just laid there."

I looked over and saw the two EMTs had rolled him over and begin CPR. "Damn," I thought. No pulse, no respirations . . . . I hurried over and verified the situation. He had a huge red spot on his forehead where it had struck the pavement, but other than that, no trauma was noticeable. Dr. Edmonds drove up in his red tiger striped Hummer and got out. He was curious. He said we appeared to be doing alright, so he just backed off and watched. During CPR the driver is very busy. I sprang into action. I got the stretcher, backboard and straps. Hurry, hurry, hurry I thought. I got the straps on the backboard and moved it up near the man's side. On the count of three, roll him," I said. They did and I moved the backboard under him. Hurry, hurry, hurry, I told myself. I secured the straps. I was rushing around, moving very quickly. They continued CPR.

We were in the smaller Rescue-One and decided to leave the stretcher behind (the police said they would get it). We loaded the backboard with the man strapped to it onto the floor. One EMT at his head to use the bag valve mask to ventilate him, and the other beside him continued compressions. Hurry, hurry, hurry, I kept thinking. I slammed the doors and hurried around and jumped in. I was about as hyped as a person could get. I put my foot on the break, shifted the automatic into drive and stomped on the gas, spinning tires and leaping forward in a burst of energy. The two EMTs screamed. The EMT at the patient's head flew over the patient crashing into the back door, hitting it just about the time the other EMT landed against him. Then the patient slid feet first toward the back door. He was strapped but apparently not a good as he could have been. His feet dug into the flesh of the two EMTs lying at the back door. The top strap now was at the patient's throat, choking him. I realized my mistake and slammed on the breaks and everything shifted again. Now the two EMTS were lying on top of the patient. He didn't seem to notice.

"I'm sorry guys . . ." It didn't sound like enough. It wasn't.

"What the hell is wrong with you?" yelled the male EMT. He and the female EMT were trying to untangle themselves from the rather awkward position in which they found themselves. They got off the man and worked themselves back in place and resumed CPR.

"Slow it down for Pete sakes!" yelled the female. I looked in my mirror and saw Dr. Edmonds had seen the entire thing. He had had a ring side seat as he stood behind the ambulance and had seen the three people pile up on the back window in a wadded up mess. He looked surprised. I was so ashamed. I let up off the break and slowly accelerated. I was so flustered. I didn't see the car driving down the street. I pulled right out in front of him. He squealed his breaks as he slammed to a stop. I pretended I didn't see and drove on.

At the hospital we unloaded the man and took him into the ER. I didn't mention the trip the poor guy had taken. He didn't seem any worse for wear. He still wasn't breathing.

I walked outside and cleaned the ambulance. Dr. Edmonds drove up along with the police officer. The two of them removed the stretcher and wheeled it over to me. I loaded it into the ambulance. The officer stood there with a smirk on his face. Dr. Edmonds just stood there in his usual somber way. Then he said, "That was interesting." I felt so stupid. The report was done and we returned to service. I got another lecture about my driving. I had to just take it, they were right. I could have killed them. The autopsy showed the alcohol, being roughly removed from the bar and being thrown into the ambulance back door had not caused his death. He had had a massive heart attack and nothing we could have done would have made a difference. I drove the ambulance many other times after that but I never repeated that mistake again. I am a creative person and so I make new and different mistakes, but not this one.

"THE ARSONIST WORE PINK"

       Christmas was only two days away. Maurice had taken off work that day. He, the boys and I were driving to Phoenix to spend the holiday with our family. We were carrying out our luggage when our pagers sounded. I looked at him, he looked at me. During the holidays there is a mass exodus out of Page. Anyone with an out of town family leaves. The PFD was seriously understaffed this time of year. We put the suitcases down and ran for our vehicles. Over my shoulder, I called out to the kids to stay at the house and we would be back in a couple of hours. They understood and walked back into the house. I went directly to the scene and he went to the fire station and responded to the scene on a fire truck.

       The trailer was a double wide, long and burning like a blow torch when I arrived. I had been to a lot of fires and had attended a lot of fire training drills and was cross trained in Fire Command. I had gotten good at second guessing the orders given by command. By this time I had commanded a few house fires. I figured since it was so involved, and we were so short of men, this would be fought from the outside. I was very surprised when Chief Nelson gave the order for the first in team to take search and rescue. Maurice (my husband) and Capt. Keller entered through the back door dragging a hose with them. Timmy Alto stood at the back door (without any protective gear) holding a charged backup line. There should have been two men on the line by the back door in full turnouts, Scott packs and face masks. If something went wrong, the two men would enter with the hose and assist or rescue the two men who were inside. With Wonder Boy standing in street clothes holding a small hose, he wouldn't be much help if something happened. I had a bad feeling about this.

       The front windows were made up of small squares about eight by eight inches. Molding strips framed each pane of glass. Some panes were already cracked from the heat. I stood with a large crowd across the street, directly in front of the trailer. It turned out to be a bad choice. I knew better but to tell the truth I couldn't see the back door from where the ambulance was parked. I wasn't thrilled that the Chief had ordered men into a structure that I didn't think should have firefighters inside. I wanted to see the exit.

       Suddenly the flames leaped and the front windows exploded. It was in slow motion. I saw the glass shatter and the wood molding strips catch fire. They flew through the air toward me, slowly spinning. I was wearing a turnout coat but everything else was civilian attire. I couldn't outrun the flaming debris. I spun around and ducked my head. I felt the pieces hit my back and the back of my legs. I reached up and felt to see if my hair was on fire. It wasn't. I checked my pant legs. No fire. I stomped on a piece of burning wood lying at my feet and moved to the side but I kept my view of the door. Something was wrong. This structure wasn't burning in the normal expected manner. Most house fires progress in a predictable pattern, this wasn't "normal." I began to become very concerned.

Inside the trailer was getting interesting. Maurice had been in many burning structures by this time. He was an experienced firefighter and he knew this structure was burning strangely. They put out the fire down the hall as they traveled toward the living room. The floor was weak and they were concerned about falling through. The fire was big. Maurice wondered what in the world he was doing inside this trailer. It was a complete loss five minutes before they arrived. They were fighting a losing battle.

Maurice's knee slipped on the floor and his arm shot out. Hot coals ran up his sleeve. He turned the nozzle of the fire hose up his sleeve and turned it on. Cool water shot up his arm and cooled his burns. He turned the hose back on the fire. Maurice turned and looked over his shoulder. The flames had erupted again and the hallway was engulfed by flames. Their exit no longer existed. The living room was a complete ball of fire. Maurice pulled on the hose and literately dragged the captain up to him and pointed behind them. They were trapped. I will never forget the way I felt when I heard the radio traffic. It was garbled and hard to understand. "Fire . . . behind.......trapped......"

My heart sunk to the bottom of my feet. I am sure I drained of color. The trailer was completely on fire. Only two small windows on the south side didn't have flames licking out of them. The firefighter, Don Parks, had just driven up in the second engine and had been getting out tools and extra bottles off the engine, tossed an ax on the ground, grabbed two Scott Bottles and cursing as he ran for the trailer. EMT Ken Connors, the ambulance driver was also a firefighter and he was in turnouts but doing EMT duties spun around and ran for the back door. No orders were necessary. They knew what they had to do.

I stood my ground, heart beating at two-hundred beats a minute cool sweaty palms and a ringing in my ears. Maurice was trapped in a burning trailer. My worst nightmare was now a reality. I stared at the side of the trailer, waiting for a helmet to break through the window and let the people on the outside know where the two men were inside. No helmet, no radio traffic.

Inside, Maurice as always was cool under fire. He and the captain were looking around. They saw the dim light of a window near them. He and the captain worked their way to the window. Both had full intentions of exiting through the window (small as it might be).

Ken charged up to the back door and snatched the hose from Timmy's hands, shoved him aside and dove into the open doorway with turnouts on but no air bottle. He opened the hose and water sprayed out. Parks stepped over Timmy who now sat on his butt on the ground. Parks slipped on a tank and took over the hose while Ken put on the Scott pack. No words were spoken, it wasn't necessary, they knew what to do. Two firefighters were inside and the exit was now solid flames. They had to open up the escape route. Together they crawled into the inferno, and started knocking down the fire.

There was no more radio transmission from the trapped men. The men inside knew their fellow fight fighters would be entering with a hose through the back door, and hopefully could knock down the flames in the hallway. Maurice and Keller then saw the flames doused. They abandoned the tiny window exit and worked their way quickly back down the hall. Maurice and Keller crawled toward their fellow firefighters with a vengeance. As Maurice progressed down the hallway, he could feel the floor of the trailer flex. The danger of falling through was serious. To fall through a trailer floor almost always meant injury and the risk of being stuck. Suddenly through the black smoke two firefighters (Connors and Parks) appeared and the four backed out the door.

"F-3 to the back door." That meant someone was hurt. I ran toward the back door of the trailer. I saw the men dressed in full turnouts, backing out the door. I went up to the men and escorted Maurice and Keller back to the ambulance (medical welfare sector). I took Maurice's coat off and his forearm was bright red. I moved away and allowed Lupe (EMT) to put cool water on his burn and bandage him. I turned my attention to Keller. He wasn't injured but he was exhausted. After Keller and Maurice got their second wind, they stood up and returned to work. The trailer soon burned it's self out. I found the owners standing in the crowd. The man was wearing jeans and nothing else. It was a cold December day. I walked up to him just as a neighbor who actually didn't know him brought him some socks, boots and a flannel shirt. I introduced myself to the man and his wife and three year old daughter.   "What happened?" I asked.

"My wife got up and lit the fireplace. She came back and dressed. Our daughter picked up the lighter." Now, this lighter was a long handled lighter that people use to light fireplaces. Some people call them torches because they are butane fueled and shoot a flame out the end. This brand didn't have any safety locks, just push the button and flame shot out the end. "She took it to her room (the first one off the living room) and started to shoot it like a gun. She set fire to the bed the drapes her toy box everything." I pictured this tiny little Angel standing spread legged in her bedroom and firing the flame thrower like a little Rambo-ette.

"My wife walked down the hall and opened the girl's door and saw the whole room on fire. She grabbed the girl and ran to our bedroom and screamed the trailer was on fire. I yelled for her to take the baby and run. I jumped up and slipped on my jeans. I was only a few seconds behind her, but the wall to my daughter's bedroom was burning when she ran by but it had burnt through as I made my way past. I reached the phone in the living room and dialed 911. I gave them the information. I turned around and the living room was on fire. I ran outside as the flames reached the ceiling."

"Is my dolly all burned up?" the little girl asked with wide eyes.

I hesitated. I looked up at the trailer. No way was that doll was anything but a blackened ash. The girl was young, but not stupid. She already knew the answer to the question. "I think so" I said.

"But now I don't have a dolly." her quivering lip stuck out. Tears formed in her eyes.

The mother looked up. "Our Christmas tree and presents are gone too, aren't they?"

"I'm afraid so. I don't think there will be much left." I found the truth was always best.

One wonderful thing that I have seen over and over again, total strangers stepped in and offered to help. This young couple didn't have relatives in the town and a total stranger took them in. Actually two more offered as well. Three hours later I left the scene. I drove immediately to the store. I walked the toy aisle and found a dolly with long blond hair and a pretty dress. I bought a dolly baby bottle and checked out. I drove back down to the fire and found the little girl and gave her the new dolly. She took the doll and squeezed it to her and smiled up at me. I felt good. I didn't tell anyone about this till now with the exception of my husband and the store manager that later donated other toys to the girl. Neighbors came forward and clothes and household items were collected. The insurance bought them another trailer. They began over.

Two other firefighters were injured before the fire was completely extinguished. The floor caved in twice and one fire captain was stuck up to his waist in a smoldering trailer (Tanner). He was pulled back out by two other firefighters. Another firefighter injured his knee as he fell through the weakened floor.

The girl was too young to be held accountable for the fire. I think back on it now and it still bothers me. I still don't know why the chief made the call to send two men into that building when it was too far gone and we were so shorthanded. The chief was usually fairly good at calling fires, but I guess everyone makes a bad call once in a while. A number of people, including myself, all agreed the trailer had burned in a highly unusual manner. It didn't burn in the expected way. It was strange. Later, on investigation it was discovered there were mainly two reasons for it burning in an odd way. The first reason was that trailer had an unusual floor plan that allowed the flames to expand in unexpected ways. Secondly, the fire was actually multiple fires, started in various places by a tiny girl dressed in pink and armed with a small blowtorch.

Maurice, the boys and I left a few hours late and arrived in Phoenix after dark. Maurice's burns healed well, but if you look carefully at that Christmas pictures, you will see the bandages on his forearms. Firefighting is dangerous. My job was also dangerous and Maurice let me do it because he knew I loved it. I knew he loved being a firefighter and I could never ask him to quit, regardless how nervous it might make me when he fearlessly enters the next fire. But from a personal level, fires were a lot more fun before it was my husband crawling through the flames.

HAY, WHAT ABOUT ME?

It sounded bad, and it looked bad as we pulled up. An old Ford pickup had left the main street of town and hit a retaining wall head on. The truck had to have been traveling at least twenty miles over the thirty-five miles per hour speed limit, perhaps more. It was a bright cloudless day, a beautiful eighty degrees in downtown Page, Arizona. We had no way of knowing it was going to be downhill from here on.

My EMT partner got out and hurried to the pickup with me right behind him. I looked around him and saw a woman sitting in the passenger seat. She was about twenty-two years old, pretty and covered in blood. She had not been wearing a seat belt and when the truck hit the wall, her body had lunged forward and her forehead had smashed into the windshield. The skin on her forehead was cut clear to the bone and hung open. Blood poured from the wound, down her face, past her broken nose, past her broken teeth and shredded lips and down her chin and flowed onto a white t-shirt with little brightly colored fish pattern.

My partner backed away and let me in. The woman was moaning and I had the bandaging supplies. He went for the backboard and c-collar. "Hold still, "I asked her as a firefighter moved into the truck from the driver's door. He took her head in his gloved hands and held it still. She had hit the windshield hard and it was possible she might have broken her neck. I quickly bandaged the wound and controlled the bleeding. I began to check her out. She was holding something in her arms. I reached for it thinking it was a blanket. She clutched it to her breast and made it perfectly clear, and she wasn't going to give it up to me.

My partner, the EMT/driver came up behind me just as I moved the blanket and a tiny foot was exposed. It was a baby. She was holding a baby! I tried to get my hands on the baby, but she moaned and pulled away. The baby was tightly clutched to her body. I moved the blanket, working around the semi-conscious mother's refusal to let go of her baby. The baby was dead, very dead. It was obvious that no amount of CPR or advanced life support was going to save this tiny baby. The unrestrained mother had been holding her infant in her arms and when the truck crashed her and the baby went forward. She crushed the baby into the dashboard with the weight of her body. "963," (deceased) I said quietly to my EMT partners. I estimated the baby to be about three months old.

The EMT/driver, backed away and backed into the driver of the pickup, the baby's father. He turned around and faced the man. Both men were tall and about the same size and age. The most striking difference was the fact that the EMT was cold sober, and the man was about as drunk as a person could be and still stand upright.

"Hay, man, what about me?" the drunk asked. He had a tiny cut over his eye with no other noticeable injuries.

"You son-of-a-bitch." My partner had just lost it. "You just killed your baby and maybe your wife and you want me to give you a band aid?" His voice rose in righteous anger. The police officer stepped between the men.

"Back off," the officer said. The EMT's fists were clinched at his side and his face was red with anger.

I tried to ignore the drama taking place behind me. The baby was dead. I could do nothing about that. I decided to not make a big deal about it. I just continued to care for the woman. Together with an off duty EMT and a firefighter we managed to get a c-collar on her neck and back boarded the woman, still clutching her dead baby to her body. She wasn't completely conscious and thankfully didn't really understand what was happening, but her basic motherly instinct was still functioning and she wasn't about to let go of the tiny infant in her arms. When we were ready to move her to the stretcher and I looked around for the driver. He was nowhere in sight. The officer was putting the cuffed driver into the patrol car. I turned to the other officer and asked, "Where's my driver?"

"He's sitting in the ambulance." The look on his face told me to let it go. I didn't quite understand what had happened, but whatever we were going to do, it would be without him. The officer offered to help and the four of us moved the woman, now strapped to a backboard, onto the stretcher and moved her to the ambulance. I had asked about the driver of the pickup and was told he wasn't hurt and was "going to jail."

I had my hands full with the woman. She wasn't doing well and as I took another set of vital signs I began to worry. The ambulance lunched forward and we were off. I continued care for her. She was put on high flow oxygen, and a set of vital signs were taken. The wound on her forehead had bled through and I added another layer of 4x 4's. I ignored the tiny bundle in her arms. It wasn't that long ago my youngest son was that small and helpless. I know the woman should have been wearing a seatbelt. I know the baby should have been in a car seat, I know the sober woman should have never got in the car with her drunken husband, but still, I felt a sense of sadness. I knew she would probably live and in a few hours she would ask someone about her baby and then she would receive the most horrible news a person could ever hear.

We reached the hospital quickly since it was only a few blocks away. The driver jumped from the driver's seat and opened the back doors. He unloaded the stretcher and we hurried into the ER. I had not had a chance to warn the staff about the baby and the doctor glared at me when he realized I had transported a dead baby into his ER. That was a no-no to beat all no-no's. As two nurses pounced on the seriously injured woman, the doctor grabbed my arm and dragged me away.

"What the hell did you think you were doing? The baby's dead!" He was mad.

"I know that. She wouldn't let it go and I wasn't going to participate in a tug of war on the main street with two-hundred people watching me wrestle the dead baby from her arms. You do it." I walked away.

After the call we all sat down and vented. It's called "defusing". The EMT/driver was still mad but had calmed down. In all my years working with him I had never seen him loose it before. We are all human and understood. He said what we were all thinking about the drunken man. He will wake up in jail and not remember how he got there or why he's there. There will be a threat of a trial and then a plea bargain. He will get a few years in prison for vehicular manslaughter. His wife recovered. I wonder if she was waiting for him when he was released from prison.

I'M GOING TO KILL HIM!

One of the challenges of being a volunteer EMT is the "on call" element. An EMT may wear the pager on their belt, waiting for it to go off while at work or at home. To stop whatever you are doing and leave immediately isn't always as easy as it may sound. The EMT may be in the middle of cooking a meal for their family, in the shower or in the middle of disciplining their teenager. They must be organized and have their shoes, jumpsuit (or uniform), and car keys handy.

Genie Slater was a small woman, perhaps a hundred pounds of sexy, aggressive, femininity. She had a fiery temper and sometimes it got the best of her. One day, her pager went off. She grabbed her jump suit, shoes and car keys and ran through the kitchen door into the garage. "Shit!" she yelled. Her car sat up on blocks, both front tires were off. She forgot her husband was repairing it and had left to get some parts. She rushed, in complete panic, through the garage hoping he was in sight, either coming or going. The garage door didn't work and her husband had sealed the garage with a thick, clear plastic. She tore a hole through the plastic when she burst through it like "superwoman" and rushed into the driveway and looked both ways. Her husband was nowhere to be seen. "I have got to get to the fire station," she said out loud. "Damn him!" Genie was raging mad as she stood in her driveway without transportation. The minutes were ticking off and she was several blocks from the fire station. There was no way she could run and make it. "There has to be another way," she thought.

A pickup with two elderly Navajos was slowly driving down the street. Genie rushed out into the road and waved them down. They stopped. She didn't explain, she just threw open the door and yelled. "Move over." The startled Navajo woman did and Genie got in. The Navajo man looked over at her with confusion. Genie looked at them. "Well, get going. Take me to the fire station." She bent down and started to put on her shoes. The man put his pickup in gear and they were off.

In the traditional Navajo culture, if someone needs something, you are obligated to provide what they need, if you can. This strange, unknown Anglo woman had made it clear she need a ride, so although surprised, they respectfully provided her a ride. They were somewhat uncomfortable with the fact that they didn't know her and she was white. They were elderly traditional Navajos living on the reservation and seldom had contact with Anglos. They grew more uncomfortable as she loudly expressed her anger at her husband putting her in this situation. "I'll kill him, so help me he's a dead man! They didn't know anything about what had happened and her anger frightened the gentle elderly couple.

"I'll kill him, so help me I'll kill him....." she was mumbling. She then turned and saw the two strangers peering over at her with growing fear. "Damn, now they think I'm a crazy woman," she thought. They pulled up at the fire station and she jumped out. "Thanks," she said as she slammed the door and ran into the station. The elderly couple continued on their journey with a story to tell about the crazy white woman who commandeered their truck and may have killed her husband. No, her husband didn't die but he was punished.

JASON & FRIDAY the THIRTEENTH

"It's Friday the thirteenth and Jason is back," the young boy said.

"Oh shut up. I think you have your movies all mixed up," his mother jokingly said. She was Susan Eldon, an EMT and her son was teasing her about her coming duty shift on Friday the 13th.

At the Fire Station she mentioned the comments of her son, and every one took up the chant. For days we joked about the coming Friday. Maurice, my husband, Susan, and Patrick Simpson were on duty. All of them had had a week of teasing and Jason comments. Jason and Michal Myers were insane mass murders. They wore hockey masks and chopped up people in the movies, just in case you have missed the two movies (Friday the 13th and Halloween) and the ten sequels.

That night, very late, the pagers went off. I was on an airport transport that evening. A patient was being flown to Phoenix. We picked up the air crew at the airport, transported them to the hospital. They were in the process of evaluating the patient. We stood around and waited. When they were finished, we would transport the crew and patient to the airport for the flight. I heard the page go out and listened to radio traffic as my husband, who was now an EMT, and his two partners responded to the 911 call. The three reported to the Page Boy Motel. They hurried to the room where a man was reported hurt. No other information was available.

The hotel had outside walkways leading to the rooms. The crew, with equipment in hand ran upstairs and stopped in front of the room. The door had a glass window. Bloody finger prints streaked the window from the inside. The thin cotton curtain blocked the view into the room. The door was locked. All three thought, Well, Jason is back and he's mad. It's funny how all three had a different point of view. Susan was standing in front of the door, a bad place to be if guns were being used. She was

315

thinking, "If I could just get this door unlocked I could help that poor man inside."

Maurice, a firefighter, was thinking, "If she would just move, I could kick the door down."

Patrick, a more experienced EMT was looking up and down the motel complex thinking "Where's a cop when you need one." He used his radio to request police. The officer arrived and the door was opened by the manager.

The room had been trashed. There had been a party. The floor was so deep in beer cans, wine bottles and whiskey bottles that it was hard to walk. The EMTs had to kick aside cans and bottles searching for the floor that was completely covered. Then they saw him. A man lay sprawled in the floor. His face was a bloody mess. Susan went to him while the men searched for Jason. He had left. The young man, age twenty-two had been hit in the face with a beer bottle. The jagged glass had cut his face and eye. The patient was covered in blood. The carpet was soggy and squished when walked upon. His blood loss was great. He was put on oxygen and his face and eye was bandaged. Very quickly he was back boarded and loaded on the stretcher. He was moved to the ambulance quickly and transported code-three. Whatever care he received, it was given en route. He lived, but later lost his eye after a valiant attempt to save it failed.

Two months later I went on a call to the same room. There had been another party. When I entered the room it was as if history was being repeated. The room was littered with beer cans and whiskey bottles just as my husband had described the last 911 call to this room. I cautiously searched the room and then I saw two feet sticking out into view. I slowly walked over and looked down. A man in his mid-twenties was wedged between the double bed and the wall. He was lying on his back. He was dressed in jeans, t-shirt and work boots. The man was known to me. He was the older brother of the man who had lost his eye in this same room two months ago.

It's dangerous to kneel down beside a man who might wake up and grab you by the throat, so I kicked the bottom of his foot and called out, "Are you alright?" He didn't move. My partner stood nearby while I stepped around the man and reached his neck. I felt for a pulse. There wasn't one. I noticed he was cold to the touch. I lifted his arm and on the underside there was lividity. The blood had pooled. He had been dead for a number of hours. We called the police and turned the call over to them. The investigation showed no foul play. The young man had died of acute alcohol poisoning. He had drunk so much alcohol that he passed out and stopped breathing. It appeared that the others at the party didn't notice he wasn't breathing for a long time and when they did, they called 911 and ran away. Jason was never found.

TOTAL EVISCERATION

Out of the many calls I went to as an EMT, a few stand out in my mind. The one involving a man named Ray Farmer is one I will never forget. I was packing to leave for Phoenix. I was running late as usual. My pager sounded with a report of a car accident down by the golf course on Tunnel Road. This was odd. It was a dirt road used as access to the golf course and the tunnel. The golf course entrance was only a city block down the road. Then a guard hut stopped all but authorized workers from a construction firm that was doing a large renovation of the tunnel that led through the sandstone cliffs to the base of the Glen Canyon Dam.

I stopped what I was doing and hurried out to my car. "F-3, 76" (en route to the scene) I called into my portable radio. I lived very close to the area and knew I would beat everyone there. I drove quickly and ignored the guard that made a feeble attempt to stop me. I just drove on through. I couldn't see an accident, but off to the left I could see a small crowd and several vehicles. The area was perhaps three-hundred yards off the road to the south. Car accident? I didn't think so. I radioed the correct location of the incident, whatever it was and drove my van as close as I could, then I got out and walked. I saw a man running up to me. He was very excited. His eyes were wide, showing a lot of the white. His spoke with an excited elevated tone. "Before you go up there," he said as he approached me, "You need to know, his . . . . guts are hanging out." I shook my head in understanding, thanked him and continued on. He trotted along beside me, taking my first aid kit to lighten my load.

The day was overcast and it had rained earlier that day. The terrain was rough. The desert was spotted with smooth boulders, half buried, flat sandstone rocks and desert bushes. The closer I got the more confused I was. The two vehicles I could see looked fine. What had happened here? I couldn't imagine that this was a car accident.

There were perhaps a dozen men standing around a man lying on his back in the sand. The man was wearing a heavy yellow rain jacket, jeans, t-shirt, belt and boots. He was of average height and weight. He appeared to be around thirty-five years of age and had hair that was slightly reddish in color. He was moaning and moving his head about. His eyes were open but they weren't focusing on anyone or anything. He was

317

confused and frightened.

I stood for a few seconds looking him over. The man was right, his guts were hanging out. A large deep gash went from under his arm pit and down his side to the belt. "So that's what a lung looks like" I thought as I saw a small gray organ inflate and deflate. As he lay on his back, his arms were flung outward and his yellow raincoat laid spread out on the sand. His intestines where spilled out on the inside of his rain coat. Thank goodness they weren't in the sand. He appeared to have been field dressed. Car accident? No, something else had happened here.

I knelled down. "What happened?" I asked as I put oxygen on him and turned it up all the way. Twelve men started to talk at once. The victim and another man had come down to burn some trash from the construction site. Unknown to them, when they stuffed the trash in the fifty-five gallon barrel, somewhere in the mess were some blasting caps and a roll of detonation cord. The two men stood around watching the trash burn. Suddenly the barrel blew up. The metal that formed the barrel became shrapnel flying in the air. A large chunk hit Ray and cut him open from up under his arm down to his belt. The other man wasn't hurt. He ran for help. I heard the ambulance go 10-8. I picked up my radio.

I hesitated. How could I describe the magnitude of this man's injuries? The medical term for intestines protruding is an evisceration, but this was more than a "loop" of intestines protruding from a wound. I didn't want to be too graphic, but they had to be prepared. I keyed the mike, "I have an adult male that was involved in an explosion. He has a TOTAL EVISRATION. This is a mast suit, O2, backboard, load and go."

"Rescue-two copies." Later I was told that the way I have emphasized *total evisceration*, had gotten the point across and the image that flashed before their eyes was exactly what they found when they arrived.

A sheriff arrived and asked what he could do. I handed him the scissors and told him to cut the man's cloths off. I took another pair and started on his shirt. The man was growing visibly weaker. His buddy talked to him but he didn't seem to hear. He was dying. I knew his chances were very slim. With an evisceration, a patient has less than a fifty-fifty chance and that is if they are injured within five minutes of a trauma center. The nearest trauma center was two-hundred and thirty miles away. We cut the clothes off, but left the rain coat on. I examined him and found several other deep cuts to his upper chest, but nothing that appeared to be serious. I looked up as a park ranger arrived. Usually they are more of a hindrance than a help but this time I welcomed any help I could get. Technically, this was NPS territory and he was in charge but he appeared more interested in the team work approach. I moved to get a blood pressure as he checked his eyes with a pen light.

The ambulance pulled up and the EMT's jumped out, each carrying several pieces of equipment before it stopped rolling. I pumped the cuff up to one hundred, I doubted it would be much higher and got a weak sound around sixty. Surly that couldn't be the systolic. This man was still moaning and mumbling. Normal pressure for a man such as him would be around one-hundred, thirty over sixty. I pumped again only up to one-hundred again and listened carefully. It was hard to hear because everyone was talking and moving around. "Quit!" I ordered and silence descended on the scene. All eyes were on me as I stared at the needle, watching it drop. Again, only a faint weak sound at sixty. I took the stethoscope out of my ears and looked up. "I got sixty over zip. (translated to mean, I couldn't hear the diastolic aka bottom number).

"Shit," someone commented.

"Get me the MAST suit," ordered the ranger.

"Can we put a MAST suit on with the open abdominal injuries?" I quietly ask the ranger.

"What do we have to lose? It can't hurt, not at this point. And we have to package him for transport."

I agreed. O'Riley was an inexperienced EMT. He and I started to put the inflatable trousers on our patient. I looked into O'Riley's eyes and could read his thoughts. This was the first time he had ever been called to do something this important. He looked worried. "Don't sweat it, we did this in drill just three days ago, remember?"

He smiled and new confidence took hold. "Yeah, we did." He started to work connecting up the hoses. I set up the rest. I looked up at the ranger. We were not to put protruding organs back in, but to move this man would require just that. He read my thoughts. "We'll just use the MAST suit to kind of hold it all in one place," he said. I agreed with him however unorthodox it seemed. We had about six to seven feet of intestines to package for transport.

The three of us put the MAST suit under him. I reached across and touched the intestines. They were slimy and gray. I tried not to think about what I was doing as I scooped them up and tried to pile them on the man's abdomen, but they slipped off and fell to the rain coat again. I wet them down and took sterile dressings that wouldn't stick to the intestines and lay them on top of the pile. I didn't have near enough bandages. Finally we decided we had little choice, we gently wadded the intestines up and we soaked the big abdominal trauma dressing in normal saline we had available and placed the dressings on top. We then wrapped the MAST suit around and fastened the Velcro. There was very little blood at the scene so we pumped the legs up a little. We then pumped the abdomen up,

319

ever so slightly, just enough to hold the organs in place. The man was quickly loaded and the ambulance speeded off. I stood watching them leave. He wasn't going to make it. I was surprised we got him loaded still breathing.

I took a deep breath and called the hospital. "We have a level one trauma three minutes from your back door. There was an explosion. He has a complete evisceration, sixty systolic. MAST suit lightly in place, with high flow oxygen." At the hospital, they knew me well and trusted my reports. The nurse signed off quickly and made two quick phone call and one paged announcement. The entire staff including the cleaning lady met the ambulance. All available doctors in town came. Two ran from their office across the field and arrived at the same time the ambulance slid into the parking lot.

Back at the scene, I tried to look it over and see exactly what happened. I had not realized how much this call had affected me till I noticed my hands were shaking. I looked out in the desert. Not five feet from me lay a large chunk of rusted metal. It was roughly the size of a dinner plate but shaped like a triangle. Shreds of flesh and blood hung from the sinister looking piece of shrapnel.

"That's what did it," I said to the park ranger.

"Yeah. Talk about being in the wrong place at the wrong time. Come on," The ranger picked up my jump kit and I carried my oxygen bottle and suction unit. We walked in silence to our cars.

"Thanks for your help."

He smiled, "No problem. Now I have to go back and hash out whose jurisdiction this is. It's a bit in the gray area." He opened his door and took out a clip board. I left the scene.

I could have driven off, finished packing and left town. But I had to see this through to the end. I drove to the hospital. As I walked into the emergency room entrance, I was surprised to find he was still alive. The tiny room was full of people. The EMTs, nurses, the doctors, and several people I didn't even know. I stepped into the room and the smell of sticky blood assaulted me. Blood was everywhere it pooled on the floor at the doctor's feet. They were having problems and slipped more than once. I left and found a large amount of towels. I slipped into the room and scattered them about. They absorbed the blood and gave some traction for those working on the man.

The victim had an IV running in almost every available spot in his body. Several of the plastic IV bags had blood pressure cuffs around them to force the blood into him faster. Dr. Edmonds drew short straw and worked to clean the intestines and reattach them inside. He worked in a sterile field and tried to maintain sterile conditions, but he was in a

320

crowded ER room, not a surgical suite. This was basic life and death battle and no one in the room expected to win.

Air Evac from Phoenix was called. DPS sent a unit to Utah to meet a Kane County Highway Patrol Officer who was speeding code-three toward Page with more blood. I helped the respiratory therapy bag the man while she hurried off to get something. He looked horrible. His eyes were shut now and he didn't move. I stood at his head, depressing the bag every three seconds. We were trying to hyperventilate him. He still looked gray. The respiratory therapists came back and took over. I moved down and helped a nurse start another IV in his foot.

"What's his pulse?" asked the doctor. I took it at the femoral artery, and gave him the bad news. It was obvious that the man was in deep shock and we were losing him. I ran out of things to do, and I left the room. I was just in the way. I stood outside the open door and became the go-fer. Then I noticed a man sitting in the hallway in a wheelchair. He held his head in his hands as he leaned forward. A man stood beside him, his hand on his shoulder.

"Is he hurt?" I asked the man standing beside him. He shook his head "no" and motioned me aside.

"He's the man's buddy. They were both down there. He thinks he killed his friend because he didn't check the stuff well enough before they burned it. He disappeared and I found him at his trailer. He's hurtin'."

I went to the man and kneeled on the floor in front of him. I questioned him a little and was convinced he wasn't injured. He looked up at me with eyes that radiated pain and guilt. "Ray? How's Ray?"

I choose my words carefully. "He's been seriously injured. He's still alive and the doctors are preparing him for transfer to a Phoenix Trauma Center." I couldn't lie. He had seen his friend and he knew it was bad. I just tried to stick to the facts but not go into any detail. "There is a better place we can wait. I'll show you." He stood up and walked back the waiting room/chapel with me on one side and his friend on the other. He sat down on the couch.

The man looked up, "Ray's from Showlow. He's got a wife and three kids......" His voice trailed off and he buried his head in his hands again. I left him with his friend.

Ray was tough and a fighter. He seemed to rally. The Air Evac crew arrived and Helen, a flight nurse took charge. Soon he was loaded in the ambulance. Everyone felt relieved to turn over the responsibility to someone else. Complete fatigue set in as the adrenalin rush left our bodies. A nurse and the cleaning woman remained in the ER and started to clean up the blood. It had actually flowed out into the hallway.

I went and told his friends and left. As I was getting in my car, I heard radio traffic that caused me to freeze. "CPR in progress, Rescue-One's 76 to the hospital."

"Damn!" I said as I turned and hurried back into the hospital. I found the staff in the lunch room. "He's coded, they're doing CPR and on their way back." With a great deal of cussing and complaining, everyone sprung to action. They ran down the hallway and frantically started to prepare the already wrecked ER for his arrival.

The ambulance pulled up and in a matter of seconds. Ray was back in the ER. Again they did battle. I took a turn at chest compressions because the crew was tired. It was an inspiring site to watch everyone work together giving a hundred percent. An EMT took over compressions and I helped here and there and went for more supplies. Heart beat was restored. had apparently been nicked in the initial explosions and the small tear grew larger and finally he just bled out into the chest cavity. CPR was useless. He had no more blood to move around his body.
Dr. Kern called the code (ordered that the crew stop CPR and declared the man dead). The EMTs stopped CPR. The flight nurses sat down and looked at the man that so valiantly struggled to live. Dr. Kern actually wiped away a tear.

I heard a radio massage that told everything. "Rescue-One, 76 to the hospital, will you call them and have someone meet us with a key." The key was to the morgue. Ray Farmer was dead.

THE WRONG ADDRESS

I was sitting in an empty classroom with my son's teacher. I hated parent/teacher conferences. The teachers had that knack of pouncing on some insignificant thing and nitpick it to death. If there was a learning issue, they never took the blame. Somehow it was always the child's or the parents fault. I wasn't responsible for teaching my son math. I paid the teacher to do it. I helped with the homework when needed. I did my part. If the child is having a problem learning, it's the teacher's inability to give my child what he needs to learn math, not mine. With my attitude I am certain the teachers hated the conferences as much as I did.

My pager sounded, "Man not breathing....." I looked up at the teacher. Her face was full of surprise. Her eyes were wide and she appeared speechless (at last). "I'm sorry. I'm on duty, I have to go." I got up and hurried from the room. Saved by the pager! I was Rescue Chief and had my own vehicle. I usually responded first and took care of the situation until the ambulance arrived. I rushed to the scene.

I pulled into the residential street lined with doublewide trailers. "832" was the address. Most trailers didn't have a number, some did but they often were out of order. The problem with trailers is that they are mobile and therefore move around sometimes. I noticed the fire chief's car parked in front of a blue and white trailer. I parked behind his car and leaped out with jump kit in hand. I hurried up the stairs. The front door was standing wide open so I ran in and came to a sudden stop.

On the couch watching television was a "thirty-something" man and a woman. On the floor were two kids of middle school age. All four looked up at me with a strange, surprised look on their face. "Did you call for an ambulance?" I asked. All four shook their heads "no." "Sorry" I then realized that I had the wrong house. I turned and left the house. I could feel their eyes follow me as I hurried away, hoping no one else saw me barge into the wrong house.

I reached the street as an officer pulled up. He rushed into the trailer next door. That seemed a good sign so I followed. As I walked past the car in the drive way I looked in. There were about fifty small "TB" syringes. They lay scattered about the passenger seat and on the floor. Stuck in the seat was a syringe with a needle and a tourniquet lay on the dashboard. It didn't take a genius to know what was going on. Respiratory depression due to drug overdose, most likely heroin. There were few heroin overdoses in Page, but when I had gone to paramedic school in Phoenix I got to see a lot of them. I rushed into the trailer. The patient was a male about twenty-eight years old, tall and reasonably attractive. His long brown hair hung about his face and gave him a certain "bad boy" look. He was dressed in jeans and a white t-shirt. He was sitting at the kitchen table, swaying back and forth and would have fallen off the chair if the pretty woman standing beside him hadn't held him in the chair. The officer and fire chief were trying to get oxygen on the man.

"What happened?"

"I don't know." She looked about nervously.

There wasn't time to play games. "Look, I saw the syringes in the car and the tourniquet when I came up the driveway. What did he take?" The police officer looked up at me surprised. Guess he had missed it.

"He's trying to quit." She looked down at her feet. "He wanted me to go get him some needles, I said no. He went and got some."

"What did he take?" I asked again.

"Heroin."

I looked up and through the window I saw the ambulance drive up. I got on the radio, "Don, just bring the stretcher." He was breathing on

▶ Confessions of a Paramedic

his own and we had him on oxygen." I had decided to not give him Narcan to reverse the Heroin at this time. Most addicts don't appreciate coming back to the real world so abruptly. Often they became violent. Since he was somewhat awake, breathing and the hospital is only a few minutes away, I wanted the crew to concentrated on maintain his airway and respirations. I turned him over to the crew's capable hands. I told them I thought he would be alright for the transport but warned them to be prepared for full respiratory arrest just in case I was wrong. They made it with two minutes to spare. He stopped breathing in the ER.

The officer and I walked outside the house. He looked at me, "Now show me the syringes." We stopped beside the car.

"There," I said indicating the entire front seat of the car. "He was hurting so bad he didn't wait to get in the house. He took a hit here in the car. See the syringe impaled in the seat? It must have been the good stuff or we wouldn't have been called." Heroin comes in many different strengths and seldom does the user know the potenticy of the drug until they shoot it up. This leads to a lot of respiratory suppression and deaths.

"Where did he get these many syringes?" he asked.

"I don't know, ask the woman." He shook his head and went back inside. Someone selling Heroin and/or syringes and needles was about to have a bad day.

DON'T CARE TOO MUCH

I will never forget Mildred. She changed my life. I first met her when her husband was ill. They lived in a trailer park. She reminded me (physically) of my own mother, thin, hair that once had been black and now mostly gray and blue eyes that showed an intelligent mind. The crew loaded her husband into the ambulance and headed off to the hospital. The husband wasn't dying and she said she would come to the hospital in the morning. It was about one o'clock in the morning.

I was just leaving when she had an acute asthma attack. I found her inhailer (medicine) and put her on her husband's oxygen. She improved. She then asked me to stay for coffee. I was tired and sleepy, but I stayed. Her husband was blind. So was my father. She told of the problems of living with a blind husband. She told me her dream of seeing Hawaii. She wanted so bad to go, but he said he couldn't see so why go. She wouldn't go without him and he didn't suggest she do so. She had had cancer four years before but seemed all right now.

As I sipped the warm coffee, I noticed the smell of gas in the trailer. I called F-2 (the Assistant Fire Chief) to come check it. It was a leak in her heater and he turned it off. She said she would have it repaired the next day. We all went home. I only got a few hours sleep before the alarm sounded the next morning.

Over the next year, I would go off and on to that house. I liked Mildred. She was such a smart, soft spoken woman. She told me she had been a nurse in a mental ward. She talked of her patients with real love and caring. Her husband beamed with pride of how good a nurse she had been. She showed me her embroidery. It was beautiful.

Then we started to get calls on her. Her cancer was back in her lungs. Her husband passed away and Mildred fought the battle alone. Her daughter wanted her to stay with her in Cottonwood, but Mildred wanted to stay in her own home. I watched the woman die a tiny piece at a time. I hated to see her suffer. I would be called and she would be unable to breath. I would put her on oxygen and talk her into calming down. She would relax and soon she could breathe again. We would take her in and after a day or two, she could go home again. And in a couple of weeks, we would be called again.

One day she looked up at me with the kindest eyes and softly said, "Dear, don't care too much. It hurts. You do know I am going to die, don't you?" Yes I knew and I did care too much, but it was too late to change now. She died one cold snowy night in the Page Hospital with her daughter at her side. She never got to see Hawaii. One simple dream, within her reach and she never saw it fulfilled. Life is not fair.

In 1990 I visited Hawaii. I couldn't stop thinking about Mildred. As I looked over the green velvet hills with primeval foliage and the magnificent Pacific Ocean beyond, I thought of how much she would have loved to see this. I didn't feel sadness though. I realized that my friend would have only felt happiness that her words had helped me see that if you want to do something bad enough, do it. Do it before it's too late. I loved Hawaii and would like to think that somehow she got to finally see Hawaii through the eyes of her friend.

NATIONAL PARK ~~SERVICE~~ CIRCUS

Team work is essential at an emergency scene. Inter-agency cooperation is important. This story illustrates one particularly awkward call were PFD was to interface with NPS on a serious emergency where team work went down the tube. I swear I am not exaggerating the following story. A real slap-stick performance, similar to a Charlie Chaplin Movie happened at the main launch ramp at Lake Powell on a warm summer morning. Lots of visitors to the lake were crowded at the main launch ramp, all trying to get their boats in the water. One man, about sixty-six years of age, sat down on his trucks bumper and began to rub his chest and left arm. He grew sweaty and pale. His breathing became labored.

"Are you alright, George?" his wife of forty-four years asked. No, he wasn't alright. George was having a heart attack. She called for help.

Now, at this time, the *park*, as the rangers referred to it, didn't have an ambulance, but they had a medic who I will call *Ranger X*. Ranger X strutted around with a "god complex." He was the kind of man nature never intended to have any power, wear a badge and certainly never carry a gun. Little did I realize three of the PFD EMTs would be staring down the barrel of his gun in a few months. He was not suited for such endeavors, but unfortunately, life had a sense of humor and he was now a paramedic, wearing a federal park ranger uniform, with a badge and gun. Many of the rangers have the same complex, but Ranger X was on a power trip to beat all power trips.

Page Ambulance responded to the scene and arrived to find Ranger X leaning over an overweight, retirement aged man and seven other rangers watching him. The man looked unconscious. I walked over and commented, "Where's your monitor and drug box?" I was planning on going and getting it out of his patrol car. "I was at a meeting and I forgot it." Ranger X said. Now, for the record, without a monitor, defibulator and drug box, a paramedic becomes a basic EMT, just like me (at the time). I bent down as Ranger X struggled to get a blood pressure. It was his third try. I felt the patient's carotid artery, and didn't find a pulse. "There's no pulse." Ranger X looked up at me surprised? (Now we know why he couldn't get a blood pressure, there wasn't one.)

"Begin CPR" I said as I started chest compressions and another EMT started to bag the man. Now, CPR isn't hard to do. You actually have to make few decisions, just to begin or stop. Follow the steps and it's easy, but I was to learn that if the NPS is involved, it can become a comedy of errors. Everything started to happen at once. There were eight EMT rangers there. They too, had been at the meeting attended by Ranger X. It was their area, but we were the ambulance company and since Ranger X was a "basic" today, it should have been our patient. At least without his drug box he couldn't repeat his performance of two weeks before when he was so hyper that instead of just gently pushing the plunger of a syringe to remove the air, he shoved the entire plunger in and Epi squirted all over a

326

bus while the man having the heart attack in the resort parking lot suffered the delay without lifesaving drugs while he got another syringe of Epi.

Now, Park Circus jumped into "action". They all began to run about in circles, everyone talking at once, everyone giving orders. There is an old saying that applied; we had "too many chiefs and not enough Indians." My crew and I were doing CPR. A number of rangers ran to the ambulance to get the stretcher. It went downhill from there. They pushed the stretcher up to the patient and ran over his fingers. Putting the man on a backboard is simple, roll him over, slip the backboard under him, and roll him back on. Strap him to the board, load on the stretcher wheel to ambulance and load patient. How I wish it had been that simple. I got tired and a ranger took over compressions. My partner was bagging the patient. With everyone yelling orders and no one was listening. It was awful. We stumbled over each other, tripped on the straps that Park Service had decided to not use, bumped into each other, and the team doing CPR just pumped on, trying to not miss too many beats.

We started rolling him to the ambulance, stumbling over each other. I hollered and insisted they stop and let me strap the man down. They reluctantly stopped long enough for me to snap the buckles. The exodus to the ambulance continued like a silent movie with Charlie Chaplin scurrying about. It got so bad, my crew and I just backed off and let the horde of rangers handle it. At the back door of the ambulance, all the rangers let go of the stretcher and climbed into the ambulance. The stretcher started to roll down the boat ramp. I and the other EMTs stood in shock for a second looking at our patient start down the ramp. I started running and so did the other EMTs. If we didn't catch him, he would be launched into Lake Powell, still strapped to our stretcher and he would sink like a rock.

I ran my little heart out, pumping my short legs with vigor I didn't know I had. We caught him a few feet from water's edge. It was frightening. We started CPR again and began working our way up the ramp to the ambulance again. We loaded him inside. All the rangers got inside all eight of them. There wasn't room for me. By this time I wanted nothing to do with this mess so I just got up front in the passenger seat and we drove to the hospital. All the way there, all eight rangers continued to shout orders and no one listened.

At the hospital, I got out slowly and the rangers exploded out the back and while running over each other feet with the wheels of the gurney as they rolled him into the ER, all yelling at once. I slowly walked into the ER and stood by the door watching. A nurse walked up to me. She asked what was happening. I told her "Just look . . . it's a joke. They almost launched him stretcher and all into the lake. I want no part of this." She went to assist the doctor that stood trying to listen to eight people all giving him a report at the same time. The man died.

MY SON STABBED ME

Domestic violence isn't always between two adults. They are not always married, living together or dating. Around five-thirty in the afternoon, Page Fire received a request for an ambulance. It was a "reported stabbing," at Seiko's Trailer Court. The trailer court was old and run down. By this time it was old and run down. It had been there since the early construction days of Page. When the community changed from a construction camp to an incorporated city, the park was "grandfathered in" and wasn't required to upgrade. There were no actual roads, just packed dirt with a layer of dust on top. There didn't appear to be any rhyme or reason of trailer placement; it appeared as if a giant had taken a handful of trailers and tossed them about. The trailers were old and poorly maintained and most were rentals. Junk and trash lay about and children ran barefooted everywhere.

I was on my way home from the PFD Office when the announcement was broadcast over the radio. I picked up my radio, "F-3 is 76," (Rescue Chief is en route to the location). I turned the car around and within three minutes I pulled into the trailer court. I slowed down and creped through the unorganized maze of homes. Children darted here and there. Two five year olds ran out from behind a rusty parked car making me stop as they ran in front of my car.

I noticed flashing code lights to my right and headed that way. I stopped in back of the patrol car. "F-3 is 97," (Rescue Chief is has arrived at the location.) I got out and grabbed my jump kit as the officer inside the forty-two foot green trailer came to the door and motioned me inside. Usually I am very cautious when entering a stabbing incident, but the police officer had motioned me inside and I erroneously assumed the scene was safe. I later wished I had directly asked him about scene safety.

I entered and immediately to my right was the living area. I could see a woman in her early thirties lying on a couch, on her back. She had her forearm raised to her forehead. I could see she was breathing and conscious. She was wearing a t-shirt and jeans. My eyes moved to her right thigh area that was covered with bright red blood. I moved to her side and knelt down. "I'm an EMT with the Page Fire Department, can I help you?" Permission to touch the patient has to be obtained.

She opened her eyes and said to me, "Yes."

I quickly dug into my jump kit and withdrew my scissors. "I have to cut your jeans." She nodded permission. As I cut a wide circle around the entry point. This was a crime scene and I didn't dare cut through the slit in her jeans made by the knife. I continued to ask her questions. "What happened?"

"I was sleeping and I felt pain in my leg and I woke up. My son was standing over me with that steak knife." She pointed to a knife lying near the doorway.

"What's he wearing, how old is he?" asked the officer.

She appeared to be short of breath when she answered "sixteen and wearing a red t-shirt......"

She closed her eyes. I took a hand full of four-by-fours and applied pressure to the wound. I got the bleeding slowed down, but I couldn't stop it.

The officer looked at me "Sharon, I'm going to look for him, you ok?"

"Yeah, I'm ok." I heard Rescue-One come on line and they would be here soon. I turned my attention to the woman. I slipped an oxygen mask on her and turned it up all the way. I took my hand and reapplied pressure to the wound. I reminded myself of bleeding control before vital signs. I then noticed the sofa was soaked in blood. It squished when I touched it. Blood trickled out from under the sofa apparently the blood was leaking through the sofa and out into the rug on the floor. The bleeding was more serious than I thought. She was in serious trouble. The knife appeared to have hit an artery and she was going to bleed out if she didn't get to the hospital soon. I had wound the roller bandage tightly but not quite tourniquet tight. My hand applied pressure and it seemed to be enough. The active bleeding had stopped, at least as long as my hand maintained pressure.

The woman opened her eyes and looked up at me. With sadness in her voice she spoke in a soft tone. "He was such a good boy until school got out. He ran wild this summer. I don't know what went wrong with him." I said nothing, what could I say? I could hear another officer arrive in the area and the two officers began looping the trailer court in search of the boy. I had told the officer I was ok, but I reconsidered. The scene wasn't safe. The front door was wide open and the boy who had just stabbed his sleeping mother could return at any minute. I touched the stun gun in my pocket and planned for the worst. If he returned I planned

329

on using my radio to request help from the nearby officers and with my stun gun, I could probably scare him off or disable him.

I heard Rescue-One go en route. My husband, Maurice was one of the crew members on the ambulance. I keyed the radio, "Rescue-1, F-3."

"F-3, go ahead."

"This is a load and go. The scene is not safe. Bring the stretcher in with you, no need for the backboard." If it wasn't safe for me, it wasn't safe for them either.

"Rescue-One copies."

The crew quickly arrived and charged into the room. "She was stabbed with a steak knife in her right thigh as she lay sleeping. I got the bleeding stopped, but you have to apply direct pressure to maintain it. She lost a lot of blood. The sofa is soaked completely through. The person who stabbed her is still on the loose, so hurry it up. Whatever you do, do in the ambulance." My husband, an EMT, took over holding the pressure to the wound. The others and I got her on the stretcher. I kept an eye on the open door, expecting at any minute for the boy to return.

The crew moved her to the ambulance just as an officer shouted over the radio, "I see him, over here Mike!" The radio was quite for a couple of minutes then as the ambulance pulled away I heard, "We got him, Code-4."

I went back inside and collected my equipment and picked up the trash we had left behind. An officer stuck his head inside, "You ok?"

"Yeah," I pointed to the knife that lay on the floor. "There's the knife he used. And the piece of jeans with the knife hole in it is laying on the couch."

"Great!" The officer went back to his car and got a camera. He came back in and began snapping pictures. I left.

The boy later said he was "just so mad" at his mother he couldn't control himself. He hated her and wanted her to shut up and stop "disrespecting him." The mother lived, but her young son was in serious trouble. I don't know the outcome of this incident. Page is isolated and had few resources for such behavioral problems at the time. What did exist believed in just handing out mood altering drugs and ignoring the real problem. I hope the family got the help they needed, but I have serious doubts. I suspect the boy went to jail and that would solve nothing.

DON'T SHOOT! DON'T SHOOT, IT'S ME!

This particular duty shift I was stationed in Tuba City and was partnered with Rick Stone. He and I worked well together. He was an exceptional EMT and I kept encouraging him to become a Paramedic. Quarters was a double wide trailer on a large dirt lot on the west side of Tuba. In Arizona, especially in the rural areas, many people carry guns for personal protection. In the middle of nowhere it may takes hours for a police officer to arrive so we have to take personal responsibility for our protection. My husband had just given me a new gun for my birthday. I was proudly showing it off to the other EMT's and Paramedic. They all carried guns in their cars and the gun lay on the bed stand next to their bed. Most EMT drivers on the reservation carried a gun behind the driver's seat in the ambulance. I carried the gun in my car and it lay beside by bed, but I didn't take it in the ambulance, I had pepper spray and a stun gun. I had grown up with guns in the home and had been taught how to handle them safely. I was a pretty good shot and felt comfortable around guns and most of my friends and family felt the same. I know this sounds strange for someone living back east, such as New York City, but customs differ across America and it works for us in the Southwest.

We ran two crews a shift out of Tuba City and we were free to wander about Tuba during slack times. When I arrived for duty I was told the lock on the back door was broken. I wasn't happy to hear that. Later that night the other crew was on a long range transport to Chinle and would be gone for hours. Rick Stone had left to visit a friend. I was alone. I didn't mind that but a locked door gives me a feeling of security. At least I could hear someone ripping off the door if it was locked and I would have some warning. I locked the door to the women's bedroom, but I wanted more warning so I devised my own burglar alarm. The back door opened into the small laundry room and beyond that was the door that opened into the hallway that led from the living room to the men and women's bedrooms. I took a round cake pan and hung it on the door knob of the inside hallway door. On the floor below it I put two round cake pans. The idea was if someone came in the door the cake pan would fall on the floor and make a noise, alerting me. I expected Rick to return in a few hours and to enter through the front door. I crawled into bed and went to sleep. It was a slow night and no 911 calls or long range transport was paged so I slept well.

About two hours later, Rick drove up and parked near the rear of the trailer. For some reason he decided to enter through the back door. He opened the back door and entered the laundry room then reached for the door leading to the hallway. When he turned the handle and started to open the door, the cake pan dropped and hit the two pans lying on the floor. The noise was loud. He later said he immediately knew what I had done. He wasn't familiar with my gun training and all he could think of was the big handgun lying beside my bed and where the bed was placed in the room, I would have a direct shot, through the hollow bedroom door to where he stood. He spun around and ran for the back door, yelling loudly, "Don't shoot! Sharon, don't shoot, it's me, Rick!" I sat up in bed at the sound of the pans clattering at his entrance. Immediately I heard Rick yelling. I got up and opened my bedroom door in time to see him run out the back door with his hands up in the air, still yelling, "Don't shoot, don't shoot, don't shoot Sharon don't shoot! It's me, Rick!" I was impressed; Rick was really making good time across the large back yard.

I began to laugh. "You can stop screaming, I won't shoot you." I yelled to him as he had reached the middle of large dirt lot that served as a back yard.

Rick stopped and turned. "You and your big ass gun scared the crap out of me!" (Or something similar to that). I was laughing standing in the doorway. The lights of our neighbors were turning on. I expected the police to drive up anytime. Rick walked back and we went back in the trailer. "All I could think of was that gun."

"I would have never shot through a door. My father taught me to always identify my target."

"I didn't know that!" It was hard to get back to sleep that night and just as soon as I drifted off my pager sounded and I had to get up.

As I said at the beginning of this book, "everyone remembers an event from their point of view." This isn't any different. Rick and I agree on the details of this event. We both think it's funny and both he and I have told the story a number of times. In Rick's less dramatic version he is a bit more dignified and not as frantic, but my version is more exciting and I believe closer to what really happened. Rick doesn't entirely agree. Sorry Rick, my book, my version.

NEVER TRUST ANYONE

The boy was found leaning up against the wall that surrounded the high school. He was a big kid, 235 pounds. His sandy blond hair hung in his eyes. He was doubled up moaning that he had food poisoning. An off duty EMT, Patrick Simpson had been driving by with his family and saw the boy and had stopped. He called the ambulance. The boy kept moaning and appeared to be in a lot of pain.

EMT Roger Nelson had arrived as a first responder by the time our two person female ambulance crew pulled up to the scene. Roger was with Simpson and they were acting strange. I didn't know why, but I knew them both well enough to realize that there was something they weren't telling me. I knelled beside the boy and took his vital signs. They were normal. Upon questioning, he admitted that he didn't have food poisoning, that he had taken some pills in an attempt to kill himself. He was seventeen years old and he wanted to die. "How utterly stupid" I thought. But I didn't say it. "What did you take?" I asked.

"I don't know. I just some big white pills I found in my Mom's bedroom."

"Where are the empty bottles?"

". . . . On the table by the front door."

"Where do you live?"

"I don't know the address. It's a white trailer in Vermillion Trailer Court (It has several hundred trailers in it) and there's a refrigerator sitting on the patio."

I looked up at the officer. "I need to know what he took. Could you go over to his house and bring the empty bottles to the hospital?"

"Sure, if I can find it." He stomped off. He wasn't happy to be given the assignment of looking for the needle in the haystack. We walked the boy to the ambulance, with him clutching his stomach. I got in and was surprised to find Simpson also getting in. He smiled. "I'll ride with you, ok?"

"Sure," I said. There was defiantly something else to this. I felt uncomfortable. This call was early in my career. If this had happened later, I would have handled it differently, but it didn't and I soon regretted my actions. The boy was polite to me. He appeared to hurt a great deal and I had complete sympathy for him as I mothered him. We arrived and soon he was in the ER. I told the doctor what we had. We left the boy with the nurse awaiting the arrival of the police officer with the pill bottles. I stepped out in the hallway and stripped the sheets of the stretcher. Simpson left and the other male EMT stood in the doorway watching the boy. "Why?" I thought. I went about my duties. Then I noticed I didn't ask the boy his birth date and I needed that for my records. I walked back in the ER. He sat up on the gurney, still holding his stomach.

I wasn't sure what had happened, but this boy appeared different than the one we had in the back of the ambulance. He was agitated, restless, and starting to become less than cooperative. "I want to get of here," he said in an assertive man's voice, the boy was gone.

"The doctor will be here in a minute. You need some treatment then you can leave."

"I want to leave NOW!" he yelled. The male EMT, the nurse and the doctor appeared in the doorway. I wasn't too street smart in those days and I was standing beside him, only inches away.

"I'm getting out of here and I'm leavin' now!" he took out of his pocket a knife and held it threateningly toward me. In reality it was only a four inch pocket knife, but in my eyes it was a two foot machete. The lights gleamed off the blade. I was in trouble. Run? No, I was too close for that. Fight? No he was a really big boy. Talk your way out of this? Yes, I was a good talker, talk it would be.

"That's a nice knife, where did you get it?" I asked in a casual tone, as if I was too stupid to understand he was threatening me. Now, on paper it sounds like a stupid remark. But I thought it might give him a second chance to rethink his impulsive action. A chance to back down before this got out of hand.

"I've had it awhile," he said, also in a casual tone.

"Why don't you let me keep the knife for you, until they are through here?" Damn I thought, I sounded like a moron.

The boy looked at me. I was old enough to be his mother. I didn't appear to realize I was in danger, or maybe, he thought, "She trusts me and doesn't believe I would hurt her." I smiled a stupid smile. The others held their breath. The boy pondered this incredibly stupid, but nice woman and his one last chance to back down from very serious criminal charges. "Here," he said as he handed me the knife.

"Do you have any more?" I asked.

"Yeah, sure." He reached back and withdrew another knife, this one longer.

"That's it?"

He smiled, "Yeah, that it."

"I'll put these in the office. You can get them when you leave." I turned and walked with heart racing but slow normal pace from the room out the side door. I didn't stop till I got the knives down the hall and into the office. My hands shook as I laid them on the receptionist's desk. I took a deep breath and pondered my lack of basic intelligence.

"I should have searched him at the scene. Damn it! The two more experienced EMTs on the scene should have searched him." I felt weak. The picture of the knife only inches from me was fresh in my mind.

At this point, things started to go downhill. Roger entered the ER. He walked up to the kid, but his manner wasn't fatherly, it was authoritative and a bit pushy. He looked down and saw a dog's choke chain threaded through the boys back belt loops (if it was swung, it could be a weapon). Without saying anything, he grabbed the chain and jerked

334

it out. The boy went nuts and grabbed the EMT's throat. I walked down the corridor, unaware of the new problem. Roger and the boy wrestled on the table with feet, arms and fists flying. The nurse grabbed a piece of the action, trying to help subdue the boy. As they fell to the floor, someone's foot hit the large overhanging light and caused it to swing wildly back and forth.

The two men fell to the floor taking the nurse with them. I walked into the door way just in time to see the nurse with her skirt drew up over her head, her pink panties with little butterflies in plain sight and the two men on the floor grunting and groaning. I don't know why, but I stood there trying to suppress the urge to laugh. It was funny. The nurse rolled free and Roger maneuvered the boy under him. He turned around while sitting on the patient's chest and yelled. "Call the police!"

I turned and ran down the hall, grabbed a phone and dialed dispatch. "We need a police officer at the hospital ER. The patient is violent and a fight is in progress." I slammed the phone down and ran back down the hall. The scene was still a circus, but Roger now defiantly had the upper hand. The boy's head was banging on the floor and the nurse had managed to smooth down her dress and slipped a pillow under the boys head as the EMT tried to keep him pinned to the floor.

The police officer sent to find a white trailer with a refrigerator on the patio, came with the empty bottles and a night stick. The boy had taken a laxative, nothing that would kill him. The officer drug him to his feet and with help from two other officers, arrested the boy and took him to jail.

Roger smoothed his shirt down and his hair. "I was worried about him at the scene. He was arrested last night for assault and hurt one policeman in the process. I guess he's out on bail."

"Why didn't you tell me? Why didn't you search him before putting him in the ambulance?"

"I forgot," he said sheepishly.

"You almost got me killed." I stormed off. This was only to be the first of several times he almost got me killed, usually it was his reckless driving, but other times . . . . . Well, at least he never got the job done.

335

NATIONAL PARK ~~SERVICE~~ SECURITY

Over the years, I have managed to work well on a professional level with many agencies. The one and only exception is National Park Service at Glen Canyon National Recreation Area. The following is a previously untold story of conflict between two agencies, NPS and PFD.

There are good men and women who work for the National Park Service, but they usually don't stay long at Glen Canyon. In my many travels across America I found only the National Park Rangers in Washington D.C. to have come close to having the same degree of negative attitude found in most GCNRA rangers.

The Rangers I came in contact with as a child were helpful people. They educated visitors and did whatever they could do to help the visitors enjoy the great outdoors. Today these rangers are called "Interpretive Rangers." They are seasonal employees. The "real" rangers (full time) have become police officers with an attitude. Many parks across America still show that positive attitude. Lake Powell Rangers have a different approach. Visitors are considered annoying by most of the rangers. I know this because they have heard them say so. I once heard the Head Ranger say to the Superintendent, "I wish we could string a chain across the narrows and keep all the $&%*^%& tourists in Wahweap Bay. That way we could control them and have the rest of the lake to ourselves." That attitude prevailed for far too many years. I had to interface with them during my years as an EMT and as Rescue Chief of the Page Fire Department. I struggled to maintain a working relationship. It was an exasperating situation. Most of the time I managed, but sometimes it wasn't to be.

Highway 89 runs through the western edge of Lake Powell Recreation Area. Although there is a great difference between a recreation area and a national park, the difference is lost on the rangers. As PFD Rescue Chief, I struggled to try and maintain a working relationship with the agency, but this was the last straw. I was at the fire department going through my mail. I noticed a short letter from Glen Canyon Recreation Area National Park Service (GCNRA NPS). They were giving us notice that Page Fire would no longer be allowed to drive through the "park" code-three. There would be no exceptions. Red lights and sirens were now considered "sight and sound" pollution and would not be tolerated.

After some phone calls and a little research, I found out the highway wasn't NPS's responsibility. It belonged to the Utah State Highway Patrol and the Arizona Department of Public Safety. Roughly the roadway and to the boundary fences on each side of the highway was considered State land, "not park land." All agencies, except GCNRA NPS, said I could drive the ambulance code-three as long as the patient's condition warranted it.

I called the Superintendent of the Recreation Area and told him what I had found and told him Page Fire was going to drive the ambulance whatever code was best for the patient. I was told NPS would not allow lights and sirens. We were at a stalemate. The supervisor of the local Arizona DPS (highway patrol) told me to call him if NPS gave us a problem. I notified our EMT's about the situation. I told them to disregard NPS and do whatever was best for the patient. I also told them if they interfered in appropriate transportation of a patient to call me on the radio. Battle lines were drawn.

It didn't take long. PFD Ambulance was dispatched to Big Water, Utah, a small community eighteen miles north of Page, for an unknown medical. I was on standby at the football game. Gordon Taylor was driving the ambulance and he speeded code-three through the corner of the recreation area. They met with no resistance from NPS as they sped to the scene driving through the southern corner. Upon arriving, the male patient was in distress. He had been ill for several days and now his fever was raging and he was incoherent. The crew decided due to the patient's condition and long transport time, a code-three return trip was warranted.

I was monitoring the radio as I watched the football game. I heard Ranger X come on the air. "What does Page Fire have?" the park dispatcher said she didn't know. The ranger then said "They are breaking park protocol by going code-three. I'm going down to the highway and stop them. I want to check out the patient and see if he's really that bad." Now a little background is needed at this point. The ranger was a paramedic, and the ambulance crew were basic EMTs. But the paramedic had not gotten medical control yet and didn't carry a drug box or defibulator. A medic without a drug box cardiac monitor/defibulator is a basic EMT. I will agree that the patient survey is done at a higher level, but if they don't have the tools to do paramedic work, what good does it do to take the time to get a paramedic evaluation when the patient could be at the hospital before the paramedic was finished with his examination.

Gordon said he saw the ranger's car sitting beside the road, and then the vehicle pulled into the road. The ranger's vehicle wasn't large enough to block the entire road but the road block was obvious. Gordon called me, "a ranger has used his vehicle to form a road block. What do I do?" He told me later that he had no intentions of stopping and letting the ranger get in and ask a bunch of questions, and then decide how we were to transport that patient. The man needed immediate attention and delay in transport might make a difference. Gordon simply called me to cover his ass when the shit hit the fan.

I was mad, very mad. "Gordon, don't you dare stop for that idiot. Your first responsibility is to the patient."

"Rescue-One copies" Gordon told me later, he believed the ranger overheard the radio traffic, and decided to back down. The ranger backed his vehicle off the road and just watched as they sped past him en route to Page Hospital. I expected to get a phone call the next day but not a peep. We had won round one.

Little did I know round two would involve a ranger stopping a PFD ambulance two weeks later at gun point. The patient with a fractured ankle was terrified, the EMTs on the call were shocked and I was mad as a wet hen. I wrote the story with full intentions of including it in this book, but no matter how I edited it, I just can't make it ready for publication. Even after the passage of time, I can't tell it without getting mad all over again.

To make the overview as politically correct as I can make it, the situation with NPS had reached a point of no return. I informed them they had no jurisdiction on any Arizona or Utah highways and we would use lights and sirens if the patient's condition called for it. I informed them DPS would be called to respond to the scene if another road block was set up by NPS. DPS knew about the situation and they were not on NPS's side. I also insisted either they put a leash on Ranger X or PFD would no longer back them up on medical emergencies or fires within GCRA and they were on their own. It became nasty but in the end, PFD ambulances were no longer subjected to this kind of abuse of power again. It was the end of sound and sight pollution. There were no more roadblocks and Ranger X kept his gun holstered. He transferred before the years end but the attitude remained.

The rangers didn't bring out their weapons again until November 19, 1995 when the NPS issued orders for rangers to fire upon the unarmed Arizona National Guard who were on their way to the Grand Canyon, if they attempted to cross park boundaries. (see the Arizona Republic Newspaper.) At Lake Powell the NPS put up roadblocks and manned them with rangers armed with shotguns. They threatened to shoot anyone who tried to enter the Recreation Area. My husband was pulled over and threatened with arrest because he had "looked" at the roadblock as he had driven past. The rangers were afraid the locals from Page would storm the roadblock. Even the rangers admitted there had been no threats but they feared the worst because they were not that well liked in Page. But that's another story to be told by someone else since it does not involve EMS.

THE EIGHT HUNDRED POUND GORILLA

The Page Lake Powell Chronicle ran the following stories, it was only the tip of the iceberg. "December 23, 1983, The Safeway grocery store in Page, Arizona was set on fire by an arsonist. There was $10,000 damage done."
"January 11, 1984, another fire was reported. At 8:10 pm, Safeway employee Shirley Bloomfield was notified by customer that there was another fire in the store. She dialed 911 then notified employees who grabbed six fire extinguishers but were not able to put it out. Page Fire arrived and extinguished the fire. An investigation is being conducted."

It was a very dark and cold January evening, around eight o'clock at night. Patches of snow lingered around the corners of the Safeway Grocery Store parking lot. No one noticed the person on the potato chip isle. He lingered, looking up and down the aisle. He wore a thick black coat and the hood covered most of his face. He reached up and grabbed a large bag of potato chips. He held a lighter under them and instantly flames engulfed the bag. He tossed it back up on the rack and quickly left the store.

Flames leaped up, licking at the tall ceiling. Shoppers continued to push carts up and down isles; no one noticed the flames that were quickly devouring isle number three. Heat rose upward and activated heat sensors. The sprinkler system sprang to life. Cold water sprayed down on shoppers, children, and employees alike. Screams erupted as the cold water drenched the running people as they ran in circles and finally finding focus and heading toward the front door. Then an employee saw the flames. Six employees found fire extinguishers and rushed toward the fire while another employee phoned 911.

My husband, Maurice had the PFD Attack Truck that night. It was a Dodge heavy duty, around a ton truck. It had a water tank, hoses and other firefighting equipment. It was a first fire responder vehicle. It was designed to arrive first, give a report to responding units and begin the firefighting process. Our pagers sounded in stereo that evening and we both leaped up. Maurice was out the door first and was driving off in the attack truck as I ran out the front door.

Back at the grocery store it was getting interesting. The six employees attacked the flaming potato chips with fire extinguishers, but it wasn't enough. The extinguishers ran dry and the flames continued to leap and dance around. The fire grew. The employees ran. The night air was freezing cold and it hit the dripping wet customers and employees as they streamed into the parking lot.

Firefighter Maurice Holbert drove up behind the building. He could see the back door was open. He believed it had been left open by an escaping employee. Black and brown smoke poured from the doorway. He keyed his radio, "Attack-One is 97 (on scene). Heavy smoke showing out the back door." Maurice put on his turnouts, Scott bottle and mask and entered in search of the electrical box. The air tank on his back fed him clean air as he felt his way through the heavy smoke. Suddenly he took a breath and his lungs filled with bitter tasting smoke. He reached down with his gloved hand and found the hose that connected his tank to his mask had fallen off. He fumbled with gloved hands and found the hose and reattached it to the mask. Clean air began to flow again. Maurice realized that the box wasn't where he thought it was and turned to leave when he ran into Captain Tanner and another firefighter with a fire hose. The box was found and electrical power was shut down.

Maurice joined them. They were searching for the fire. Heavy black smoke descended from the ceiling down to around four feet from the floor. Visibility was poor. The experienced firefighters believed the fire had not spread beyond the initial site. They continued to search. Suddenly a loud noise caught their attention. It was a cardboard display unit. As I shopper I have always hated them cluttering the aisle with a display of an item. I know they are trying to ignite the impulsive shopping urge, but they still clutter the aisle. The cardboard base became wet from the sprinklers and folded to the side, dumping Pacante sauce all over the floor. Red salsa exploded as the glass jars broke.

Outside the burning store, I arrived and staged a safe distance from the front door. I looked around for those that may have been injured. I quickly found there were no injuries, but there were dripping wet people quickly turning into human popsicles. I moved the people over by the ambulance. I divided them into two groups, group one were shoppers who were uninjured, and didn't see anything and group two were employees. The shoppers were in a hurry to just go to their cars and leave. The ambulance crew arrived and quickly verbally checked them out in the warm ambulance and took their names and addresses. They were allowed to go to their cars and go home after signing refusal forms. I climbed in the ambulance with six employees. They were dripping wet and I gave them blankets and turned up the heater.

Maurice and the other two firefighters continued searching for the fire. Suddenly loud popping sounded as the bean dip reached a high temperature from the fire and exploded. Tanner was hit by hot flying bean dip. His uniform saved him from burns. They found the fire and turned the hose on the flickering flames. The fire monster died quickly.

Outside in the ambulance I questioned the employees and discovered none were injured. Their only complaint was the freezing cold. I asked them what they knew about the fire. None had seen anything and there were no security cameras. The manager was called at home and they then took turns calling their family. Most needed a ride because their purses were still in the building with their car keys.

The fire was now out. The smoke diminished and now the mess was visible. Water stood deep in the aisles. All cardboard displays that cluttered the aisles had collapsed. One firefighter smelled like whiskey as he had wadded through a broken Jack Daniels display on aisle nine. Another firefighter smelled of pickles. It was an odd situation. The Fire Chief climbed into the ambulance and finished questioning the employees. They were allowed to leave when the manger arrived. No one knew anything. It was frustrating. The fire was set intentionally; there was no question about that.

When the fire was over and everyone returned to the station an eight hundred pound gorilla stood in our mists. No one said anything but we all were thinking the same thing. We were reasonably sure who had started the fire but not one of us was willing to put our thoughts into words.

A member of the fire department had a teenage child that was suspected of sitting a number of dumpster fires. There was no real proof, but a number of people had reached the same collusion independently. The fires always occurred after school, during fire drill, or when the member of the fire department was not at home. The teen had been seen often near the dumpster fires, just watching. Firefighters and police had been staking out dumpsters trying to catch the armorist in the act, but it didn't work. It appeared as if the culprit knew when the stake outs were in place. The teenager hung around the fire department. This seemed strange since the teen and his parent fought loudly and often about everything. The teenager also asked a lot of questions that caused a number of people to remark on it being unusual. We all had children and recognized this wasn't normal behavior.

Another coincident that disturbed us the most was the fact the teenager had been in unofficial attendance when a firefighter demonstrated at fire drill how easy it was to set a bag of potato chips on fire with a simple Bic lighter. A week after the drill demonstration, a small fire was set at Safeway, but the fire went out on its own. The sprinklers were not activated and only a half burned bag of corn chips was found by an employee. Now, two weeks later, a second fire was set and it was obvious the arsonist had learned from his previous mistake. This time, the fire may not have destroyed the building, but it had done serious damage. We were lucky no one was injured or killed.

A few days later Safeway reopened. Most PFD personnel ignored the gorilla while I and others struggled with our suspicions. There was no real proof, just a firm gut feeling and circumstantial evidence. Was that enough to accuse someone's teenager of being an arsonist? Arson is a serious crime. Then, without warning, the member of the fire department turned in their resignation, packed up and unceremoniously left Page. The dumpster fires stopped. The gorilla disappeared, and the Safeway arson fires stopped.

HAPPY NEW YEARS!

Snow had fallen on the city of Page earlier that day. The city sat on Manson Mesa and overlooked the Lake Powell from a thousand feet higher elevation. It was a dark night. No moon was visible in the overcast sky. Nine miles to the north of town, Lake Powell's water lay deep and dark with a smooth black surface. No breeze blew, just a bone chilling cold. A thin layer of ice covered the marina and moored houseboats.

Sheri was enjoying herself. She and her husband had driven for six hours that day from Phoenix, Arizona in the van full of friends. They had decided to usher in the New Year with a party on their houseboat. It had sat unused for months and was docked at the Wahweap Marina. Tonight the boat was brightly lit. Sheri and her two female friends had cooked a wonderful meal and everyone was starving. The three guys were standing outside on the deck, smoking.

"I told them it's time to eat, but they don't appear to be moving." Cindy said. She and the others were thirty-something, upper middle working class.

"Well, I bet I know how to get them inside," said Sheri. She bent down and removed the casserole from the oven. The fragrance of chicken, mushrooms and other good things drifted through the cabin. She took the oven mitts and lifted it. "The guys can resist anything but temptation, she said as Cindy and Lizzie laughed.

Carl, Ray and John stood finishing up their cigarettes when the door opened and Sheri walked out on the deck. She was smiling and holding the fragrant casserole. "Does this look interesting?" She asked as she moved it around letting the men smell the meal.

"I'm through," Ray said as the tossed the cigarette down on the icy deck and crushed it with his shoe.

"I was getting cold anyway," said John as he sniffed the dish.

"Then follow me, men," Sheri said as she turned and started toward the cabin door. Suddenly her shoes slipped on the ice, her feet went out from under her and she went down flat on her back and the casserole dumped chicken, rice, mushrooms and thinly sliced carrots all over her chest, face and hair.

"Shit," said her husband Carl, "Sheri!" He rushed to her, slipping and sliding, but not losing control. He and John kneeled beside her. "You ok? Sheri?" Carl asked.

Sheri opened her eyes and brushed the rice from her face, "I don't know." The men helped her up as dinner fell to the deck. Sheri was assisted into the cabin. The woman took her to the bedroom to change since she had food all over her.

As she undressed with her friends assisting her, she began to notice pain. "My neck hurts, and I think I may have broken something, my left arm is throbbing."

Cindy tossed the soiled clothing in a plastic bag. Lizzie looked at the arm. "I think it might be a good idea for us to take you in to the ER to be checked."

"I'll be ok," Sheri said but she soon discovered new painful spots.

The men looked up as the women came back. "Now what's for dinner?" asked Ray.

"Beer and chips?" answered Carl. "Everything else is trash."

"We have salad and green beans and rolls," offered Lizzie.

"Maybe we could order some pizza," offered John.

Sheri sat down carefully and rubbed her shoulder and neck. Carl noticed her discomfort. "Honey, why don't we get you x-rayed, and then while we are in town, we can get some pizza."

Sheri sighed, "I'm sorry guys. I didn't want to spend New Year's in the ER waiting room. But I think I really did hurt something."

"That's not important now, let's get you into town. We'll all go," Cindy said. Sheri stood with help and stiffly slipped on her coat. She then slowly shuffled toward the door. It was obvious she was in pain. Carl secretly began to really worry about her. She cautiously scooted her feet across the icy deck. The deck rail gate was opened by John and he stepped off the boat onto the dock. "Come on," he said as he held out his hands.

Sheri stopped and looked down, the eighteen inches between the houseboat and dock looked like a mile. Sheri was afraid of water. She took a deep breath and stepped off the boat. Suddenly, her feet went out from under her, again loosing traction due to the ice. She made a valiant attempt to gain the dock, but again her foot slipped, John grabbed for her but only managed to deflect her back toward the boat and off balance. She screamed, Cindy screamed, Lizzie screamed and Carl screamed. It was ciaos as she slipped and her head hit the rail. Then her body hit the deck and she slid, and slipped between the boat and dock, into the wet, icy, darkness.

Sheri could not swim. She feared nothing more than water. Now her nightmare had come true. She was submerged in the coldest, darkest fifteen feet of water she could have ever imaged. She stiffened and sank like a rock. "I'm going to die," she thought. She couldn't move her arms or legs, she was frozen in fear.

The three men, without spoken word, dove into the lake. They tried to not pay attention to the bone chilling coldness. They could see nothing in the blackness. They waved their arms around, feeling for Sheri. "How deep is the lake here?" thought Ray as he continued to dive deeper.

Carl could only think of his wife. He was frantic. He then felt something, hair? He grabbed a handful and pulled. It was Sheri. Her long hair had fanned out and now turned into a perfect handle. Carl started swimming back up. He broke the surface and with the help of his two friends and the women, they managed to drag Sheri back onto the icy deck of the boat. She just lay there, gasping. She rolled into a fetal position and began to violently shake. The men got out of the water and immediately they picked up Sheri and all six of them hurried to the heated cabin. Sheri was again stripped and redressed in dry clothing. The men toweled off and changed clothing. "I don't think I will ever be warm again," said Ray. The others agreed.

Ok, let's try this again, if she didn't need it before, she really needs to be checked out now." Carl was really worried about her. Sheri now walked stiffly with strange limp and listed to her left. It appeared to take considerable effort for her to keep her balance. "You ok?" he asked.

"NO!" Sheri's easy going temperament had disappeared. She ached from top to bottom and she couldn't take a deep breath. She knew she had cracked at least three ribs and she was dizzy now. It was hard to focus. Again, the group started out.

With great effort, Sheri was safely transferred from the boat to the dock. "Thanks guys, I can make it now," she said. They let go and she instantly slipped. Her feet flew forward and then up in the air, her head flew backwards, and she went down, slammed back first on the icy dock. Her head went smack. She almost lost consciousness as she struggled to stay awake. Sharp pain went from the back of her head down her spine and exploded at her tail bone. She screamed in agony.

344

Her friends could not believe it. Cindy took her cell phone out and dialed 911. Carl bent down, "DON'T TOUCH ME!" Sheri screamed. "DON"T TOUCH ME!" She lay still. "I really hurt myself this time." She began to cry.

"I don't think you should move," said Cindy. I called an ambulance. Obviously we couldn't get the job done."

I was up watching TV. There isn't anything else to do in Page on New Year. Maurice was trying to stay awake until midnight. The boys had gone to bed. My pager sounded. I was surprised. With it being so cold and damp, few people were out. Those living on the reservation were snowed in and the town people were all in their warm homes or out of town celebrating. I slipped on my shoes and grabbed my keys. "Happy New Years," I said as I went out the door. Maurice smiled.

The ambulance had to travel a bit slower due to the icy road, but made good time being the only vehicle on the road. We pulled up to the marina dock. We got out, put a backboard on the stretcher, stacked the jump kit on top and carefully started slipping and sliding down the dock. Monica was an EMT and could not swim. She leaned over to me "Sharon, remember, if I go in the water, come get me, I can't swim." I told her I would, but boy I hoped she managed to stay on the dock. The water looked cold.

We approached a group of people. That part of the dock was dark. Only a faint light flickered about twenty feet away on a tiny pole. "What happened?" I asked. Five people started to talk at once. I managed to figure out the unbelievable story of Sheri's New Years Eve tragedy. Poor Sheri!

I kneeled down and the cold ice seeped through my uniform. Sheri, can you hear me? She opened her eyes and answered. "I'm so.... cold......." Her voice trailed off. I could image since she lay supine (on her back) on the layer of ice that coated the dock as a silent gentle snow started to fall. She wasn't shaking anymore. Her core temp had dropped into the dangerous zone. A near frozen tear lay on her cheek.

We quickly applied a c-collar and log rolled her onto the backboard. We lifted the board and Sheri yelled out "DON'T DROP ME!"

I could understand her concern. "We won't drop you," I said, hoping it would turn out to be the truth. We put the board on the stretcher and it slid a bit, but stayed on the dock. We strapped her to the stretcher. I had the vision of her and the stretcher sliding into the dark water, her strapped to the board. "No, No, Sharon, none of that," I said to myself. Her friends, husband and we three EMTs slipped and slid back to the ambulance. It was parked on the launch ramp that had a slight incline and

345

it took great effort to safely get her loaded into the ambulance. I hopped in and began examining her. Her speech was slow and sluggish. She told me she hurt all over. When questioned for details, it seemed her most serious area of pain was her neck, back of her head, her ribs, left arm and left hip. She began to cry again. We had covered her with a fuzzy blanket and turned on the heater, but I wasn't going to warm her any more, fearing cardiac arrhythmias.

At the hospital she was x-rayed. Three fractured ribs, one cracked ulna, badly bruised hip, and a concussion. The knot on the back of her head was huge. She was sick to her stomach and developed a horrible headache. The clock struck midnight. Everyone wished everyone in the ER a "Happy New Year." Sheri was unimpressed. She spent New Year's Day in the Page hospital. She was heavily drugged with happy pills. The next day she was carried to the van by her husband and friends. I am sure she slept all the way home. It was a New Year none of them would forget.

WHERE'S HIS WEDDING BAND?

". . . . . . . CPR in progress." The radio went silent as Cheryl and I climbed into Rescue-One. Doug clicked on the siren and lights and we pulled away from the station. At the stop light a tourist stepped out in front of us. Doug slammed on the breaks coming within inches of flattening the man. He never turned or looked at us. He just continued on across the street.

"He's not wearing ear phones. How could he have not heard us?" Doug asked.

"Maybe he's deaf."

"That's all the more reason to look both ways." We turned onto the main street of town. It was called "Seventh Avenue" at the time but later its name was changed to "Lake Powell Boulevard." We quickly arrived at a local motel.

"It's room 210," said Cheryl, an EMT.

I thought to myself, "Of course he would be on the second floor of a motel with no elevator. I bet he weights three hundred pounds as well." Part of front desk clerk training must include evaluating a guest's health, weight and age. Young healthy athletic individuals get ground floor rooms. Those who are overweight, older and looking ill are put on the top floor. If the hotel has an elevator the guest's room will be as far from the elevator

346

as possible. And of course, most hotel elevators aren't big enough for a stretcher. We climbed the stairs lugging our equipment, walked down the long outdoor baloney. We found the room and entered. The patient did indeed weight near three hundred pounds. He was lying on the bed, on his back. A police officer straddled him and had his arm halfway down the man's throat. "What are you doing?" I asked as I entered the room.

"I blew his damn teeth down his throat." The officer then removed his hand and the teeth grasped firmly.

"Get him on the floor," Doug ordered and we all complied. I started chest compressions. Cheryl used her bag valve mask and gave him breaths. Without his teeth in it was hard to maintain a seal but she managed to get a good seal and delivered the breaths on time. The man's wife stood in the corner of the room crying and trying to make a deal with God. Doug went for the stretcher. He had problems dragging it up the flight of stairs but he got the job done.

I was in the zone, fifteen compressions, wait for two breaths, then resume compressions again. CPR has changed so many times since I began this career. Today this sequence is out dated, but at the time it was considered the standard. I kneeled on my knees beside the man's upper body. My two arms were stretched out and elbows locked. My fingers were laced together and I was throwing my weight into each downward stroke. It was hard work. Then I felt it. It was subtle. When I leaned back his chest didn't immediately rise back in place. Then it did, almost a beat off. "Any change?" I asked Cheryl.

"No."

I continued CPR. Then it happened again. "Stop CPR" I said. I took the stethoscope and listened. He was breathing and he had a heartbeat. "We have a pulse and he's breathing!" I announced. Now I was a new EMT and this was the first time I had restored a heartbeat. It wasn't what I had expected. I don't know why, but I expected him to open his eyes and look around. This man didn't. His eyes remained closed.

We quickly got him on the backboard and on the stretcher. Just as we reached the top of the stairs, I checked again and he wasn't breathing and I couldn't find a pulse. "Begin CPR." Again we did CPR. About two minutes later he took a ragged breath and his heart started up. We hurried down the stairs. We loaded him and as the back doors closed again, he went into arrest. His wife rode in up front in the passenger seat.

When we pulled up at the hospital's back door, the doctor was waiting for us. He opened the back doors and announced, "He's dead."

I was shocked! I missed a beat but then blurted out "He's breathing, he has a heartbeat!"

"Oh," said the surprised doctor. "Well, then . . . . bring him on in." We quickly unloaded him and wheeled him into the ER. Before we could gather our gear he went into full code arrest again. CPR was begun again. Advanced Life Support was begun. But finally, his heart wouldn't restart and all attempts to revive him were stopped.

I felt mixed emotions. I was thrilled we had restored his heartbeat, but then he had the nerve to die. It kind of took the glory out of it. I was new at the emotions of an EMT and I wasn't sure how to look at this call. I finally came to the conclusion that we had done everything we could and it was just this man's time to die.

Two weeks later the Fire Chief called us all in, including the police officer. "Remember CPR at the Lamp Lighter Motel? Well, I got a letter from the man's wife. She says we stole her husband's wedding band."

EMTs and Paramedics in the course of our duties move freely about a person's home. We enter the bedroom and bathrooms; We open medicine cabinets and dig through purses and wallets. Honesty is a necessary part of what we do. To be accused of theft is a big deal. "We didn't take anything," the officer said. We all agreed with him.

"I believe you, but the problem is how do we prove it." The chief had a point. How do you prove yourself innocent? Innocent until proven guilty only applies in a court of law. In the real world innocence often has to be proved. We all felt insulted and a bit frightened. We didn't take anything, but she thought so. It's a strange feeling to be in this situation. We all worked so hard to save her husband. Between shoulder blades and the tops of my hands ached for days afterwards. I lay awake at night going over that call, trying to find something I could have done differently. And now she accuses me and the others of stealing his wedding band. We were being wrongly accused but there was little we could do to change her mind. The fire chief wrote a letter to her lawyer stating no one could remember him wearing the ring and it was not found in the ambulance or jump kit. I doubt the letter impressed her or the lawyer.

Then another letter came threatening to sue the department. It was turning ugly. Our lawyer wrote their lawyer professing innocence of our crew and asking to see the proof if the other side did indeed have proof that the crew had stolen the jewelry. This really bothered us. Part of us was sorry the widow didn't have her husband's wedding band. Another part of us were indigent that we were accused of theft. We were all honest people and were well respected in the community and now we stood accused of theft. It hung over our heads like a black cloud. It was never far from our thoughts. We were frustrated and worried. Our reputation and the Fire Department's reputation were at stake. I knew I hadn't taken the ring and the other three people wouldn't have either. I had seen these people under pressure and I trusted each of them with my very life. We were innocent regardless of how it might appear.

Finally, six weeks after the man's death a handwritten letter arrived. It was from his wife. She said she went through his suitcase again and found the wedding band. She believed he took it off before showering that evening. She apologized for accusing us and thanked us for our attempt to save her husband's life. The biggest box of Whitman's Chocolate candy I had ever seen was with the letter. If felt good to be exonerated.

THERE MUST BE A FULL MOON TONIGHT

Mary and Henry Brown had been married for fifty-three years. They had led a good life. Henry had been a good provider and Mary had been a good mother of four and grandmother of ten, and a great-grandmother of two. Today they were on an adventure.

It was a little after two in the afternoon when they arrived at the Lee Ferry's boat ramp. They parked and got out. A small fishing boat had just been pulled from the water and tied down to the boat trailer. Two men climbed into their pickup and drove off. A slender young man named Joe, a local river runner stood at the water's edge, fiddling with a large raft, the kind used to run the rapids with groups of tourists. He didn't look up as Henry and Mary walked up nearby.

It was a hot August day, not a cloud in sight, no breeze, just blue sky and a huge fiery ball of heat and bright light shining down. The Colorado River rapidly speeded by, eager to travel through the beautiful Grand Canyon that lay just ahead. Henry stepped to the edge of the water and snapped pictures of the east wall of the canyon on the other side of the river. He loved taking pictures. "Smile, Mary," He said. She giggled and posed for the picture. Henry still saw the beautiful young girl he had fallen in love with fifty-five years ago every time he looked at his wife.

They followed the sign and found the trail head. It was a two mile trail with the river on their right and an eight-hundred foot rocky sandstone cliff on their left. Neither of them had ever been much of an outdoors person, but both were enjoying this day. Neither knew this was their last day together. It was probably better that way. Hand in hand they walked down the dirt trail. On their left they came upon the old mud brick houses that had once been the home of the Lee family. In the 1800's The

349

Lee family ran a ferry across the river as the Mormon families were traveling down the "Honeymoon Trail" from Salt Lake City to Tuba City and Mesa Arizona. "Stand by the house," said Henry. Mary walked over, turned around and smiled. As Henry took a few pictures, she noticed she was beginning to perspire. Thank goodness she was wearing her dark navy blue polyester pant suit. The perspiration wouldn't show. She also realized she should have never worn panty hose.

They continued their walk. Mary became very thirsty. Her mouth was dry. Neither she nor Henry had brought along water to drink. "Oh well," she thought, she would get a big glass of iced tea at the Marble Canyon Lodge Restaurant when they finished their little outing. A mile down the trail Mary quit sweating, her skin turned flushed, and she became nauseated. Her pulse increased and she was beginning to develop a headache. She wanted to go back to the car, but then she was distracted and smiled as she saw Henry down on his knees snapping a picture of a cactus flower. She could go on a little further. He was having such a good time. They continued to walk down the trail. It grew more beautiful. But Mary had developed a severe headache and was struggling to not throw up. She staggered, the world was fuzzy, and she struggled to keep her balance.

Henry noticed something was wrong. "Mary? Are you ok?"

"No, I don't feel well . . . . I'm sick . . . . my heart is pounding, I . . . . I . . . ." she mumbled, then fainted. Henry reached for her and lowered her gently to the ground.

"Mary? Panic was in his voice. He couldn't wake her. "Oh no!" His worst fear was coming true. She was having a heart attack! He yelled "Help, help," and looked around. No one was on the trail. They were completely alone. He slipped his hands under her arms and dragged her off the trail. He propped her up in a sitting position on the large flat rock. "I'm sorry Mary, I'm going for help." He reluctantly left her and ran head long down the trail back toward the parking lot, screaming "Help, someone help me, my wife's having a heart attack!"

Joe was a river runner. He was also an EMT and volunteered at the Page Fire Department. He looked up at the sound of Henry screaming. He secured the large raft he was readying for a float trip and hurried toward the screams. He found Henry, near breathless, running toward him. "What's the matter?" Joe asked.

"My wife. . . . . . (gasp) is having a heart attack . . . . That way." He pointed down the trail. Joe took off running down the trail. Henry followed at a slower pace, gasping in an effort to catch his breath.

Joe told me later he had prepared himself for CPR as he ran down the trail, going over the compression and respiration rate and ratio. As he

350

sprinted down the trail, he keyed his radio and called the National Park Service Ranger (NPS) assigned to Lees Ferry. "Bill . . . . Heart attack on the west trail . . . . get over here ." Bill responded in his SUV painted the disgusting green that was a favorite color of NPS.

Joe was surprised when he found Mary. "She was leaning up against this big flat rock, her head was laid back her arms flung outward." He ran to her side and felt for a pulse. It was weak, thready, and very rapid. Her skin was hot to the touch, red and dry. He had lived his life in the desert of Arizona and knew instantly, this wasn't a heart attack. It was heat stroke. "Sharon, she was laying there, frying in her own juices on that hot flat rock. You could have cooked an egg on that rock." He later told me.

Joe knew her brain cells were rapidly dying. Henry arrived just in time to see Joe heading for the river with an unconscious Mary cradled in his arms. "Hay, what the hell are you doing?" Henry shouted as he saw Joe leap into the cold Colorado River with Mary in his arms. Henry wasn't medical, but even he knew this wasn't the treatment for a heart attack.

Joe hit the cold water and prayed the temperature of the water wouldn't cause Mary's heart to stop. It didn't. Joe was a good swimmer and he kept Mary's head above water. He looked up and saw Henry was having a hysterical fit. "Its heat stroke. I've got to cool her down," he tried to explain, but Henry didn't believe him. About that time Ranger Bill arrived.

Bill looked down in the water at Joe and the patient. "Heart attack?"

"Heat stroke. She's really bad." Bill was a big man. He bent down and with no difficulty lifted the woman from the water. He checked and found a weak, rapid heartbeat and labored respirations. Joe climbed out of the river.

Bill got on his radio and called his dispatcher. "Get Page ambulance heading this way. We will head toward Page and meet them somewhere around Bitter Springs." The dispatcher made the call. Bill and Joe carried Mary back to the parking lot and loaded her into the ranger's vehicle. Henry followed, still confused about what was happening and worried beyond belief. The ranger's vehicle wasn't an ambulance, but this wasn't that complicated. Cool her off any way possible.

I was busy at the Fire Station in the ambulance bay. I had my left leg precariously perched on a small step ladder. My right knee was up on the driver's fender of Rescue-Two. I was balancing with my left hand and my right arm was extended outward. My fingers closed around the dip stick and I withdrew it just as the sound of my pager echoed through the metal building. "Beeeeeeeeeeeeeeeeep!" sounded the pager on my belt. I loved my work, but the timing sometimes was horrible. I had tried several times that day to complete the vehicle inspection, but I kept being interrupted. I shoved the dip stick back in the slot and climbed down. I shut the hood and went to wash my hands. By the time the driver arrived I was ready to go.

I rode shotgun as the ambulance pulled out of the station into afternoon traffic. Most people pull aside and let us past, but some don't. We quickly got through town and turned south on Highway 89. It was pedal to the metal time. Highway 89 is a narrow, two lane highway with very few pull offs. If vehicles from both directions pulled over as far as they could, the ambulance could squeeze through by straddling the yellow line. There wasn't much room and an element of trust was required, but we passed car after car in this manner and each time it worked.

Then, up ahead we saw the trailer. It was half of a double wide trailer being pulled by a large truck. It was creeping up the six percent incline of the Little Cut at a rip roaring fifteen miles per hour. There was not a passing zone. Time was a serious factor. The driver, Jake, looked over at me. "Get around him if you can, but be careful," I said. He slowed down. With red lights flashing and sirens blaring we roared ahead at fifteen miles per hour. The truck driver saw us, but there wasn't anywhere for him to pull over. "Frustrated" is the only word that comes to mind. I scooted around in the seat as I listened to the radio traffic. Bill had called in they were pulling out of Lees Ferry, heading our way. Jake finally took a deep breath and pulled out into the oncoming lane. He floored the accelerator and the ambulance leaped ahead. We zipped by the truck now crawling at a snail's pace. A curve was ahead. I said a prayer, hoping there wasn't a semi coming around that curve heading for us. There was, but we managed to get around the truck and trailer and slipped back into our lane with five feet to spare. The truck driver was wide eyed as he speeded past us.

I held on as we speeded around the tight curves and finally reached the top. For five miles we had a relatively flat road. We made good time. Then we entered the Big Cut and it was a seven mile downhill roller coaster ride, 6% grade, tight curves, old bumpy road and slow vehicles in our way. The guardian angel assigned to our ambulance had tattered feathers but managed to get us to the bottom of the steep hill safe and sound. I got on the radio "Where are you Bill?"

"Mile Post three."

"We are pulling off at the next wide spot in the road, meet you there," I said. "There, on your right." I pointed out a graveled pull off. Jake slowed down and pulled off the road and came to a stop. Up ahead we could see the ranger vehicle speeding toward us.

"I see you," he said on the radio. They pulled off and parked near the back of the ambulance. We got out and walked up to the ugly park service SUV. Joe was driving. He leaped out and opened the back hatch. Out jumped Bill. Bill was a good looking, big muscular man. I was surprised to see he was dressed rather oddly. He was still wearing his boots, dark green pants, and belt. His ranger hat was on his head, and no ugly gray shirt. He looked good, but strange somehow.

As the two EMT's unloaded Mary, Bill walked up to me to give his report. He explained she was in serious trouble. "I took my shirt and wet it down. I covered her with it. She's so hot to the touch."

"Well, that explains the new uniform," I said.

Rick laughed, "Its cooler, but I don't have a place to pin the badge." He laughed again.

We walked to the ambulance and saw them load Mary. "Where's her husband?"

"POV." (driving his private vehicle) "Good luck."

I jumped in the back and looked down at my patient. She was in her mid-seventies. She had been pretty once, and was still an attractive woman. Her hair was damp as well as her clothes. I almost fell when Jake spun the ambulance around and floored the accelerator. I cut her clothes off, down to her underwear. The EMT wet her down, dribbling water all over her, soaking her hair and body. The water ran off the stretcher onto the floor. I activated cold packs and placed one behind her neck, under her armpits, at her wrists, groin, behind her knees and at the soles of her feet. Blood vessels are close to the surface at those locations and my hope was that the cold packs might cool down the blood as it passed by.

My partner began to fan her. I turned the air conditioner down as cool as it would go. Her skin was so hot to the touch, the water quickly evaporated. I dribbled water all over her again and we continued to fan her. I checked her vital signs twice during the trip. They were not good. I was a Basic EMT at the time so treatment was kept to the basic level. I called the hospital and gave them a head's up on what we were bring in. They said they would be ready for us.

"Hang on! Jake yelled. The ambulance swerved left then right. "Damn tourist &#%$*!$%!" he said with feeling as he whipped the ambulance back in the correct lane. I didn't know exactly what happened, but I didn't hear grinding metal or breaking glass, so I guess it turned out ok.

We arrived at the Page Hospital Emergency Rooms back door and were met by a doctor and two nurses. The Page Hospital was small. It had

24 beds and a two room ER. At that time as you entered the ER entrance to your left was the regular size ER room, to your right is a much smaller one and had once been a storage room and before that the only dentist office in town. My partners unloaded her while I gave an update on Mary's condition. It wasn't good. They had set up an ice bed. It is an inflatable oblong container that looks like a child's swimming pool. They had filled it with ice and laid two sheets over it to protect the patient's skin from direct contact with the ice. We lifted Mary onto the ice. She didn't open her eyes, she didn't respond in any way. Her eyes stayed half open, seeing nothing.

The doctor started his exam as the two nurses started two IV's of cold normal saline. Vital signs were taken. We helped them for a little while then I went down to the break room and started our paperwork while the two EMT's cleaned the ambulance. Water was everywhere. It was a real mess.

About twenty minutes later, I finished all the paperwork. I got up and wandered leisurely down the hall. I stopped by the ER and looked in. Mary lay on ice, not moving, barely breathing. Her husband stood by her side. He looked down at her with tears in his eyes. He was in a personal hell. The two nurses and two doctors were running around, each trying desperately to fend off the grim reaper that now stood in the corner of the room staring at Mary.

Then I noticed, Henry, the patient's husband, reached up and rubbed his left arm and shoulder. He let go of Mary's hand and leaned forward, bracing himself on the gurney. I didn't like what I saw. "Are you alright Mr. Brown?"

He turned, his face was a pale color, and he raised his right arm and began rubbing his chest. "I'm alright. . . . . just take care of Mary."

"Mr. Brown, something's wrong. Do you have chest pain?"

"I . . . . . . .well, it's a little hard to catch my breath." He was breathing fast, and his distress was now obvious.

"Guys, I need a little help, (they ignored me) then I said the two magic words, "chest pain." Instantly two doctors and three nurses looked up. I stepped up to him and moved him across the hall into the tiny exam room. One of the doctors followed me. I got Henry onto the exam table and adjusted it in a sitting position. I cranked up the oxygen to high flow and slipped a non-rebreather mask on him. The doctor put on EKG leads. The doctor and I stood looking at the monitor. Now I understood why his chest hurt. At the time I couldn't read an EKG, but it was too fast, irregular, and at times an ugly blip would appear. That couldn't be good. If it wasn't stopped, he would have a serious heart attack. The doctor began barking orders and I jumped to his commands. A nurse broke away from Mrs. Brown and took over my duties. I was glad she showed up I was

354

a basic EMT at the time and well over my head. I went outside and walked up to the EMT's. They were ready to go. We got in. As the driver started the ambulance we saw a small car slide into the front parking lot. Two men leaped out and began to drag a young man out of the car. All three men were covered in blood. That got our attention. The oldest of the three men saw us, he screamed "Help, help!"

My two partners ran over to help, one turned and yelled back to me, "severed jugular!"

I turned and ran into the ER yelling "severed jugular at the back door!" Two critical patients in a two room ER made it full. The hospital had called in another nurse and she came running around the corner and tossed a sheet on the gurney in the hallway just as the EMT's drug the third patient through the back door. I ran to help them as the nurse prepared the stretcher. The patient was a skinny Navajo teenager. Blood covered his clothing; his eyes were open wide, His eyes were filled with complete terror. We laid him on the stretcher. The nurse and I bent down to examine the jagged, nasty looking gash located on the left side of his neck Dark red blood flowed abundantly from the open wound. No way was a dressing going to stem the flow of this blood.

As we all started to work on the boy, his uncle began to explain. "I was auguring with this other guy and Jimmy stepped in between us trying to break it up. Then that bastard lunged at me with a broken beer bottle and Jimmy got it in the throat." The other man stood silently, wringing his hands, staring at the young boy on the stretcher. Jake took his blood pressure and found it very low and a very rapid pulse, both signs of hemorrhagic shock caused by serious blood loss.

The other EMT ran to the ambulance and got our jump kit and an oxygen tank. He soon had the boy on high flow oxygen. The nurse was sitting up an IV. I slipped on gloves and tried to use a dressing to stop the flow of blood, but it didn't work, not even a little bit. I took a deep breath and reached into the wound. I felt around applying pressure here and there until the flow of blood slowed down and stopped. The beer bottle had cut the jugular vein. It's a very large vein in the neck. I had managed to apply pressure to the vein and thus control bleeding. I realized my fingers were deep inside the boy's neck and the only way to fix this was to have a surgeon stitch the vein closed. Page is very rural and we didn't have a surgeon at the time. In one way the boy was lucky. If his carotid artery had been cut he would have died. But the jugular is not under as much pressure and under the right circumstances can be managed.

The uncle and his friend left and went to the office to sign in the boy and call his mother. The nurse got the IV going. My fingers were cramping and she took over holding pressure to the vein. Just as I stepped

355

away from the stretcher, shaking my hands trying to restore circulation, the door to the ER exploded open. Two large Navajo men stormed in with fists clenched and angry expressions on their face and shouting. Had they come to finish the job?

The two male EMTs hurried to meet them. They were determined to keep the men from the helpless boy as he lay on the gurney. The nurse couldn't move. She was holding pressure on the wound. I picked up my radio and in an excited voice screamed for police backup as I watched the two EMTs exchange 'push-shoves' with the two men. This was getting nasty.

My husband was at home and over the scanner he heard me call for the police. I was usually calm and concise when speaking over the radio. But this time was different. Maurice at once recognized panic in my voice and he knew all hell had broken loose at the hospital. He rushed to my rescue. My knight in shining armor burst through the ER door and joined the two EMT's facing the angry men. The nurse and I decided to run. We pushed the gurney down the hallway with the boy looking back and forth at us with a worried look. We were almost running, where I have no idea, but heading there at top speed. Her fingers were still embedded in the boy's neck and I struggled with the radio, oxygen tank and IV as we shoved the gurney down the hallway. She and I were both covered in blood and we must have been quite a sight to behold because people stared at us as we zipped by. I didn't know it at the time, but Maurice and the two EMTs managed to back the two men out the back door.

I heard over the radio that the Page Police arrived (every officer on duty including the police chief). The Sheriff arrived, then two National Park Rangers, two DPS Officers (Highway Patrol) a Navajo Police Officer and one off duty Utah Highway Patrol Officer. They were outside and had called in a code-four, indicating the situation was under control. We turned around and slowly rolled the boy back to the ER hallway, hoping a doctor could leave the heart attack or heat stroke patient and maybe help with the boy.

Maurice and the EMTs came back inside. Maurice was an EMT and he relieved the nurse and held pressure on the boy's jugular vein. One EMT took vital signs again while the other replaced the now empty oxygen tank with a full one. The doctor caring for the heat stroke patient came out and asked Maurice to remove his fingers. He checked over the wound and we all noticed the blood started to flow again. The RN was ordered to relieve Maurice and apply pressure again. The doctor went in search for equipment. He had great expectations of doing a little surgery to repair the severed jugular. He came back, gave it a try. It didn't work He tried again, it didn't work The doctor left to call for Air Evac to fly the boy to Phoenix

Children's Hospital in Phoenix. The RN, Maurice and I took turns holding pressure. The boy finally spoke. He looked up at us and weakly said, "Thank you."

Blood was started on the boy and he was wheeled, far more slowly this time, down the hall to a room. There the RN and the doctor took turns holding pressure for over an hour and a half. The plane arrived from Phoenix about ninety minutes later. The air crew tried a few things and finally agreed that holding pressure was the only thing that worked. The RN and paramedic took turns all the way to Phoenix holding pressure and then all the way in the ground ambulance to the hospital. The surgical team was waiting and took the boy straight into surgery.

Two more medical air transports arrived. One took Mrs. Brown and the other flew Mr. Brown to a Phoenix area hospital. The two men went to jail, the RN and doctor's hands cramped in a claw for the rest of the day. The EMT's and I went back to the station, restocked the ambulance and went home. Maurice went back to the house, and the uncle meekly accepted the initial wrath of the boy's mother, his own sister.

We got word about three days later that the boy, Jimmy, had made it and would be as good as new. Mr. Brown, the man with the heart attack survived, but sadly, his beloved wife, Mary, didn't.

SEPTEMBER 11, 2001

This was a sad day in American History. I was asleep when my husband woke me up informing me that "terrorists just flew two planes into the World Trade Center." I jumped up, instantly awake. I knew what this meant. I hurried into the living room and saw on television the flaming towers. Excited reporters, who knew very little, were trying to explain what was happening. My sons were in town, putting a new roof on our house. We all sat and watched as the horror unfolded. Then someone said the building was going to collapse. People began to move away, then, slowly at first the towers folded upon themselves and fell as we watched in shock. We saw people running down the streets, covered in concrete dust. I said at the time the people should be holding cloths to their faces to keep the fiberglass and concrete dust out of their lungs. Even the simple face masks some of the police officers had put on were not good enough. Some people and many rescuers would later have serious lung problems that resulted in lifetime disabilities and at times cancer and death.

Toward afternoon, my Page Fire Department pager sounded. I responded down to the station. Our Fire Chief Vince Martin and Assistant Chief Lawrence Kindle was there and the people from fire and rescue arrived. The chief said we were going to an alert status. No one knew what to expect next. He said we were to watch closely our uniforms and ambulance. Terrorists could gain access to anywhere with two men in EMS uniforms driving an ambulance. We were told to watch for anything that looked strange. We were told to keep pagers on, approach scenes with heightened awareness. I left with an uncomfortable feeling. New York is a long way away, but now it was here in Page.

A week after the attack, I was working in Tuba City. My son, David, answered a knock on the door. A Page Police Officer stood there with a serious look on his face. "Do you know where your mother might be?" he asked.

"No," said David. He knew I was out of town for a few days working, but he didn't know when I left or when I would be back. He went and got his dad. The officer again asked where I might be. My husband came to the door and said I was in Tuba, working.

"When did she leave?" Yesterday, he answered. He and David were very confused. They were accustomed to odd things happening since my job was somewhat different, but the questions didn't make sense. "Have you heard from her since she arrived in Tuba?"

Maurice was now a bit worried. "Yes. She called last night."

Then the officer filled in the blanks. I had sold my car a few days ago. The car was parked in front of A-Automotive repair shop. The car's new owner had driven it there to be repaired on Monday. But the police thought it was still my car, and they knew they had not seen me recently, and the car was parked near the fire station. Police were very nervous and this didn't look right to them, and they were keeping a protective eye on fire and rescue people due to the threat of terrorists. They came up with a possible kidnapping. My husband told them we had sold the car and I was safe. He thanked them for their concern and they left. This was only the beginning.

TUBA CITY AIRPORT Early October, 2001

The female security guard pulled up to the Tuba city airport, unlocked the double gate in anticipation of the ambulance that was due anytime. They were meeting the Air Evac plane that would be landing soon. The airport was thirteen miles west of Tuba City. When the grant to build the new landing strip had been obtained, the Hopi and Navajo Tribes couldn't agree on where to build it. The Hopi's wanted it in their nearby village and the Navajo's wanted it in Tuba City. The two tribes have never played well together so they decided to build it in the desert away from either community. No one was happy.

It was just a landing strip with a lighting system housed in a small block structure with a generator. The lights were activated by the pilot going to a pre-set channel and clicking the radio microphone three times. The system was simple. Security from the hospital (thirteen miles away) would arrive and unlock the gate. The ambulance would arrive and the plane would land. The ambulance would take the air transport crew to the hospital. They would pick up the patient and the ambulance would drive the crew back to the airport and the patient would be loaded on the airplane and they would fly the patient to a larger hospital. It would take a total fifty-four miles driven by the ambulance and twenty-six miles driven by the guard to ship one person to a higher level of care. But it didn't seem to matter, the Navajo's were happy the Hopi's didn't get their way and the Hopi's were happy the Navajo's didn't get what they wanted.

The runway ran north and south. About a fourth mile from the south end ran Highway 160, east and west. About a quarter of a mile west ran Highway 89. The security guard was a Navajo woman around twenty-six years of age. She stood five foot four inches tall and weighed about one hundred and forty pounds. Her black hair was worn long. She took her job seriously. She looked up as a black car turned off the highway onto the small road leading to the airport. It stopped about two hundred feet from her. Two men got out. One was black and one was a man of mid-eastern descent. She tensed. The black man approached her with the brown man lingering behind. The mid-eastern man began snapping pictures, a lot of pictures.

She had seen pilots get out and snap a couple of pictures before, pilots like to collect snapshots of airports. But this group didn't look like pilots and twenty-four or so pictures of a small, uninteresting runway was overkill. She became very uncomfortable. "Hello," the black man said. "Waiting for an airplane?"

"Yes, an Air Evac plane is landing soon."

"How big is an Air Evac plane?" he asked.

"Kinda big."

"How far do you think a plane like that could fly?"

"I don't know." She was beginning to get worried. He began to ask all kinds of questions. She remembered the briefing they had received after Sept 11th. Terrorists love airplanes. Air Evac planes could be used by terrorists for a number of things and all were bad. Were they here to high-jack an airplane? She became frightened. She decided to try something, "The ambulance will be here any minute."

The man looked around quickly, as if looking for the ambulance. He then smiled and said, "We have to be going now." The two men climbed into the car and drove off. She radioed immediately and reported the men. Her supervisor arrived, followed by Navajo PD, and two black cars with two FBI agents. The reservation is "Federal" and the FBI had jurisdiction. The NPD and the FBI quickly found out the details and left to find the men. They were located by the NPD unit at a bead stand by the dinosaur tracks, about four miles east of the airport and about two hundred yards north of the main road.

The Navajo PD Officer that arrested them told me later that the black man was driving and became verbally abusive when approached. The officer slammed one onto the hood of the car and the man growled, "You have no idea who I am." It was a cold and chilling comment. Another NPD unit arrived and arrested the passenger. The FBI arrived and found one man in the back seat of one NPD car and the other in the back of the second NPD car. The FBI took over. The men were transported back to Tuba PD for questioning. The NPD officers were debriefed.

The ambulance arrived at the airport and the guard told them the story. The plane arrived. Then the FBI arrived. The ambulance and the air crew drove off as the security guard and the planes' pilot were hustled off for questioning by two men in black suits. When the ambulance crew picked up the patient at the hospital and were ready to leave, the FBI drove up and let the pilot off.

I came on duty the next morning at eight. A few hours later we were notified of a transport. There was a lot of illness on this side of the reservation and the Tuba Hospital was full. They had to ship out by ground and air due to the lack of beds. As we drove up to the airport to pick up the air transport crew, I noticed some things had changed. Number one, there was a black van sitting in the desert across the highway from the airport turnoff. It was new and had tented windows so we couldn't inside. It just sat off in the desert. I noticed it had a few antennas most vans didn't have. Then I noticed a small black helicopter. It hovered off the southwest corner of the airport, just a few feet above the ground. It too had tented windows, no tail number and no markings. It was there, day and night, whenever we came out to the airport. It had a sinister look about it with small missiles attached to the skids. I realized they were there for National Security reasons, but it was intimidating none the less.

360

A transport plane arrived and we met the crew. We were to take them to the hospital where the patient waited. As they got off, the first thing they saw was a pickup sitting by the east fence, about one hundred feet away. Two men leaned on the hood, rifles held high across their chest. It was the female security guard's brother and husband. They were there to protect her and us. We knew them and so we smiled, and waved. We then went about our business. I actually liked them being there. The helicopter was to keep terrorists from high jacking the plane and our protection was of low priority as far as their mission was concerned. The two Navajo's were there to protect the guard and us. I felt much safer.

After two weeks, the van and the helicopter disappeared. We never found out anything about what happened to the men who were arrested. The FBI refused to tell us anything.   Even the NPD didn't know what happened to the men. They said an unmarked Lear Jet landed at the airport to pick them up. No one ever saw them again. They are probably sitting in a cell at some undisclosed location at the time of this writing.

I began to be more aware of how vulnerable we were sitting in the middle of nowhere waiting for an airplane. The planes were big and would make large missiles in the hands of a terrorist. Hopefully, they have lost interest in Tuba City airport or any other small airport around the United States.

The RELAY YARD EXPLOSION(& Home Land Security)

September 11, 2001 everything changed. New procedures were devised to protect possible targets. The Glen Canyon Dam and the Navajo Generating Station were two targets that were on "the list." We were aware the radical Muslims knew about the two because of "intelligence" and a few odd happenings.

For the first year or so, National Park Service, and the Department. of Public Safety (in most states known as the Highway Patrol) took turns guarding the bridge and dam. Once, two mid-eastern men were seen taking pictures of the dam, but were not snapping pictures of areas most tourists photograph. They looked nervous and uncomfortable. When the NPS approached them, they ran for their car and sped off. Of course all kinds of radio traffic erupted, and every law enforcement officer north of Flagstaff started looking for them. They were not found. Finally the police received a few reports here and there from people that had seen them. Apparently they drove away from the dam and drove quickly through Page and headed east on Highway 98. They stopped along the road long enough to take pictures of Navajo Generating Station from various angles then disappeared. This left an uncomfortable feeling, but the mystery remained unsolved.

On April 20th, 2004, I was on call at the fire department. A loud explosion occurred. We were sitting in the high school parking lot and we had not heard or seen anything out at the dam. We had just been released from a false alarm pulled by teenagers. The report we got was "the dam called and requested an ambulance because a transformer blew." Well, my mind went right to patient care. It's a hazardous material situation due to the PCB's (mixed in the oil) in the transformers. Also, was someone working on the transformer when it blew? I dug out the guidebook for haz mat and begin looking up the proper guide. It tells us everything we ever wanted to know about handling PCB's.

The driver, Donald O'Reiley and EMT Fran, were up front and I was in the back. I heard Donald call and ask for a better location. I began reading out loud from the guide so they would know what we were going to do. Donald drove across the bridge and immediately turned left and started up a steep gravel road leading to the relay yard up on the hill, across from the visitor center. Donald slowed down. Up on top of the hill, by the gate to the relay yard sat two DPS cars. "Now what do I do?" asked Donald. "One is motioning me to drive on and the other is telling us to stop." I looked through the opening and said, "Stop." I saw the two officers, one of which was DPS Sergeant Dean Baker. He withdraw from the car, two assault rifles (M-16's) and tossed one to the other man. I then understood. This was more complicated.

DPS couldn't communicate to us over the radio because PFD had a new frequency and had withdrawn permission for DPS to put the frequency in their patrol cars. Our Fire Chief, Lester Cane was a control freak and wanted to limit access to Fire Department radio traffic and he had changed everything as far as radio communications was concerned. Previously we could talk to them and they could talk to us, but he didn't play well with other agencies, especially DPS and he severed communication between agencies. Now DPS had to call their own dispatcher and have them phone Page Dispatch and relay information or requests. Then the Page Dispatcher would call the DPS dispatcher and relay the PFD end of the transmission. It was a dangerous situation, but the chief was in control and that was all that counted, at least to him. DPS was concerned about the communication issue and PFD's Chief was concerned about the power issue.

Because of the PFD Chief's control issues, we sat on the gravel road unsure what dangers faced us. I could see Dean trying to talk to us over the radio. We just waited. Then he found a common radio frequency not often used and heard him say "Page Fire, we are treating this as tactical, (Medic One) stage at the (Dam) Visitor Center parking lot." Donald told him we copied and started to turn around and suddenly NPS's ambulance and fire truck drives up close behind our bumper.

I got out and walked back to the NPS ambulance. "This is a home land security issue, we have been ordered to the visitor parking lot. I don't know about you guys." Paul, an I-EMT from Big Water Utah and NPS ranger said they had heard the radio transmission and was also going to move over to the parking lot. He said we could turn around first and he would follow.

I got back in Medic-One and we slowly turned around, which wasn't simple since it was narrow, gravel, steep uphill road. At the visitor center we parked up next to a rock cliff that sheltered us from the relay station. Dean and the other officer slowly walked around outside the fence of the large relay station, rifles in hand. No evidence was found of entry into the yard. The two officers waited to enter the station until an employee got there to escort them since touching the wrong thing could kill you.

I looked up when I heard the siren blaring. PF Chief Lester Cane was rushing to save the world. Instead of pulling into the parking lot, he turned onto the gravel road and drove up and parked behind the police cars, got out and strutted up to Sergeant Baker. Now, there is no love lost between these two men. Dean's wife, Mary, use to work for the Fire Department and Lester ran her off with his unreasonable behavior. So when Lester walked up to Dean, Dean lost it. I am certain Dean couldn't believe Lester's arrogance. Without question, Chief Cane had to have heard the radio traffic. This was DPS's jurisdiction and any other agency that is involved is expected to follow orders. Dean had trouble believing how incredibly stupid Chief Cane was for entering an unsafe zone. If this had indeed been a terrorist act, Cane would have been in serious trouble. Few would have cared if Chief Cane had been shot by a sniper terrorist, but the paperwork would have been horrible so Officer Baker loudly and firmly ordered Chief Cane to leave the area, which he did. He came over the staging area, didn't say much, just sat on the engine step and quietly waited. He was very mad. We left him alone.

Phillip Yates, with the Bureau of Reclamation, a relay man, opened the gate and the three men entered the yard and investigated. They decided it looked as if it was not an act of terrorists and the explosion was "normal" equipment failure. No haz mat response was needed since the oil under the transformer was still on the concrete pad and no one had been exposed. We were released and drove back to the station.

What happened wasn't known until later that evening. At SRP's Navajo Generating Station (around seven miles to the east) there is a very large relay yard. Oddly, the generating station gets all its power from the dam and the two relay yards are connected. The transformer at SRP "went to ground" and blew up. Why? Well sometimes a snake or a large bird will cause the short. Also, equipment failure sometimes occurs. This actually isn't that uncommon according to my husband, Maurice, who was a relay man in Phoenix. The short back fed up the wires to the relay station at the dam had caused the transformer to blow up.

Even though it wasn't terrorists, it seemed appropriate action at the time. We are all uneasy about the threat. It has been reported that the dam has been mentioned in e-mails between known terrorists. Homeland Security believed terrorists are eyeing it with interest because it would be spectacular if the bridge or dam were blown up. Also, the generating station provided power to southern California and if they could disrupt power to southern California, it would make the six o'clock news. At this time we all continue to walk softly and carry a big stick.

PUBLIC REACTION

Public's reaction to the 911 event was intense and very emotional. A lot of people, including firefighters, police and EMTs were murdered that day. The general public realized the people who died were trying to help others. I was use to not being thanked for what I did. Sometimes people thanked me, but usually they were in the middle of the most awful thing that had ever happened to them and they would forget normal social niceties. Sometimes they would later write a letter or send a card, sometimes we would meet on the street and they would thank me, but in general, "thanks" was not a normal occurrence.

After 911, things changed, for a time. I remember being in Flagstaff a week after that horrible day. My partner and I had delivered a patient to Flagstaff Medical Center and we had stopped at Wal-Mart on our way back. I was in full paramedic attire, navy blue t-shirt with "Action Medical, Paramedic" printed on the back and over the left front pocket. I was wearing dark navy blue medic pants (sort of like cargo pants) and had a pager and radio on my belt. We walked into the store and the door greeter said "I just wanted to thank you for all you guys do." She smiled. We were surprised, but managed to gracefully accept her thanks. As we walked through the store, man, woman and children would walk up to us

364

and thank us for our service. It was nice to be recognized in this way. The average person's eyes had been opened by the heroic efforts of those in public service in New York and were taking the time to let us know they respected what we did and were thankful we were doing it.

A few days later we went into a Circle K store and the guy behind the counter said "My brother almost died in a car wreck about a year ago. I never told the EMT's thank you. I just want you two to know how much it means to have people like you. Thanks." It was obvious he meant every word. I thanked him and started to pay for my coffee, but he refused to accept our money. I was moved.

For months afterward, it happened often. It was nice to have complete strangers come up and thank me. Adults would approach us and say thank you. Children would smile and point at us and wave. Then as time went on, the public display of gratitude became less and less. Today, nine years after the event all we hear in the media concerns the dead fire fighters but no mention of the EMS personnel that died that day. It is rare to be acknowledged publicly by the general public. I'm not upset, but while it was happening, it was a good feeling.

THE CORN GAS STATION FIRE

All fire departments have a "Big One." This is the one incident that they talk about for years, the one that tested their resources, skills, training and bravery. Page Fire Department's "Big One" was the Corn Fire. It happened October 27, 1986. It was a Monday morning. It started out like any other morning. I am not a morning person. I had been up for three hours but at 9 am I was still struggling about the house in a semi-comatose state. The day was beautiful, the sky clear and the sun bringing warmth to an October day.

Suddenly a loud, deep boom broke the quiet morning. I watched in horror, as the large front window of my house appeared to bow inward and quiver as the shock wave hit it. I was surprised when the glass held. Nick-knacks on my shelve rattled about, the dog jumped up and stood looking about confused. There was no doubt in my mind, something big had exploded and it was nearby. I rushed to the front door, slipped on my shoes, grabbed my car keys and my radio and rushed outside. I had no idea where I was going, but I knew soon, very soon, the radio would come to life and I would know.

As I rushed to my car the voice of the fire chief blared over the airway. Usually he is calm over the radio, but today his voice had an edge to it that alerted me to the seriousness to the event. "...Phillips 66 has just had an explosion. Page a full call out..." Phillips 66? I got in the car and started it. I searched for the gas station's location in my memory. Yes, the corner of Lake Powell Blvd and North Navajo. No, they tore it down and built a 7-11 convenience store. Phillip 66? Oh yes, Corn's Tires (and gas station) on the corner of Aero and North Navajo, two blocks east of its old location. I turned on South Navajo and looked up. I could see a dark black smoke rising straight up in the windless sky. It looked bad. I tried to image what could have happened. Nothing I thought of was good.

To backtrack just a little, this story actually started three days before, on Friday afternoon. The Corn's (father and sons) had discovered that they had under built. They needed more storage space. In an effort to correct that oversight, they decided to build a little storage shed on the back of the station. Nothing too fancy, just a small enclosed room to store the tires.

That same day, a little after five o'clock, a member of the Page building department (who would prefer to remain nameless) was driving home and noticed construction activity behind the station. He knew they had not applied for a building permit. He made a mental note to check on what they were doing first thing Monday morning. When Monday morning arrived he decided to make a few calls and handle a few small items of business before going over and checking on the unauthorized construction project. The building inspector ended up spending the first hour of work on more pressing business.

"Timing is everything," I once heard. Maybe, maybe not, but this time it defiantly played a part. Now, a gasoline tanker drove up to off load fuel. The driver fitted the hose into the underground tank and started to pump. Now, when an underground tank empties, fumes fill the empty space. When liquid is pumped into the tank, it pushes the fumes out. A vent pipe is always placed above ground to allow the fumes to safely vent into the air. Guess where the shed was built? They built it around the vent pipe. Oh, they left a few inches above the roof, but not enough to vent the fumes anywhere except down into the shed. It was cool and the fumes fell downward and filled the shed and lay patiently waiting for an ignition source.

At the same time the gasoline tanker was pumping, a propane tanker, with the capacity of 6,000 gallons of propane arrives. Now there is no rule prohibiting both from off-loading at the same time, so the driver connected to a 1,000 gallon propane tank and begins to pump liquid propane into it. Mr. Corn smelled something about this time, inside the building. Now remember, timing is everything. He got up and walked to the back of the store, sniffing. He opened the back door that opened into the new shed, just as the pop machine kicked on. Presto, ignition. The fumes that hung on the floor exploded and moved as a fiery wave, outward. The percussion of the blast knocked seventy-two foot long double wide trailers off their foundations across Aero Avenue. Nearby trailer's front doors and windows exploded inward as the wave hit them. Debris was thrown over seventy feet in all directions.

Children screamed and mothers went in frantic search for their young. On the north east corner sat the Warner's nursery. Their plate glass window shattered inward, spraying glass into the store and knocking over plants and displays as the employees dove for cover. Remember, timing is everything? Well a local man had just filled his gas tank. He replaced the nozzle and then dropped his gas cap on the ground. He bent down just as the explosion roared to life. Flames and derbies sailed over his car. He was completely shielded by his car and wheel. He didn't ask any stupid questions. He just got in his car and peeled rubber and drove away from the now flaming gas station his gas cap still in his hand.

The fire station is only a half block from the fire. Chief Nelson arrived to find the building smoking and flames quickly growing. The main thing that caught his attention was the double trailer tanker truck with hose still sticking in the filler opening in the ground leading to the underground tanks. The driver was struggling to quickly remove the hose. "Get the truck out of here!" yelled the chief. The driver needed no encouragement at all. He was now so hyper and wired with adrenalin that he could have picked up the truck and carried it away from the pending explosion but instead he leaped in his truck and roared forward climbing over tin and boards and pulling two blocks down before he parked his rig and sat down with quivering hands to ponder his life and the near loss of it.

The Assistant Fire Chief Timmy Alton, one Engineer, (Stan Links) and one firefighter, (Mark Teak) rushed to the screen. The Fire Chief and Assistant Fire Chief and I, the Rescue Chief, were full time, but all the others were volunteers and most of our firefighters worked during the daytime. The number on the initial responding engine wasn't near enough to do the job. Chief Nelson became the captain and Assistant Fire Chief Alton was demoted to firefighter. They now had one engine fully staffed; it was reminiscent of David rushing to fight Goliath.

Police descended upon the scene and set about evacuating people from the street behind the flaming gas station and the trailers across Aero Avenue. One young officer a new one fresh from the academy who's name

I wish I could remember, noticed a hand move and reach feebly up from under a pile of debris and flip the switch on the propane truck to kill it. I don't know why but the dead man switch had failed. The officer wadded into the scattered wood and tin in an effort to get to the injured man lying beside the biggest bomb you can image, a propane truck with a capacity load of 6,000 gallons (according to Black Mountain Gas). He reached the spot and heaved the sheet of metal off and picked the timber off the man. He looked down at the man. He was sixty-one years old and an employee of Black Mountain Gas. His face and hands were cut and bruised by the flying debris. A severe laceration to his arm was bleeding. His leg was shattered and badly angulated. The officer looked up at the burning building and the huge tanks and tanker truck. It took him only a split second to say to hell with all the EMS training that preaches against moving an injured person without trained help and equipment. He grabbed the man heaved him up over his shoulder and carried him away from the fire. He gently laid the badly injured man in the middle of Aero Avenue.

As I drove to the scene I listened to the radio traffic. It sounded bad and appeared to be getting worse. I drove by and had to swerve around pieces of plywood in the road. I looked and saw the man on Aero laying still. I headed that way. Suddenly my radio came to life. "Sharon! Get out of there!" I looked up and could see the Fire Chief. He motioned me back the way I had come. I looked up and saw his concern. I had stopped in direct line of the huge propane tank that was being heated by the flames from the burning building. If it blew, it would blow from the ends and I was in direct line of what could be the "missiles path." The tanks were taller than a man, and longer than a full size pickup truck. I complied by moving my car and parking in front of the restaurant, Bella Napoli.

I parked my car and got out. I stood looking over the situation. It was grim. The two propane tanks were above ground, one was 1,000 gallons and the other was 500 gallons. The LPG truck was parked near the larger tank. PFD had battled to have them moved but finally the city attorney who was barely adequate and could never hope to achieve anything but mediocrity had decided to grandfather them. Now I could see the flames licking out the windows of the station and wrapping around the tanks hugging them sharing its warmth and heating the liquid inside.

I thought, "This is bad." I could see for the first time we were facing a horrible test. There was only two choices, fight it or give up and run. To fight meant to gamble everything and everyone's life on winning. To lose meant to die. Our second choice was to give up and let it blow. Run? Evacuate? To evacuate was a fantasy. I could see at least a hundred people milling around watching the fire. The area on three sides was heavily populated and there was no way to evacuate in the time we had between now and the pending explosion. If I was to go by the book, a quarter mile radius, maybe more, should be evacuated. With a handful of officer s and hundreds of homes, many businesses, and the main street of town in the "fire ball zone" I just didn't think we had time to even try to evacuate. This was either going to work or it wouldn't. If it didn't, I wouldn't be around to be yelled at.

I watched as the four men rushed about setting up a hose to cool the tanks. I understood firefighting techniques. I could see that the chief was going to fight. Did I want to be part of the battle? I wasn't sure I did. For the first time in my career I seriously considered just turning around and leaving. To die by fire wasn't the way I wanted to go. I stood looking that kind of death in the face. I could be dead in the next few minutes. I don't mean to be melodramatic, but I could die in a ball of orange and yellow fire as my flesh burned and fell from my bones. I could..... No this was the job I had promised to do. So many lives depended on this working. If they were going to fight it so was I. Maybe I could move the "command post out of the pending fire ball's range? No, the fire station was too close to the incident and if I was to be of any help, due to the serious shortage of man power, I had to be there on site, not hiding out of danger's way several blocks away. I shoved the vision of the pending fire ball into the back of my mind. I looked around. I could never hope to evacuate all the stupid people that were flocking to the excitement.

What could I do to help the four desperate men, struggling to get water on the heated propane tanks? I looked over and could see men and women skidding into the fire department parking lot and rushing into the station. I looked at the people that now blocked Navajo, the street that ran in front of the fire. I decided the best thing I could do was crowd control and start organizing the responding fire and rescue personnel. If I could clear the way for responding rescue equipment that would speed up the entire process.

"Command . . . . Dispatch?" The radio had came to life. No answer. The Police Dispatcher was trying to contact the Fire Chief. I couldn't see a single policeman except the one sheriff that stood in the middle of the street watching. I was only one person and I would need help.

I saw the local newspaper reporter wandering around the fire scene snapping pictures. I had ran him off from more fire scenes than I could count, but this time I ignored him. He wasn't in anyone's way and I just didn't have time to chase him down and run him off.

"Sharon is there anything we can do to help?" I turned around to the sound of my name. There stood the biggest SOB north of Flagstaff. J.B. Reighman, NPS Superintendent of the Glen Canyon Recreation Area. He and several rangers had walked up from the district office three blocks away.

I had never liked the man, but any port in a storm. "You have uniforms and are easily identified as authority. I need you to clear these people back to give room for the responding fire engines and ambulances. We are going to set up here in the street."

"Which people?"

"Those people across the street (I pointed to the large group of people that had gathered in the parking lot of the shopping center that had been evacuated) need to be moved back. So do the ones in the street."

"How far back?"

Try to get them to leave the area. If they won't get them out of the way of responding fire units; they have to be moved back to the corner west of the fire station (Lake Powell Boulevard and Navajo)"

"You've got it." J.B. turned and assigned his men to the task." He then turned back to me after they left. "Sharon ....the tanks?" I knew what he was asking. I don't think all of his men completely understood the seriousness of the situation but he obviously did.

"Hopefully they won't blow. If they do, we don't have a prayer." I know that wasn't what he wanted to hear, but it wasn't the time for lies. He shook his head in understanding and walked away to help his men. I never liked the man and probably never will but at that moment I respected him.

"Command . . . Dispatch?.........COMMAND . . . DISPATCH!" Still no answer from the Fire Chief. I could see him moving around the area but he didn't answer his radio. I saw Sam the engineer of the only fire truck at the scene struggling with the hose. He had got it connected to the hydrant and was spinning the crank to allow the water to rush into the hose .I relaxed a little. Water to cool the tanks would postpone the coming explosion and just might by enough time till additional engines could arrive.

"We just might win this one after all" I thought as hope suddenly appeared. I waited for the hose to grow round with water. The hose lay flat. Something was wrong . . . . very wrong. Sam straightened up and ran like a gazelle to the engine. He keyed his radio.

"Engine one to Command!" he yelled into the radio. No answer. He tried again no answer. "Command in the blind, we have no water the hydrant is dry." He threw the radio down and leaped from the engine.

"Damn!" I said out loud. I stood helpless watching as Sam ran to the hydrant and disconnected the hose and ran dragging it behind him to another hydrant. The firefighter that held the nozzle was getting baked well done. Mark held a dry hose nozzle in his hand and knelt only a few feet from the 1,000 gallon tank. The propane truck with another 6,000 gallons of propane sat only feet away from the flames. He could only watch the flames lick the tank and truck and heat them up. Doubt filled his mind and soul. Sam broke records in connecting the hose to the second hydrant. I watched in silence prayer as he spun the wrench on top. Water sprang forth from below and ran quickly down the hose filling it and leaping forth from the nozzle. Precious, cool water, praise the Lord!

The tanks sizzled as the cool water hit them. Steam fogged the air. One of the Corn son's (I won't name him in this piece) walked up to me. He had stood in the crowd watching the firemen struggle to get water. He had expected the water to go on the burning building. When it hit the tanks instead he went berserk. He was thirty-seven years of age, a large man with a known temper. We had had difficulties with him before when his home had a small chimney fire. "What the hell are they doing?" he yelled as he charged toward me waving his arms.

"They have to cool the tanks."

"The building's on fire not the damn tanks!" He walked up invading my personal space, "The f......... tanks will cool if you put out the damn fire!" A Note for all non-fire fighting people, every fire fighting book will tell you to cool the tanks first (because of the explosion danger) then with additional help put out the fire. I tried to explain that that was the best way to control the situation. All he could see was his families building. A young woman, his current girlfriend walked up and tried to calm him down but it didn't work. I noticed he was burned on his arm but he violently refused any treatment.

"See that window?" He pointed to the west front window. Flames were roaring out of it with a vengeance. "Well, just outside that window is a five-hundred gallon propane tank and it's completely engulfed by the flames." (The tank was about six foot long and about three foot tall)

I keyed my radio. "Command . . . . . . F-3" again no answer. I tried a couple more times. I could see him but I couldn't raise him on the radio. "Command . . . . F-3 in the blind, there is a 500 gallon propane tank engulfed in the flames coming from the windows on the west side of the building." I looked back at the station. The second engine was pulled out on the apron and responding firefighters were climbing aboard. I knew they were copying the radio traffic and they now knew about the tank. I keyed my radio, "Engine Two?"

"Engine 2," responded Captain Earl Tanner.

371

"Your assignment is the tank on the west side of the building, under the window. Get water on it." If command wasn't answering the radio, someone had to make assignments. I had gone through all the fire commands training and had actually handled a couple of small house fires, but this was a major event and I sounded far more confident on the radio than I felt at that moment. The crowd had been moved back by the rangers and the rangers stood guard. Whatever anyone would say about the local rangers, mostly bad, they could take orders and did that well. I again, silently, thanked J.B. for getting involved.

I could see second degree burns to the Mr. Corn's son's face and head. "Will you let me treat your burns?"

"Hell no!" He put his arm around his girlfriend and together they walked across the street and disappeared into a real estate office. I could see the way was clear for the next engine. I mentally made a note of where I wanted the ambulance to park when it arrived.

"F-3 dispatch." I answered. "We can't get F-1 to answer" she continued. "I got a call from the school . . . . they want to know if we want them to release the firefighters that teach for them?" Only one week prior to this the Fire Chief and I had talked about the deal we had struck with the school and the power plant. Only for the "Big One" would we have them call their employees that were firefighters/EMTs away from their jobs. The negotiations had gone on for almost a year and wasn't really liked by the school or the plant but accepted as their civic duty. They reluctantly agreed to the plan. I was told to never put the plan into action unless it was really "the Big One." Was this the Big One?

Yes, it was. But I didn't exactly have the authority to activate the system; I wasn't actually "Command." The fire department pecking order had me third in command and number one and number two were already at this fire. What if I was wrong and this wasn't the big one? Later when the tape was played back everyone laughed and joked about how it took a whole three seconds for me to assume authority I didn't have. "Yes, and call the plant and have them send their men too." I had just done something that would either get me praised or fired if I lived through this. I stood looking at the tank that was engulfed by flames. It could blow soon. No water was being put on it. Only the bigger tank was being cooled. Again I considered moving the command post six blocks away, but I couldn't abandon the men working so hard to gain control of the monster called "fire." Also, weather I liked it or not, I was "Command." If I made a wrong decision and the tanks and tanker truck blew, the six thousand gallons of propane would kill me, the entire fire department and hundreds of people.

Why won't the Chief answer the radio? Later we found out his radio had fallen from his pocket and he didn't know it was gone. For nine and a half minutes, I was command. For the non-firefighters out there, the first ten minutes is the most critical because that is the time assignments are made, trucks told where to park, and the whole system is set up and a plan of action is formulated. I decided to set up in the middle of the street. If the big tank blew, it wouldn't matter anyway.

The second engine roared past me, still trying to reach Command on the radio. They couldn't raise the Fire Chief either. The volunteers were an independent lot and they just rushed in and did what obviously needed to be down. Luckily the captain on that engine, Earl Tanner had copied my radio transmission and knew the tank was located in the flames and he was going after it, just as "Medical Control" had ordered him to do. Three men took two hoses over the tank under the window and began cooling it down.

The ambulance drove up. I had them park and wait. "Medical Control, dispatch?"

"This is Medical Control," I said.

"I have Wahweap on the phone. They want to know if you need their medics and one fire engine."

I hesitated. I didn't like it, but apparently I was now officially in Command. "Yes, have them roll."

Everything was happening at once. It's hard to put it all in order of occurrence. My personal thoughts were jumbled and brief. I was busy. I only remember shoving the fear of dying back into a dark corner of my thoughts and the brief thought of my family. My two sons were in school. "Good." It was far enough away that even if this blew, they should be safe. The only thing that bothered me was my husband. I knew that by telling dispatch to call the plant that I was involving my husband in this. Now we both could die. Who would finish raising our sons? "Stop that Sharon" I thought." No time for that now. No time."

My youngest son, Stephen was twelve years old at the time and had heard the explosion and felt the windows rattle, but was unaware of all the excitement until later in the day. Unknown to me my oldest son wasn't safely at school. His carpentry class had boarded a van and had left the school to visit a construction site, sort of a field trip. They had heard the explosion just as they were boarding the van. They had stopped for donuts at Basha's Grocery store at least that was the excuse the ex-firefighter teacher gave for stopping. The store would have been within the outer edge of the fire ball had one occurred.

David was sixteen and had spent a lot of time listening to firefighting stories. He knew a lot about the dangers. He and the others had gotten out of the van and walked to the corner to see what had exploded. David looked down the street and could see it was a gas station.

He saw the plume of smoke and the activity. He saw me walk away from my car. His thoughts were of his cameras. He was rather fearless when it came to getting a good picture. His Pentex camera was in the trunk of my car. He briefly considered how he could get his camera out without bothering me. He decided he couldn't get a picture so he would just look out for number one and get out of there. He turned to his teacher. "You can stay if you want but I'm leaving."

Mr. Charles had been a volunteer firefighter a few years ago. He too realized what had happened and what could happen. "We're all leaving," he said. He quickly got the boys in the van. They didn't go to the planned building site (located within a few blocks of the fire). He drove to the far side of the town and off the mesa to another site. He took the boys just about as far from any potential fire ball as he could and still stay within the city limits.

Maurice, my husband was sitting in his shop working on a radio when his phone rang. He answered it. It was his boss. "Maurice there was an explosion and fire in town."3 .

"I'm on my way," he said as he slammed the receiver down. He hurried from the shop and ran to his truck. He climbed in and floored the gas pedal never to lift it again until he roared into the fire station parking lot in record time. As he sped the six miles into town he said he could see a black plumb of smoke rising into the sky for two hundred feet. Maurice knew it was bad. He knew that by responding he was putting himself in extreme danger but the thought of responding never crossed his mind. He knew I was in the middle of it and brief thoughts of my safety crossed his mind. He had a job to do and he was going to give it his best shot. He also knew I had a job to do and he wouldn't interfere. As he approached town, he came upon a road construction project. The man standing in the road with a stop sign had no idea why Maurice roared up to him and rolled down his window. "There's a fire in town, I'm a firefighter and a bunch of other firefighters are behind me." The man looked surprised, but understood. He had seen the smoke rising up from town and now he knew what happened. He let Maurice through and pondered how to handle the line of firefighters speeding toward him.

Back at the scene I stood watching as the second engine company prepared to put water on the small tank engulfed in fire. I heard a man's voice behind me say, "Excuse me?"

I turned around. A short young man stood beside me. "What is it?" I asked.

"There are at least fifty people behind that building." he pointed to the two-story shopping center that had been evacuated. I knew an alley ran behind the center. If the big tank blew it wouldn't matter. But if the

374

smaller one blew, maybe they could live through the explosion if just a bit further away from the explosion. But the group stayed behind the building, they could be in firefighter's way and they were in server danger if the small tank blew.

I looked around. J.B. had returned and was standing near me. Beside him was a short, thin young man in his early twenties. He was a paper pusher. "I need your help," I said motioning to him. He didn't look like much but he was wearing a uniform he would do. His eyes grew big. His mouth opened but no words came out.

J.B. said in his most authoritive voice "Go with her and do whatever she tells you to do." The young man reluctantly followed. We walked across the street and around the shopping center. We walked down the alley. There were at least fifty to seventy-five people gathered at the end of the building. They were in a horrible place. They stood watching the excitement as the firefighters hit the flames and the tank with water. One woman held up her three year old son so he could see.

"Dumb, dumb people," I thought. "I'm with the Fire Department, everyone out of here. You are in a dangerous area." They turned and looked at me. The young ranger just stood behind me and said nothing. They began to move." Hurry. A propane tank could blow." That got them moving. The boy and I followed them down the alley. I left him at the alley's entrance to keep them back. He seem happy to be alive and willing accepted what he thought was a safe job and far enough away. Little did he know.

One of the people in that crowd was a man named Billy Woodspur "Friendly Billy's Motel." He had a camcorder and was taping the fire. He sold the tape to a Salt Lake Television Station and we made the six o'clock news. He later gave me a copy. I treasure it.

The plant was six miles away the school only one and a half but the men from the plant started arriving first. I saw my husband walk toward me. "Hi, where do I go?" he asked." Back to the station and get your full turnouts on," I said.

"I'll use someone else when they get tired," he said.

"No you won't. Go get you own on and come back." I waited. He was boss in our home. Would he take orders from me? Maurice hesitated a second and then turned around and headed back to the station. I signed a sigh of relief. I watched in amusement as he met a group of men also rushing without turnouts toward the fire. I guess they just focused on the fire and started moving toward it, without thought of taking the time to put on their protective gear. "Might as well go back, we can't do anything till we get fully dressed. It's an order." They reluctantly turned around and followed him back to the station.

"Page. . . Command." At last the Fire Chief was on the airways.

"Go ahead Command."

"Call the school and plant to release firefighters."

"That's already been done sir."

He was quite for a moment. Then he answered. "Very well." I could tell he would investigate later why it was done without his permission. Oh well, that's life.

"Medical Control, Command."

"Go ahead Command"

"We have an injured man over on Areo near Engine One. Get a crew in there. Load and go."

I turned to my EMTs who awaited orders. I knew what the Fire Chief was saying. Things were sort of under control. . . sort of. It was still a gamble. "The man is lying right over there." I pointed to the spot. Three people were kneeling around him, one was an off duty male nurse from the hospital one Sheriff's Officer and a bystander. They (Doug Alton, Mitch Riley and one other,) ran with jump box in hand as the ambulance driver slowly drove through debris and fire hoses to park as close as possible to the spot.

I stood watching as they broke all records rolling him on a backboard and threw him in the ambulance and sped off. This was the first time I had ordered someone to do something that could very well result in their death. I was amazed they didn't hesitate. They did it and did it without question. I turned around and saw park service ambulance arrive. Good timing. Quickly I told them what was happening. They parked their rig behind the Italian restaurant. It was block and would shield them from the fire ball. . . . maybe.

The volunteer firefighters were back this time fully attired in firefighting gear. I looked at them. I knew them all. They had the look of eager anticipation on their faces. They were a different breed. They loved this stuff.

I tried to contact the Chief over the radio, but there was no answer. I gave up. "Report to Captain Tanner over there." I pointed to the west side of the building. They hurried off. I had just given my husband an assignment. I prayed it didn't result in his death or injury. Captain Lenny Miller arrived with the old fire engine. I assigned him the inside sector.

A woman walked up to me. She was in her early thirties, about thirty pounds overweight. She was dressed in jeans, t-shirt, tennis shoes. Her dull brown hair hung unstyled to her shoulders. "I live two blocks away. I left my daughter at the house. How serious is this?" She asked.

"Do you have a friend down off the mesa in Lake Powell Mobile Home Village?" I asked.

"Yes," she answered.

"Well. . . . Now would be a great time for you and your daughter to go visit her." She thanked me and ran off.

Two men Mark Teak and Brody Smyth had been manning the two hoses cooling the huge tanks off. Brody had been on the second truck and had gone to help Mark with a second hose. The two men were giving one-hundred and fifty percent. The heat was horrible. It radiated through their suits. Their bodies dripped with sweat. They would swing their hose off the tanks and hit the fire as it roared through the window to cool it and then swing back to the tanks. They were melting inside their suits from radiant heat.

Finally Brody, with Mark's "ok", moved away and staggered to Engine One. He fell to his knees and then flat on his stomach. He rolled over on his back and lay there gasping for breath and unable to move. Stan's voice boomed over the radio. "Firefighter down by Engine One!"

"Medical Control copies," I said. Our ambulance had not returned from the hospital yet. I turned to the ranger medics. "Over there, by that engine." They raced to their van and hurried over. Brody was young. I was surprised to find that it was always the younger firefighters that gave out first. He was eighteen and so exhausted he could raise his arm. His feet lay still and he couldn't talk. His eyes were open but he was out it. He had given everything he had and had nothing left.

The park medics got him in the ambulance, started IVs, began cooling him and rushed to the hospital. I watched them leave. I hated it when it was one our own. "Sharon? Where do you need us?" I turned around and there stood two more firefighters from the school. I tried to call the Fire Chief again who had assumed command. But he didn't answer.

"Go to Engine one. Find out from Stan what the firefighter was doing that went down and go take his place." They both left. One took Brody's place on the nozzle and the other relieved Mark.

I turned around as I saw the National Park Service fire truck drive up. I had a bad feeling when I noticed that the men on board all had new, clean turnouts. One got off and walked over to me. "We can do whatever you need us to do, except pump water. We haven't covered that yet and none of us know how to do that."

I was somewhat shocked by their comment. I could find jobs for the firefighters, but why did they bring this huge, slow fire truck if it was of no use but transportation? I tried to not let my irritation show. These men were bravely offering to help and I could use them. "See that man with the red helmet?" I was pointing to Captain Miller who was standing in the doorway of the building. "All of you go over to him and do what he tells you to do." They smiled and walked off. I believe they had no clue to what a dangerous assignment I had just assigned to them. Oh well, ignorance is bliss.

Utility one arrived. Utility would handle assignments of individual firefighters from now on. Captains would call for needed manpower and utility would make the assignments. The truck carried extra Scott packs as well as drinking water and equipment. The system was finally in order. Command was commanding and the other pieces of the organization were now in place. I relaxed a little. The danger of bevy was less as time passed. And I no longer was burdened with total command of the incident. I now concentrated on Medical Control duties.

A man came up to me. I didn't know him. He was a member of the firefighting unit at the plant and not a member of the Page Fire Department. His name was Branson La Pole. After telling me who he was he asked to be assigned. I really was through with that, but this was different. "Do you know about Scott bottles?"

He shook his head to the affirmative. "Really now....can you put them on and take them off and know how to handle them?"

"Yes I do."

"OK, go to that white truck (utility). I want you to help the firefighters off with empty packs and on with new ones. Devise any method you want but keep the empty ones separate from the full ones." He hurried off. I must add that he did a very good job that day. He later joined the fire department and in 2002 he was made Assistant Fire Chief.

"Where do we go?" I turned around and there stood more firefighters and EMTS.

"Firefighters go to Utility one for assignments. EMTs stay here with me." I had a lot of equipment and they could use it if someone needed help until the ambulance was clear from the run to the hospital. Sherri Parish a local reality agent and personal friend came over and offered a large water cooler bottle of water and all the coffee cups she could find. I thanked her. I set up a monitoring station for the exhausted firefighters.

Inside the burning building my husband crawled on hands and knees. He couldn't see anything for the heavy black smoke. He was with Captain Tracy Homes. They were dragging a hose and were extinguishing any flames they came across. The burnt wood was black, the smoke was black, and the world was dark. The two men felt completely alone in this alien environment. They could hear the roar of the fire and the hollow sound of their breathing in the respirator. They had a pole and were using it to clear a path.

Suddenly Maurice bumped into something. He moved his faceplate close and peered at it. It was a propane bottle the type that goes on a RV. It was hot and black from the flames. Maurice grabbed Tracy and pointed at the bottle. Tracy's face mask filled with "eyeballs" as he grasped the situation. There were other bottles. They both felt their stomach flip. Hot propane bottles? This isn't good. Maurice hooked one bottle and gently lifted it out through the gaping hole in the wall. The firefighter standing outside with a hose was there as a backup if something flared up. He was quite surprised to see the blackened propane bottle appear out of the smoldering ruins.

No one needed to tell him what to do. The bottle had not quite settled on the ground before the water hit it. It sizzled as steam rose off it. Another bottle appeared suspended on a pole. He hosed it off too. So on and so on. Later the firefighter that was standing outside told me the story and said he was shocked to see a smoldering LPG tank emerge from the charred hole in the wall. He said he hesitated only a second as he watched in dismay as the tank was placed on the ground by the mysterious pole. He forgot the burning building and set about cooling the tank. He said he was beginning to calm down when a second tank appeared then another and another. He didn't know who was inside the building, but he wished he himself were somewhere else. He said he was so sure the tanks would blow and he was about to die.

"Page Command.......We have control," the radio announced. I smiled. I was going to live and so were the others. It was a good day. We had cheated death and won. The fire chief called me over. For the first time I walked across the street and into the parking lot of the station. "We aren't sure but we are missing a nine year old girl. She was in the building just before the explosion. Her mother can't find her."

My eyes traveled to the blackened hull. The roof had caved in and the sides were charred black. They were still standing but not intact. If she was in there she was dead. Morbid visions of a charred small body flashed in my mind. I had seen burnt bodies before and they were not pretty. A nine year old who had died that way was more than I wanted to face that day.

I went to check out if anyone had an idea where the girl might be. After a lot of questions it was discovered she had asked her father if she could go to grandmas (on the block behind the station). He had said "yes." He had then gone to investigate the strange smell in the storeroom. The mother knew nothing about the daughter leaving.

The father and mother had fled the building separately and both had been burned. They had wandered around lost in the crowd and finally he was driven by a friend to the hospital and the woman was driven by a policeman. It took a while but finally communication was established and the daughter was found safe with grandma.

I went back to the fire department office to call the State Fire Marshal's office. This was going to take careful investigation and an outside agency was a good idea. I walked into the office and was met by a harried secretary. It was her first day on the job and she had been left alone in the office with complete pandemonium.

I took the stack of phone messages she gave me and sat down at my desk. It was the first time I had sat down and relaxed since the explosion. I buried my face in my hands and shut my eyes. I was suddenly very tired. I opened my eyes and made the phone call to the State Fire Marshal's office. He said he had heard it on the news and was on his way. I glanced through the stack of messages. Reporters and more reporters had called including Salt Lake City, Phoenix and Flagstaff. One caught my eye. Tom Brocah from New York had also called. I tossed them aside. Reporters didn't impress me. I had grown to dislike them with a passion. They were like vultures that were attracted to death and disaster and fed upon others misfortunes. Tom Brocah? I was too tired to be impressed.

The phone rang. The secretary looked up. "It's the reporter from the Arizona Republic. He wants to talk with someone about the fire. `

I sighed. I didn't like this part of the job, but it was an excuse to sit for a few more minutes. "Transfer him over to my phone." My phone ran and I picked it up. He identified himself with the same tone the emperor of the world would use just before he expected you to fall on your knees in worship. Again I was unimpressed. After establishing who I was and feeling apparently happy with my status he began questioning.

"I understand a tanker truck exploded..."

"No. The tanker truck did not explode."

"Yes it did."

"No it didn't."

"Well then, what exploded?"

"The gas station blew up. The tanker truck was offloading at the time but it was driven away by the driver."

"Are you sure a tanker didn't blow?"

I raised my voice. "I just spent my entire morning working the fire. That's what happened weather you like it or not.

His voice became huffy. "Well why did the gas station blow up?"

"I have no idea."

"Well who does?"

"No one at this point has any answers."

"I want to talk to someone who knows something."

"You're out of luck. I'm all you're going to get. The firefighters are still crawling around the smoldering ruins. The fire is under control but the station is still burning."

"Well when will someone know what happened.

"I don't know, tomorrow . . . maybe." This sparing went on and on. He had it in his head that a tanker had blown up and just wouldn't let go of that idea. I grew tired and finally I suggested he phone Warner's nursery and Maverick Country Store for their stories. He thought that sounded great and hung up. Later in the paper he described me an "uncooperative spokesperson for the fire department." We all got a good laugh out of it. I was "uncooperative" because I wouldn't tell him what he wanted to hear. I called my mother and Maurice's mother because I knew they would hear it on the radio and television and worry about us. I kept it simple and didn't tell them everything. I just wanted them to know we were ok. I promised to call them later that evening.

I tossed the phone messages on the fire chiefs desk with Tom Borcah's on top. It's funny but none of the calls were returned. He was just as unimpressed with old Tom as I was. The story aired on the national news, but only with information received from other sources, such as Mr. Woodspur, the man I ran off from behind the gas station with the video camera. He had called the TV stations with his video and report. They paid him for the story.

I walked back to the scene. The ambulance was back and they were treating exhausted firefighters. Mark Tate was taken to the hospital for exhaustion. The report was the man hurt in the explosion had a horrible mangled leg. The three burn victims were minor and the firefighter would be all right after some fluids were pumped into his dehydrated body and his PH balance was restored.

"Medical Control," my radio came to life.

"This is Medical Control.

"We have some people with problems over here at Maverick Country Store." The man speaking was a firefighter that had been sent with two other men to investigate a "strange" smell reported by the employees of the store. They had found nothing but three women employees worrying they may be "sick".

Rescue two and I reported down the block. The women were sitting on the pavement outside the building. I listened as the EMTs questioned them. My gut feeling was they were hysterical. They apparently had seen the man drop the gas cap across the street and as they watched him bend down they saw the building exploded. They screamed and ran to the rear of the store, expecting the front window to break. It did. They stood in fear and watched from a front row seat all that had gone on. It was now settling in how serious the innocent was and how close they had come to dying that day.

I put them on oxygen and told them the oxygen would help them breath. They were to take slow breaths and let the oxygen work. They didn't need oxygen but they thought they did, so I gave it to them with some subtle suggestions they would improve. They did. I left them with the other EMTs and went to check with the firefighters in the store. "What have you found?" I asked as I came in.

"Nothing. There's no gas leak in this store. How's Brody?"

"He's going to be fine." We talked a few minutes and I left. I returned to the ambulance and the upset women. "The smell you smelled wasn't a gas leak. You are downhill from the fire. The water from the fire hoses ran a lot of water into the sewer disturbing the nasty smells. The odor was only the stirred up smells from the sewer and completely harmless." This wasn't completely true because methane gas was one of the smells but they didn't need to hear that, besides, the concentration amount was small and wasn't at risk of exploding. The firefighters felt the concentration wasn't a problem so why upset the women even more. I strongly suggested they close for the day and they did. The oxygen had healed them and they all went home to ponder the meaning of life.

Clean up was long and horrible. Melted tires ruined the turnouts and they had to be thrown away and replaced with new ones. Cleanup took twelve hours from start to finish. It was on all the news stations local and national.

The newspapers spiced it up and it appeared on radio and television. Most reports stated the tanker truck blew up. An off duty Phoenix Firefighter dropped in to tell us he had been in the crowd watching and they couldn't have handled it better. He was amazed at how well we had done with such limited resources. "...by the book it was fought by the book. Very good job." We felt good. Phoenix Fire is one of the best and a member of that fire department had congratulated us.

I went to the local newspaper and asked for the pictures a reporter had taken. I wanted to make copies. He gave them to me and asked why I hadn't ran him off like I had so many other fires. "I had written you off," I told him.

His eyes got big. "You mean you expected me to die?"

I smiled, "If the tanks had blown, we would have had a quarter mile smoking hole in the ground and no structure in town would have had windows."

"Well, he said, I remember wondering why you ignored me and then I saw the tank in the flames (under the window) and I ran away."

382

"A wise thing to do, under the circumstances," I said. I took the pictures to the local photo place and had copies made.

Overall, Mr. Corn, age thirty-seven, received second degree burns to his face and head. He was treated and released from the Page Hospital. He and his father rebuilt. Firefighters Brody, age eighteen and Mark, age thirty-four, were treated for heat exhaustion and released. The semi truck driver, Dennis Spendlove was treated for a sprained back. Bob Slasor, age sixty-one years was flown to Flagstaff Medical Center serious condition. He had a badly fractured right leg, cuts to his face and hands and a severe laceration to his arm. He lived, but never completely recovered.

As I looked back on the incident, I felt a great since of success. I had sat in so many classes learning the command system. I had put on fire gear and entered burning building (as few times as possible, since I didn't like that part of the job) I had spent hours and hours with disaster planning. All the time I expected when the "Big One" occurred, I would be Medical Control, not in command of the incident. I felt good. All that time spent in training and planning had finally paid off. I will never forget the fear, the adrenalin rush, the burden of responsibility, the sense of accomplishment and most of all the high I got from cheating death and winning. This was the big one and it worked. I will never forget it and neither will my family or anyone that had a part in that call.

THE WALLS OF JERICO

Page is located in a beautiful part of the country with red rocks, breathtaking views, and a lake unlike any other. The Wahweap Creek area is said to resemble the Holy Land. A "made for TV movie" began filming "The Bible" on the Warm Creek Road, about five miles east of Big Water, Utah (eighteen miles west of Page). Any time a movie company came to town, interesting things happened.

One small thing happened that still makes me laugh. The movie company needed some costumes made. I was asked to recommend a local woman with good sewing skills. I suggested a woman I knew who was very talented in sewing. She was a LDS member and sewed all her families clothing. She was a shy woman, quiet, polite, and naïve about the world outside the tiny town in which she lived.

She was asked to bring her tape measure pencil and paper to the Holiday Inn and take measurements of one of the stars. He played a King and they needed flowing robes of the kingly type. She arrived and was directed to the room. She was let in by the star, which she promptly recognized. He was a well-known actor and for this film, he would play a king. He smiled and welcomed her. Shyly she entered.

The star was use to Hollywood's way of doing things. He had been through so many costume fittings in the past, it didn't occur to him it was her first time. He walked to the center of the motel room, and dropped his robe. He was dressed in a small bikini brief. He held his arms out and stood still, waiting for her to take her measurements. She froze. She was a prim and proper person. Here she stood in a motel room with a barely clad man. She was so embarrassed. She awkwardly approached him with her measuring tape in hand and very quickly took measurements, carefully not touching the Star. She stammered and falling over her own feet, she fled the room.

She made the kings robes, and they were beautiful. Thankfully they were "flowing robes" and an exact fit wasn't necessary. She told me to never ask her to do that again. All her friends and family found the story amusing and she never lived her embarrassment down.

Now for the big thing, the Stunt Man. When the page went out, it made me laugh, "This is a medical emergency. We have a report of a roman soldier who fell off the walls of Jericho." We got in the "old" Rescue One (an old Cadillac ambulance). We drove on the highway into Utah and after eighteen miles we turned off into the community of Big Water, Utah. It is a bedroom community of small homes and trailers, known for polygamist Chief Joseph's large collection of wives and children. We continued through town and turned on Warm Creek Road. It was a dirt road, bumpy with ruts and patches of sand that threaten to trap a vehicle.

We reached Warm Creek. The creek flowed across the road. We were lucky, it wasn't at flood stage. The ambulance traveled down the steep incline and forded the water, then drove up the steep bank on the other side. More bumps, ruts, sand and rocks, awaited us as we slowly progressed down the dirt road. To our left were tall cliffs and strange giant piles of brown and black dirt left over from the Jurassic period when this area was underwater. My children and I had gone in search of shark's teeth in this area by straining the black dirt a number of times.

The trip was painfully slow. We then caught a glimpse of Jericho. It stood strangely in the distance. I am told the area resembles the Holy Land, and there stood Jericho of the Bible. Hollywood had built a "fort-like" structure of wood and Styrofoam. It looked like it was made of brick. As we got closer, it was obvious this movie was low budget. But, when seen on TV months later, it looked good. We had turned off our code lights and siren while on the dirt road, but we turned the back on to let them know

384

we were approaching. We were met by an excited assistant producer and production assistant. They directed us to the back of the structure.

We collected our equipment and began walking toward the back of the walled city. It was designed to be viewed from the front. From the back, the structure was two-by-fours and unpainted Styrofoam. As we walked, the producer excitedly explained the accident. "The roman soldier was standing on the wall poised for battle with the Jews that surrounded the town. An explosion went off, and the roman soldier fell to his right and he should have gone left. He landed on some wooden props and junk instead of the air bag."

"Explosion? I don't remember any bombs mentioned in the Bible" I thought. I forced myself back to the problem at hand. I then saw our patient. He was in his late 20's, tall, strong, everything you would expect of a stuntman. He was dressed as a roman soldier. He wore a white tunic top, helmet with a small feather on top, breast plate, short skirt, sandal/boots that laced up to his knees. He had a sword sheath on his belt and still held the sword in his hand. He lay on his back in the sand beside a stack of building supplies, a couple of boxes, some tools and debris left over from building the walled city. He was wide awake and wisely not moving. Beside him, giving comfort, support, and reminding him not to move, was the stunt coordinator.

As I approached, I could see an obvious inappropriate erection, a sign of a fractured back. There was no doubt, he had broken his back in the fall, but he wasn't paralyzed, not yet anyway. The bones in his spinal column were badly broken and the tiny, sharp bone pieces lay dangerously close to the delicate spinal column. The spinal cord is about the size of a piece of spaghetti and about as strong as a piece of spaghetti that needs another minute or two of boiling. It would easily separate and paralyze this young man if a bone shard were to cut it. This was very serious.

The man wasn't going to die, but he was in serious danger of living the rest of his life in a wheelchair. Also, if his back broke at the waste, the impact was sufficient enough to have also fractured his neck, so he was in danger of being paralyzed from the neck down. I knew his back was broke, and I decided to pretend, worst case scenario, his neck was fractured as well. There was no need to discuss the seriousness of the situation to my two EMT partners, because they too knew what was at stake. It was obvious the stunt coordinator also understood.

I kneeled beside him and introduced myself. I asked him to not move. I began to ask questions as the two other team members set up the backboard. He appeared to have no other injuries and had no pre-existing medical problems. I took his vital signs and they were fine.

"I think I hurt my back really bad," he said. I looked up at the stunt coordinator and could see he also believed this to be a serious injury.

"In case you are right, we will be very careful. We are going to log roll you onto the backboard. It will act as a splint, keeping your spinal column still." I said. Normally, I would have cut off his clothing down to his underwear, but his injury appeared to be an isolated injury and I was afraid to risk any additional movement. I decided to board him in complete military attire. Let the hospital worry about the breast plate and all the rest.

"I'm a stunt man, I know about broken backs......" his voice trailed off. The hint of fear had crept into his voice. He wasn't sure his back was broken, but he feared the worse. He was right, but he didn't know it yet.

I was deeply concerned about moving him. But I couldn't leave him lying on the sand in the middle of nowhere. I took his head and placed the two EMTs at his shoulder and midsection. I had the assistant producer take his knees, the stunt coordinator the backboard and the production assistant the feet. They all kneeled on the patient's left side and placed their hands on his body, waiting for the signal.

"On the count of three, we will gently roll him, as a unit, toward you, the patient's left side." I turned my head and nodded to the patient's left. "Does everyone understand?" They indicated they did. "Now, when he is on his left side, you, (I indicated the stunt coordinator) will examine his back for other injuries, don't touch the backbone." He nodded his head. He was familiar with accidents and I felt he could accomplish the task. "Now, (to the patient), you can let go of the sword. Then you can help by keeping your body stiff, like a board as we roll you." He said he understood.

I held his head, said a silent prayer and counted "One, two, and three." Everyone did great. They rolled him as a unit to his left side. The stunt coordinator did a good job of examining his back, and then slipped the backboard in place. We then rolled him back over, onto the backboard. "Wiggle your toes," I commanded. He did. I was thrilled. His spinal cord was still intact. "I want him strapped and taped with duct tape to the backboard. It's a very bumpy road and he must be firmly secured to the board, more so than usual." My team understood. We went about taping the man to the board, almost like a mummy. He almost had to ask permission to blink his eyes. After I was convinced he would not slip or move on the board, we lifted the board and with help from bystanders, we carried him to the ambulance.

"Drive very, very slow. I don't care if it's 5 mph and takes us an hour to get back to town. Avoid the bumps and ruts as best you can." I told the driver. He said he understood and we started down the poorly

386

maintained dirt road. Every bump felt twice as bad as it had before the patient was onboard. The ambulance bumped and jiggled as it slowly crept down the road. This was before Page had a helicopter for medical rescues and we just had to do the best we could. I put him on oxygen. He didn't really need it, but it helps psychologically, the patient expects you to do something and this seems to quite them down, relaxes them and helps manage pain. It's all in their head, but it works.

I noticed we had done a great job taping him to the board, he didn't slip or move. But, the board moved on the stretcher, bouncing as the ambulance would drive up a hump in the road and dip into a rut then spin wheels through deep sand. I explained to the patient and the EMT and I leaned over the patient and with our bodies held him and the backboard to the stretcher. The padding absorbed some of the shocks and we managed to hold him to the stretcher. It was hell for me. My back began to hurt, my arms ached and I feared each bump would sever his spinal cord. I frequently asked him to wiggle his toes. Each time he complied I was pleasantly surprised he still maintained the ability to do so.

Then, I held my breath as we dipped nose down the steep embankment to Warm Creek. We forded the running water then spun tires as we leaped a few feet at a time up the opposite embankment. The ambulance gained the top and after another mile of brutal dirt road, we hit the community of Big Water and paved roads. It was wonderful.

He could still wiggle his toes. I breathed a sigh of relieve. We gained the highway and sped toward Page Hospital. I took his vital signs again, they were fine. One minute he would be calm, then fear would sound in his voice and he would start moving toward panic. I would calm him down and he would relax a little, only to cycle back to fearful mild panic. I understood his fears but I couldn't tell him "everything was going to be ok," because that would be promising him something I had no right to promise. I didn't know how this would end.

When we got within radio distance, I called the emergency room and gave them a report. The stunt coordinator had left ahead of us and was already at the hospital. I didn't know it yet, but he had called Hollywood and the studios had launched a fancy medical air transport plane from California. This man needed surgeons skilled in spinal injuries. The studios were making sure this stuntman was going to get the best available medical care.

We arrived at the hospital and took him out of the ambulance. He could still move his toes when we moved him to the hospital gurney. The "rent-a-doc" from India wasn't happy the patient was still in his roman soldier attire. I told him I didn't want to chance causing more harm. The doctor chose to do the same. This was before Page had a CT scanner or

387

MRI. They managed to x-ray around the uniform well enough to confirm my suspicions. L-1 and 2 were crushed. No other injuries were found. Since his neck was ok, the helmet was removed and they gently cut off the breast plate and removed his sandal/boots. But the tunic, belt, sword sheath, skirt were left in place.

The doctor wasn't happy about the air transport being arranged without his input and permission. Doctors are use to making all the decisions and they hate patients or family to take that power away from them. He was upset and loudly announced the plane was only part of it. "I haven't approved the air transport," he said in heavily accented English.

It was apparent the stunt coordinator had done this before and wasn't going to allow some small town doctor and tiny hospital to harm his stuntman any further. "With all due respect, doctor, you are in over your head. If you continue this power trip the patient will sign out against medical advice. I am sure the ambulance will transport him to the airport to meet the plane. You have x-rayed him, and confirmed the broken back I know you are doing your best, but this hospital and you are not prepared to handle this, he needs specialized care."

"I have to arrange an accepting physician," said the doctor, hoping to regain some control of the situation.

"Dr. Vencent Monrow (famous neuro doc in California) is the accepting physician," answered the stunt coordinator.

"Well, there has to be arrangements made at the hospital and assurance that they have a bed for him,' countered the doctor.

"California UMC has a room and it's waiting for him." It was apparent the movie studio had inside pull. They just called and the plane will be landing in sixty-five minutes.

The doctor had lost all power. He was angry, but managed to control his temper. He left the ER for a cup of coffee. The staff (and doctor) was left with permission to only monitor the patient's vital signs and do the minor little things to prepare him for air transport.

When the plane landed, we took the patient and stunt coordinator to the airplane. As we loaded him into the airplane, he looked up at me and smiled. "I can still wiggle my toes. Thanks." He was turned over to a highly skilled medical team. He was still dressed as a roman soldier, minus the helmet boots and sword. The stunt coordinator turned to us. "Thank you for everything. You all were great." He shook all our hands. He climbed aboard and we stood by our ambulance, and watched the large Lear Jet take off and disappear into the horizon.

This would ordinarily be the end of the story. We often never find out what happened to our out of town patients. As time passed, I occasionally wondered what happened to the stuntman. I hoped he was able to walk and would recover. Months passed, four to be exact. One day, as I sat at my desk in the fire department office, the door opened. In walked the stuntman. He had a big smile on his face.

His eyes met mine, "See, I can walk and I owe you my undying gratitude." I got up and he walked over and gave me a big hug. I called the others that were on the call, but I was unable to contact them. He sat down and told me about what happened to him over the last four months. He said the flight was smooth. At the LA airport, he was taken by ambulance to the hospital where the surgical team waited. He was taken into surgery soon after arrival. He woke up in intensive care with his girlfriend and the stunt coordinator standing beside his bed. The surgery was successful. Recovery involved some pain, and rehab but he recovered quickly.

"I just wanted to thank you and the other EMT's. The doc in California told me I was only a centimeter away from living the rest of my life in a wheelchair. I can never thank you guys enough. Thank you." He was starting to tear up. He stood and hugged me again. I thanked him for coming in and told him we had wondered about him. I promised to let the others know about his complete recovery. He smiled again, "Well, I'm off to LA, I have a shoot Thursday. I'm back to jumping off buildings." He laughed and walked out of the office.

I love happy endings. This call made it all worth it.

THE END

ABOUT THE AUTHOR

Sharon Mozelle Mercer grew up in Phoenix, Arizona. She married Maurice Holbert and they have two sons, David and Stephen. Maurice, Sharon and their two young sons moved to Page, Arizona, three-hundred miles north of Phoenix when Maurice, who worked for Salt River Project transferred to Navajo (electric) Generating Station. Sharon became an Arizona EMT-Basic and served as a volunteer for the Page Fire Department and in three years became PFD Rescue Chief (paid staff) in charge of thirty-two EMTs. She responded to emergency calls and handled the emergency as needed until the ambulance crew arrived. In multiple patient incidents and fires she was Medical Command. She was also cross trained as a fire fighter, engineer (drives and pumps the fire truck), Incident Command, and responsible for the department's budget planning and continuing education and training program. Holbert also flew medical air transports from Page to various destinations, including but not limited to Flagstaff, Phoenix, Colorado and Seattle, Washington. She was a member of the Northern Arizona Disaster Preparedness Board and the Northern Arizona Critical Incident Stress Debriefing Team associated with Flagstaff Medical Center in Flagstaff, Arizona.

Holbert resigned as Rescue Chief for PFD and returned to school. She was accepted into the prestigious Maricopa Medical Center Paramedic Training Program (through Phoenix Community College in Phoenix) and became a Paramedic. She became certified as an Arizona Certified Emergency Paramedic (CEP), a National Registry EMT-Paramedic, and later a New Mexico Paramedic. Sharon joined the small fraternity of female EMS providers. Only 18% of the 1.1 million U.S. Paramedics are female.

Holbert's career involves working as a Paramedic in a number of different settings. Holbert has worked in a large local physicians office (with six doctors, lab, x-ray & minor surgery) and in two hospital emergency departments. She worked on the Navajo Reservation for a private ambulance company in Tuba City and Kayenta, Arizona in the remote four corners area of Arizona. At various times in her career she also reviewed the medic's reports for quality control and proctored paramedic students on "ride-alongs". Holbert also has worked in the (EMS) industrial setting by working at a local coal powered electric generating station and manning two company clinics designed to care and treat employees, one at a local resort and another at the Kayenta and Black Mesa Coal Mines. She also worked for numerous movie, television and commercial production companies as a Set Medic.

Sharon loved to teach and during her career she has taught American Heart Association CPR, First Aid and Babysitter classes. She became a part-time instructor for Yavapai and later Coconino Community College and taught EMT-Basic, EMT Refresher, and the First Responder Class for many years. She was also certified as a Pre-Hospital Trauma Life Support (PHTLS) instructor. Many of her EMT students have made successful careers in EMS. A number have gone on to become paramedics, respiratory therapists, registered nurses and physician's assistants.

Sharon's thirty year career has been exciting, demanding, and rewarding. An author just can't fit thirty years into one book. She currently is working on a second book. Check her web site (sand-dancer.com) for updates.

Made in the USA
Lexington, KY
22 October 2012